Treatment Strategies for Patients with Psychiatric Comorbidity

An Einstein Psychiatry Publication

Publication Series of the Department of Psychiatry
Albert Einstein College of Medicine of Yeshiva University
New York, NY

Editor-in-Chief   Herman M. van Praag, M.D., Ph.D.
Associate Editor   Demitri F. Papolos, M.D.

Treatment Strategies for Patients with Psychiatric Comorbidity

Edited by

SCOTT WETZLER
WILLIAM C. SANDERSON

John Wiley & Sons, Inc.

New York • Chichester • Weinheim • Brisbane • Singapore • Toronto

Library of Congress Cataloging-in-Publication Data:

Treatment strategies for patients with psychiatric comorbidity /
    edited by Scott Wetzler and William C. Sanderson.
        p. cm.—(An Einstein psychiatry publication; 14)
    Includes index.
    ISBN 0-471-11773-0 (alk. paper)
    1. Mental illness—Treatment. 2. Mental illness—Complications.
I. Wetzler, Scott, 1955-   . II. Sanderson, William C.
III. Series.
    [DNLM: 1. Mental Disorders—complications. 2. Mental Disorders—
therapy. W1 EI535 v.14 1997 / WM 400 T7863 1997]
RC480.5.T755 1997
616.89'1—dc20
DNLM/DLC
for Library of Congress   96-34774
                                           CIP

Printed in the United States of America

10 9 8 7 6 5 4 3 2 1

Contributors

Gregory M. Asnis, M.D. Professor of Psychiatry, Albert Einstein College of Medicine, Bronx, New York.

Aaron T. Beck, M.D. University Professor of Psychiatry, Center for Cognitive Therapy, University of Pennsylvania, Philadelphia, Pennsylvania.

Alan S. Bellack, Ph.D. Professor of Psychiatry, University of Maryland School of Medicine, Baltimore, Maryland.

Paul C. Bermanzohn, M.D. Assistant Professor of Psychiatry, Albert Einstein College of Medicine, Bronx, New York.

Jack J. Blanchard, Ph.D. Assistant Professor of Psychology and Psychiatry, The University of New Mexico, Albuquerque, New Mexico.

Giovanni B. Cassano, M.D. Professor and Director, Institute of Psychiatry, School of Medicine, University of Pisa, Pisa, Italy.

Imran Faisal, M.D. Research Fellow, Department of Psychiatry, Albert Einstein College of Medicine, Bronx, New York.

Tova Ferro, Ph.D. Department of Child Psychiatry, College of Physicians and Surgeons, Columbia College, New York, New York.

Jack M. Gorman, M.D. Professor of Clinical Psychiatry, College of Physicians and Surgeons, Columbia University, New York, New York.

Arthur T. Horvath, Ph.D., ABPP Center for Cognitive Therapy, La Jolla, California.

Robin B. Jarrett, Ph.D. Professor of Psychiatry, University of Texas Southwestern Medical Center, Dallas, Texas.

Gary J. Kennedy, M.D. Professor of Psychiatry, Albert Einstein College of Medicine, Bronx, New York.

Justine M. Kent, M.D. Research Fellow, College of Physicians and Surgeons, Columbia University, New York, New York.

Richard J. Kessler, D.O. Assistant Professor of Clinical Psychiatry, Albert Einstein College of Medicine, Bronx, New York.

Ronald C. Kessler, Ph.D. Professor, Department of Health Care Policy, Harvard Medical School, Cambridge, Massachusetts.

Daniel N. Klein, Ph.D. Associate Professor of Psychology, Department of Psychology, State University of New York at Stony Brook, Stony Brook, New York.

Dolores Kraft, Ph.D. Assistant Professor, University of Texas Southwestern Medical Center, Dallas, Texas.

Jack D. Maser, Ph.D. Chief, Anxiety and Somatoform Disorders Program, National Institute of Mental Health, Rockville, Maryland.

David McDowell, M.D. Assistant Professor of Clinical Psychiatry, Columbia University College of Physicians and Surgeons, New York, New York.

Lata K. McGinn, Ph.D. Assistant Professor of Psychiatry, Albert Einstein College of Medicine, Bronx, New York.

Stefano Michelini, M.D. Institute of Psychiatry, School of Medicine, University of Pisa, Pisa, Italy.

Edward V. Nunes, M.D. Assistant Professor of Clinical Psychiatry, Columbia University College of Physicians and Surgeons, New York, New York.

Mary Alice O'Dowd, M.D. Professor of Psychiatry, Albert Einstein College of Medicine, Bronx, New York.

Richard Pitch, M.D. Assistant Professor of Psychiatry (pending), Albert Einstein College of Medicine, Bronx, New York.

William C. Sanderson, Ph.D. Associate Professor of Psychiatry, Albert Einstein College of Medicine, Bronx, New York.

Paul Silver, Ph.D. Clinical Assistant Professor, University of Texas Southwestern Medical Center, Dallas, Texas.

Samuel G. Siris, M.D. Professor of Psychiatry, Albert Einstein College of Medicine, Bronx, New York.

Drew M. Velting, Ph.D. Post-Doctoral Research Fellow in Child and Adolescent Psychiatry, Columbia University, New York, New York.

Fred R. Volkmar, M.D. Harris Associate Professor of Child Psychiatry, Yale University School of Medicine, New Haven, Connecticut.

Scott Wetzler, Ph.D. Professor of Psychiatry, Albert Einstein College of Medicine, Bronx, New York.

Joseph L. Woolston, M.D. Associate Professor of Child Psychiatry and Pediatrics, Yale University School of Medicine, New Haven, Connecticut.

A Note on the Series

Psychiatry is in a state of flux. The excitement springs in part from internal changes, such as the development and official acceptance (at least in the United States) of an operationalized, multi-axial classification system of behavioral disorders (the *DSM-IV*), the increasing sophistication of methods to measure abnormal human behavior, and the impressive expansion of biological and psychological treatment modalities. Exciting developments are also taking place in fields relating to psychiatry; in molecular (brain) biology, genetics, brain imaging, drug development, epidemiology, experimental psychology, to mention only a few striking examples.

More generally speaking, psychiatry is moving, still relatively slowly, but irresistibly from a more philosophical, contemplative orientation to that of a empirical science. From the 1950s on, biological psychiatry has been a major catalyst of that process. It provided the mother discipline with a third cornerstone, that is, neurobiology, the other two being psychology and medical sociology. In addition, it forced the profession into the direction of standardization of diagnoses and of assessment of abnormal behavior. Biological psychiatry provided psychiatry not only with a new basic science and with new treatment modalities, but also with the tools, the methodology, and the mentality to operate within the confines of an empirical science, the only framework in which a medical discipline can survive.

In other fields of psychiatry, too, one discerns a gradual trend toward scientification. Psychological treatment techniques are standardized and manuals developed to make these skills more easily transferable. Methods registering treatment outcome—traditionally used in the behavioral/cognitive field—are now more and more requested and, hence, developed for dynamic forms of psychotherapy as well. Social and community psychiatry, until the 1960s were more firmly rooted in humanitarian ideals and social awareness than in empirical studies, profited greatly from its liaison with the social sciences and the expansion of psychiatric epidemiology.

Let there be no misunderstanding: Empiricism does *not imply* that it is only the measurable that counts. Psychiatry would be mutilated if it would neglect that which cannot be captured by numbers. It *does imply* that what is measurable should be measured. Progress in psychiatry is dependent on ideas and on experiment. Their linkage is inseparable.

This Series, published under the auspices of the Department of Psychiatry of the Albert Einstein College of Medicine, Montefiore Medical Center, is meant to keep track of important developments in our profession, to summarize what has been achieved in particular fields, and to bring together the viewpoints obtained from disparate vantage points—in short, to capture some of the ongoing excitement in modern psychiatry, both in its clinical and experimental dimensions. The Department of Psychiatry at Albert Einstein College of Medicine hosts the Series, but naturally welcomes contributions from others.

Bernie Mazel originally generated the idea for the Series—an ambitious plan which we all felt was worthy of pursuit. The edifice of psychiatry is impressive, but still somewhat flawed in its foundations. May this Series contribute to consolidation of its infrastructure.

HERMAN M. VAN PRAAG, M.D., PH.D.
Professor and Chairman
Academic Psychiatric Center
University of Limburg
Maastricht
The Netherlands

Preface

All too many mental health professionals fail to appreciate that most psychiatric patients meet diagnostic criteria for more than one disorder. In standard practice, the clinician reaches a diagnostic determination of a principal disorder, and then neglects to continue the evaluation, or ignores the treatment implications of a secondary (or tertiary) disorder. Typically, the clinician focuses treatment entirely on the patient's principal disorder. Published treatment guidelines and manuals reinforce this way of thinking as they consider treatments for only a single diagnosis.

Treatment Strategies for Patients with Psychiatric Comorbidity is intended to redress this way of thinking. More often than not, patients have more than one disorder, and these comorbid diagnoses have significant impact on treatment strategies and outcome. In fact, standard treatments for a given disorder are oftentimes ineffective because of the presence of a secondary diagnosis. The primary aim of this book is to describe how comorbid disorders necessitate modifications in standard psychotherapeutic and psychopharmacological treatments.

Demonstration studies examining the efficacy of psychiatric treatments carefully screen patients to identify a homogeneous group with a single psychiatric disorder. This design tends to overestimate treatment effects because patients with comorbid conditions have been excluded. A more naturalistic and valid design would identify an unselected sample of patients who present with the principal diagnosis along with a variety of comorbid disorders. Such a heterogeneous group is more representative of patients in standard practice and would give a more accurate indication of treatment efficacy.

The frequency of psychiatric comorbidity accounts in large part for why clinicians rarely administer treatments exactly according to guidelines or treatment manuals. Treatments must be tailored to meet the needs of the individual patient's comorbid presentation. Pharmacological strategies are altered as medications are combined or prescribed in nonstandard dosage regimens. Psychotherapeutic treatment is changed as specific strategies must be chosen to address the patient's entire symptom configuration.

This book is intended as a practical compendium of clinical advice and recommendations for mental health professionals regarding how standard treatments may be modified to deal with comorbid disorders. It may be read straight through or used as a reference book that the clinician may refer to when faced with difficult clinical problems.

Treatment Strategies for Patients with Psychiatric Comorbidity is divided into three sections: an introduction, which considers general issues relevant to comorbidity; a core section on treatment strategies; and a section on related topics. The treatment section has parallel chapters on psychotherapeutic and drug treatments for the most prominent groupings of psychiatric disorders. Each chapter considers treatments for the most common comorbid conditions. This organization is derived from epidemiological research on the most prevalent combinations of psychiatric disorders.

We hope that this book will contribute to a greater appreciation for how comorbidity influences treatment response among psychiatric patients.

SCOTT WETZLER, PH.D.
WILLIAM C. SANDERSON, PH.D.

Acknowledgments

We would like to thank the Department of Psychiatry at Montefiore Medical Center—our home for these many years. In particular, we thank Dr. T. Byram Karasu, chairman and Silverman Professor of Psychiatry, Albert Einstein College of Medicine, for creating a welcoming academic environment, and Mrs. Estelle Herschfeld, who is the guiding light for the Division of Psychology.

Contents

PART I
Introduction

1

Treatment Implications of Comorbid Mental Disorders

JACK D. MASER
GIOVANNI B. CASSANO
STEFANO MICHELINI

The third edition of the *Diagnostic and Statistical Manual of Mental Disorders* (*DSM-III*, American Psychiatric Association [APA], 1980) brought a paradigmatic shift, both in American psychiatry and clinical psychology (Klerman, 1990) and throughout the world (Maser, Kaelber, & Weise, 1991). The enormous success of the *DSM-III* concept is largely the result of meeting the clinical research community's need for a better diagnostic system, addressing a confluence of dissatisfaction with the *DSM-I* (APA, 1952) and *DSM-II* (APA, 1968), and meeting the need increasingly recognized in the late 1960s and the 1970s for an empirical knowledge base (e.g., see Katz, Cole, & Barton, 1968). Its success is not unqualified, however. Even after its fine-tuning through successive editions, many would say that the most current edition, *DSM-IV* (APA, 1994a), represents only a fraction of clinical reality. In *DSM-IV*, clinicians find categories defined appropriately by descriptive, observable definitions; they also find that the boundaries of

The opinions expressed in this chapter are those of the authors only and do not necessarily reflect the views of the National Institute of Mental Health. The authors thank Dr. Dan Oren for a thoughtful critique of an earlier version of this chapter. Correspondence regarding this chapter should be sent to Dr. Jack D. Maser, NIMH, 5600 Fishers Lane, Room 10C16, Rockville, MD 20857.

any given category are an inadequate match with the patients they treat. Comorbidity and the frequent presentation of atypical and subclinical symptoms are the primary reasons for failure to match patients with the *DSM-IV*'s discrete, categorical, prototypes of mental illness. Comorbidity is discussed, and then the spectrum concept is presented as an example of a complementary perspective. Interested readers are referred to several sources for broad considerations of comorbid disorders: Kendall and Watson (1989) and Klein and Riso (1993) provide a more psychological perspective, whereas a more psychiatric approach is given by Caron and Rutter (1991) and Nottelmann and Jensen (1995). Maser and Cloninger (1990) attempted to incorporate aspects of both perspectives.

DEFINITIONS

A battle over the proper terminology—comorbidity versus some other word or phrase—flares up on occasion. Lilienfeld, Waldman, and Isreal (1994) critiqued the term *comorbidity* and were answered, in the same journal issue, by five experts in psychopathological nosology (Blashfield, McElroy, Pfohl, & Blum, 1994; Robins, 1994; Rutter, 1994; Spitzer, 1994; Widiger & Ford-Black, 1994). Winokur (1990) prefers *cosyndromal* or use of the primary-secondary distinction over *comorbid.* The multiple uses of the primary-secondary distinction have been discussed in Maser, Weise, and Gwirtsman (1995), and Winokur refers only to the chronological meaning of the primary-secondary distinction.

In medical terms, morbidity conveys, at least in part, the notion of a disease process. Disease is produced by pathogens, but despite the suspicion of many, there are very few pathogens known to underlie the mental disorders described in *DSM-IV.* Cosyndromal is a more technically accurate term, and the temporal definition of the primary-secondary distinction has value; but in line with current usage, we shall continue with the term *comorbid* in relation to mental illnesses, even when there is no known pathogen.

The term *comorbidity* is derived from the medical epidemiology literature. Two definitions are in common usage. The first is Feinstein's original coinage in 1970: "any distinct additional clinical entity that has existed or that may occur during the clinical course of a patient who has the index disease under study" (pp. 456–457). Apparently, Feinstein did not intend to make a distinction between disease and disorder in this definition (personal communication cited by Spitzer, 1994).

Psychiatric epidemiologists have used relative risk as the basis for their definition: A patient diagnosed with the index disorder has a statistically defined risk of having one or more other diagnoses. The statistic used most commonly is the odds ratio, defined as the probability of the occurrence of an event divided by the probability of its nonoccurrence. An odds ratio, in a comorbidity sense, is the odds that a second disorder will occur in the group already having one disorder divided by the odds that the second disorder will occur in a group without the first disorder.

For example, Boyd and colleagues (1984) describe the odds of a person's having two unrelated disorders during the past month. In a patient diagnosed with panic disorder, the odds that the person will also have a manic episode are 24.1. Subjects who have bipolar disorder are at greater risk of having comorbid panic disorder than are subjects with unipolar depression. Confirming data reported by Savino and associates (1993) and Chen and Dilsaver (1995) showed that the prevalence of panic disorder among subjects with unipolar depression was 12.5 per hundred adults and 26 times greater than among subjects with bipolar disorder. Regier and others (1990) show that the odds of a person's having any bipolar disorder in the presence of an alcohol abuse/dependence disorder are 5.1 times greater than the odds for a person without an alcohol disorder. Among persons with an alcohol disorder, the odds that they will abuse other substances are 7.1 times greater than for those who do not have an alcohol disorder. The implication for diagnosis is clear: Given the strong likelihood of co-occurrence, clinicians diagnosing one disorder are remiss in their duty if they fail to search for others over the lifetime and in the family history of their patient. Similarly, the implication for treatment is clear: Persons presenting for treatment of one mental disorder are likely to require treatment for more than that mental disorder.

One of many clinical studies that we might cite is by Oldham and associates (1995), who reported on 200 cases of individuals seeking psychiatric treatment. Semistructured interviews were administered to evaluate the presence of both Axis I and Axis II disorders in each patient. The presence of any Axis II disorder made the co-occurrence of a mood, anxiety, psychotic, or eating disorder quite likely. Moreover, Axis I disorders did not cluster neatly with the Axis II disorders. That is, psychotic disorders were not comorbid with just Cluster A personality disorders (paranoid, schizoid, and schizotypal) but were also found among the other two personality disorder clusters. Oldham and others have documented how widespread comorbidity is between the two axes, and the clinical importance of their findings rests on the considerable extent to which Axis II disorders complicate the treatment of Axis I disorders (Reich & Vasile, 1993; Reich & Green, 1990).

COMORBIDITY AND CATEGORICAL CLASSIFICATION

Comorbidity and the classifications found in *DSM-IV, The International Classification of Diseases*[1] (*ICD-10,* World Health Organization, 1990), and similar categorical systems are inextricably related. Without a categorical classification scheme, there is no reason to discuss comorbidity. What if, instead of a categorical approach to psychiatric classification, the designers of *DSM-III* (and successive editions) had chosen a dimensional approach? The diagnostician would then quantify attributes; syndrome categories, defined by clusters of symptoms, would not exist, and therefore, could not coexist.

The *DSM-IV* disputes the claim that "each category of mental disorder is a completely discrete entity with absolute boundaries" (p. xxii). However, although its designers can make this statement with every honest intention, researchers and insurance companies act as if each category is a discrete entity. Moreover, *DSM-IV* does not provide any standardized information about the frequency of co-occurrence of disorders, further suggesting that each category is discrete. The claim is also made that "there is no assumption that all individuals described as having the same mental disorder are alike in all important ways" (p. xxii). They may differ in severity, impairment, and symptom expression, and we will focus attention on the last of these possible differences.

The *DSM-IV* uses polythetic criteria sets, which means that a given individual may present with a subset of diagnostic criteria from a larger set. Thus, a person diagnosed as depressed must have at least five symptoms out of the longer list of nine diagnostic criteria. Polythetic criteria sets, however, speak to heterogeneous clinical presentations only within a diagnostic category.

Consider adjustment disorders (*DSM-IV,* pp. 623–627) as a relatively understudied but common example seen in clinicians' offices. Adjustment disorders are not usually considered a serious mental disorder (compared to schizophrenia, bipolar disorder, or panic disorder). But as we shall see, they can be serious enough when comorbidity, substance use, hospitalization, and suicide are taken into account. Adjustment disorders are activated by a stressor causing a person marked distress and/or impairment in social or occupational settings; the distress and/or impairment must resolve within six months of the termination of the stressor. (Continuation of the diagnosis is allowed when the stressor is chronic.) What is often not considered is that adjustment disorders are usually accompanied by a variety of coexisting symptoms.

Greenberg, Rosenfeld, and Ortega (1995) probably studied a more serious cohort of adjustment disorders than most clinicians see because their sample came from inpatients at an acute psychiatric service. Among the patients admitted to this service, 7.1 percent of the adults and 34.4 percent of the adolescents had a diagnosis of adjustment disorder, often with comorbid substance use disorders, and suicidality. They also tended toward a relatively shorter period of institutionalization than a comparison group with major depression, and only 18 percent of those who required rehospitalization received the same diagnosis. Adjustment disorders do not seem very stable over time, or alternatively, they have a low diagnostic reliability among clinicians (Newcorn & Strain, 1992). It would be interesting to know whether the comorbid disorders had greater stability than the adjustment disorders.

COMORBIDITY AND TREATMENT DESIGN

The *DSM-IV* does not suggest specific treatments for each disorder category and subcategory.[2] However, modern treatment researchers—psychosocial and psychopharmacological—have attempted to design treatments tailored to specific *DSM* categories. The strategy links treatment to diagnosis, and we may expect this strategy to succeed to the extent that the targeted *DSM-IV* classification is valid. It is possible that treatment researchers will successfully design treatments that fit *DSM-IV* categories but fail to treat their patients successfully because the categories do not completely represent the patients. To the extent that comorbidity presents a challenge to the official nomenclature, it presents a similar challenge to treatments designed and targeted for *DSM* categories.

COURSE OF ILLNESS

Given the presence of multiple disorders, which disorder appeared first? What implications does this knowledge have for treatment? These questions are the basis of an important debate, one that is ultimately to be resolved by longitudinal data revealing the natural course of these disorders and the long-term outcome of treatment. Some believe that childhood separation anxiety is a prodrome (i.e., precursor or predictor) for adult panic disorder. If we knew that separation anxiety disorder or an extreme sensitivity to separation in adulthood preceded the onset of panic disorder, we could screen for that disorder, intervene when appropriate, and (theoretically) prevent the onset of panic. Similarly, if we knew that clinical or subclinical social phobia preceded the onset of depression, we could screen for the anxiety disorder and take similar steps to those described for separation/panic disorder. Knowledge about the course of illness will impact prevention and treatment, and it will enhance our understanding of the origins of mental disorders.

Because longitudinal research is complex, tends to become dated, and requires stability of investigators, subjects, and funding, course of illness is not easily studied. In spite of these difficulties, such studies have been done and data exist. In this regard, consider three data sets related to depression and anxiety: the National Institute of Mental Health (NIMH)—Collaborative Depression Study (CDS), the Munich Follow-up Study, and the Zurich Cohort Study of Young Adults. The CDS is a naturalistic *clinical* investigation of consecutive patients who sought treatment at five major teaching hospitals in the United States. Patients were periodically tracked, and at their five-year follow-up, depression was found to precede their anxiety disorders (Coryell, Endicott, & Winokur, 1992).

In a community *epidemiological* survey, Wittchen and Essau (1989) followed patients in the German city of Munich to report that after seven years, the majority of their subjects with both disorders experienced anxiety before depression. This is the opposite finding of Coryell and associates (1992). Subjects in the Munich Follow-up Study came from both the community and a cohort of former psychiatric inpatients. In Switzerland, Angst, Vollrath, Merikangas, and Ernst (1990) found that persons diagnosed seven years earlier with pure anxiety tended to develop additional depressive disorders, but persons originally diagnosed with pure depression tended to retain that single diagnosis over the follow-up period. That is, a diagnosis of pure depression remained relatively stable, whereas one of pure anxiety exhibited substantial instability as reflected in additional major or recurrent brief depressions.

There are several implications of these three sets of data, two of which (i.e., Munich and Zurich) agree that anxiety tends to precede depression. The Munich and Zurich surveys, as well as the Epidemiologic Catchment Area (ECA) study (Robins & Regier, 1991), are more likely to reflect true base rates of pure and comorbid disorders (e.g., see Tables 1 and 2 in Johnson, Weissman, & Klerman, 1990).

A second implication is that the *DSM-IV* is most relevant when its individual diagnostic categories are applied to pure depressions found in community surveys. Pure depression subjects are less likely to seek treatment and less likely to have additional mental illnesses during the course of their depression. Conversely, clinicians seeing a patient with a pure anxiety disorder (i.e., no depression or substance abuse) may expect additional disorders to appear if effective treatment for the person is not promptly instituted. The degree to which treatments are effective in preventing the appearance of these other disorders or in reducing their symptomatology when they already exist concurrently is represented sparsely in the literature and is a welcome topic of this volume.

A third implication is that mixed cases seem to have a worse outcome. Consider persons who have been subjected to confinement in an institution, be it prison or a mental hospital or a home for the emotionally disturbed. Whereas there may be several reasons for confining an individual to an institution, most people would agree that such confinement is *prima facie* evidence of a poor outcome. One might ask, to what extent is institutional confinement due to comorbidity? Mental hospitals and prisons have much higher base rates of mental and addictive disorders than are found in the community at large. For example, the ECA study revealed that about 90 percent of prisoners with schizophrenia, bipolar disorder, and antisocial personality disorder also had a substance abuse comorbidity (Regier et al., 1990). Another example comes from Wittchen and Essau (1989), who found that subjects with mixed anxiety/depression were more severely impaired in psychosocial functioning and evidenced more management problems in social roles than subjects with a pure disorder. In terms of remission rates, Wittchen and Essau's mixed group evidenced lower rates than those individuals with pure depression. An unfavorable, chronic course was found in 44.1 percent of the mixed anxiety/depression group but in only 26.3 percent of the pure depression group. The clinical study found depressive symptoms to be more severe, persistent, and recurrent when the patients had a coexisting anxiety syndrome than when depression occurred among patients without anxiety (Coryell et al., 1992; Pini, Goldstein, Wickramaratne, & Weissman, 1994). Moreover, mood congruent delusions and the delusional subtype of depression are more frequent among patients with both depression and panic disorder than in patients with depression only (Pini et al., 1994). Obsessions and compulsions clearly had the gravest prognosis when they were present in a depressed patient, but the presence of any anxiety syndrome predicted a worse outcome than was projected for patients without a comorbid anxiety syndrome.

A common limitation of these three studies is the lack of any assessment of temperament as a marker of mood vulnerability (Akiskal & Akiskal, 1992; Akiskal et al., 1995). Savino and colleagues (1993) studied 140 panic patients and showed that high rates of temperamental dysregulation often co-occur (over a lifetime) with anxiety disorders and may represent the only manifestation of a mood lability preceding the onset of an anxiety disorder. In this perspective, any data lacking information on temperamental features appear incomplete for characterizing the temporal relationship between anxiety and mood disorders. A limitation of the report by Coryell and colleagues is that it is a clinical, not a community, study. As such, it may not be a valid representation of the natural course of illness. Berkson (1946) demonstrated an often replicated rule in epidemiological research: Persons seeking treatment for a medical problem usually have an additional medical diagnosis, and prevalences recorded in clinical settings do not reflect the base rate for either diagnosis in the community. Most of the subjects entered the NIMH—CDS seeking treatment for existing comorbidities. Perhaps this particular set of patients was unusual in having their depression precede anxiety. Perhaps this progression is the more severe and drives people into a clinic. The answers are not yet clear, but the patients who entered the proband group of the Collaborative Depression Study and who were reported on in the Coryell study probably reflect what practicing clinicians see.

IMPLICATIONS OF COMORBID DISORDERS FOR THE HEALTH CARE SYSTEM IN THE UNITED STATES

As the health care system in the United States is moving in the direction of health maintenance organizations (HMOs) and as Congress has directed the NIMH to increase its allocation to research on mental health services, we add some discussion on comorbidity as seen through the perspective of an HMO.

There appear to be significant differences in the patients who select an HMO compared to those who seek treatment privately or at a major medical institution versus those meeting diagnostic criteria located in the community. Even in outcome following treatment, there is a difference between individuals treated in a mental health specialty clinic versus a general medical specialty clinic (HMO) (Hays, Wells, Sherbourne, Rogers, & Spritzer,

1995). These differences in type of clinical setting may have implications for the conclusions that can be drawn for the threshold number of criteria used to define a diagnosis. Depending on the setting, a health care professional might treat patients with subclinical symptoms or with full-blown disorders with considerable comorbidity. For example, the general medical and mental health specialty clinics might be compared for subthreshold (i.e., not meeting *DSM* criteria) and full diagnosis. Hays and colleagues (1995) studied patients in three settings: solo fee-for-service physician practices; HMOs; and large, multispecialty group practices. Depressed patients in these settings were compared with patients having such severe and chronic physical disorders as diabetes mellitus, myocardial infarction, and congestive heart failure, whereas hypertensive patients were used to control for chronicity in an otherwise healthy group. Dependent variables included measures of functioning and well-being, role limitations, social functioning, emotional well-being, and other areas.

One might expect, and the investigators found, that depressed patients in the mental health specialty clinics had more severe depression and greater limitations in functioning and well-being than patients in the general medical sector. They also tended to show better improvement than those treated in the general medical sector. General population means for these dependent variables are very similar to scores recorded from the hypertension group. Even for patients with subclinical depression at baseline, functioning and well-being were similar or worse than the general medical conditions at two-year follow-up. Moreover, while the depressives who met full diagnostic criteria improved, those with subclinical symptoms remained stable.

Levenson, Hamer, and Rossiter (1990) screened 455 medical inpatients. They found 27.9 percent to be very depressed and 27.5 percent to be very anxious, and about two thirds of this sample had both depression and anxiety. Length and cost of hospital stay were significantly correlated with psychopathology: 40 percent longer median stay and 35 percent greater mean cost for the high psychopathology group. The point is that comorbidity is costly to the health care system.

SPECTRUM-COMORBIDITY: DIAGNOSTIC AND THERAPEUTIC IMPLICATIONS

The difficulty if not the impossibility of classifying many patients with multiple disorders into one of the *DSM* categories has spawned a variety of other procedures to cope with clinical reality (Maser, Weise, & Gwirtsman,

1995). These include use of the primary-secondary distinction, multiple diagnoses, use of both Axes I and II, associated features of a disorder, and the spectrum of a disorder concept (Cassano & Savino, 1993). In this section we describe the concept of spectrum as an additional perspective for the clinical evaluation of concomitant psychiatric disorders.

The necessity of this additional conceptual tool to describe mental disorder phenomenology derived from similar observations that gave rise to other coping mechanisms: Sharply divided categorical systems of classification do not capture the complex and variable psychopathology seen in most patients. Usually this complex phenomenology is simplistically attributed to premorbid personality traits, to personality disorder, or to residual symptoms and/or maladaptive behavior residual to a previous Axis I disorder.

The definition of spectrum includes a range of subclinical and/or atypical symptoms and isolated behavioral features that are partial or subclinical expressions of a categorical disorder. These are usually overlooked by clinicians. The spectrum itself is not a diagnostic category. A good example of this concept was given by Cassano and Savino (1993), who described the panic-agoraphobic spectrum as an expansion of panic disorder phenomenology described in *DSM-III-R*. It included symptoms and behavioral features belonging to the following areas: panic attacks; anxious expectation; polyphobic features; avoidant behavior; reassurance sensitivity; help-seeking behavior; maladaptive behavior; predisposing or prodromal factors; and physiological sensitivity to chemical substances. Table 1-1 describes the main features of the panic-agoraphobic spectrum; the left side shows some of these areas, and the right side shows items that the clinician can recognize as objective, descriptive signs of those areas.

When adhering to a *DSM-IV* diagnosis, co-occurring symptoms and subclinical or atypical manifestations of other disorders that cut across different diagnostic categories are often seen as associated features of the primary disorder. However, when even a few isolated or subclinical symptoms are present, there may be significant impairment in the patient's social functioning (Klerman, Weissman, Ouellette, Johnson, & Greenwald, 1991), and the phenomenology of the Axis I disorder may be significantly modified, thereby delaying and misleading the diagnosis. For example, symptoms of an overlooked comorbid anxiety and bipolar II disorder can often be observed within the categories of borderline personality disorder and atypical depression. In these cases, feelings of insecurity and agitation and episodes of dyscontrol brought about by atypical panic symptoms co-occurring with

TABLE 1-1
Panic-Agoraphobic Spectrum

Domains	*Areas*
Subclinical and atypical panic attacks	Typical symptoms Atypical symptoms
Anxious expectation	Anticipatory anxiety Alarm state
Phobic and avoidant features	Claustro-agoraphobia Secondary social phobia Illness and related phobias Medication phobia Natural phenomena phobias Sleep phobia
Reassurance sensitivity	Help-seeking behavior Counterphobic measures Demonstrativity
Substance sensitivity	
General stress sensitivity	
Separation sensitivity	Separation anxiety symptoms Loss sensitivity
Associated medical conditions	Mitral valve prolapse Thyroid disorder

a depressive episode in a bipolar patient may be easily confused with the impulsivity and aggressivity of borderline patients. In the same way, unrecognized, subclinical, or isolated panic symptoms may bring atypical features such as mood reactivity to a depressive episode. The high rates of comorbidity between panic disorder and bipolar disorders found by Savino and associates (1993) and Chen and Dilsaver (1995) support these observations. Higher rates of comorbidity could be reasonably expected if subjects were selected using a symptomatic extension of *DSM-IV* criteria.

The impact of a mild, subtle, and long-lasting psychopathology on patients' quality of life was very clear to Sir Aubrey Lewis, who wrote in 1936,

It may be said, simply, that severe emotional upsets ordinarily tend to subside, but that mild emotional states, when often provoked or long maintained, tend to persist, as it were, autonomously. Hence the paradox that a gross blatant psychosis may do less damage in the long run than some meager neurotic incubus: a dramatic attack of mania or melancholia, with delusions, wasting, hallucinations, wild excitement and other alarms, may have far less effect on the course of a man's life than some deceptively mild affective illness which goes on so long that it becomes inveterate. The former comes as a catastrophe, and when it has passed the patient takes up his life again . . . while with the latter he may never get rid of his burden [p. 998].

Detection of subtle, long-lasting, underlying psychopathology is more difficult when it is concomitant with an Axis I disorder. Description of a clinical reality that includes a complex array of symptoms belonging to different disorders and their proper treatment led us to speak in terms of subclinical and atypical spectrum comorbidity. Early recognition of spectrum comorbidity (observed over a lifetime) leads to a significant improvement in diagnostic accuracy, choice of a more appropriate treatment strategy, management of treatment, control over the potential for substance abuse and prediction of outcome (Cassano et al., submitted). Moreover, clinical experience shows that the adoption of a proper treatment strategy covering both the Axis I disorder and the lifetime occurrence of spectrum symptoms often produces dramatic changes in the lifestyle of the patient, who feels free from psychopathological features that the clinician and even the patient believed were stable personality traits.

Unrecognized spectrum symptoms occurring at one time in the patient's life may impact his or her personality and the presentation of any psychopathology at some future time. An example might be of a young man who, at the age of 20, experiences one or two mild panic attacks. He seeks no treatment, but the attacks change his life in certain ways. Prior to the mild panic attacks, he was described as energetic, open to new experiences, and socially outgoing with a hyperthymic temperament. Following the onset of panic symptoms, he becomes increasingly pavid, dependent, socially avoidant, and worried about his health. These features become stable and traitlike. When this patient is seen by a clinician at age 40 for a depressive episode, his panic symptoms have long been forgotten, and he presents as a fearful person, somewhat hypochondriacal, and dependent on others to such an extent that he tends to avoid remaining alone. Now the recognition of distinct symptoms of the panic spectrum and the consequent adoption of a well-targeted treatment strategy become fundamental. If the clinician attempts to treat only the depressive episode, he or she will miss the main reason for the patient's 20 years of fearfulness, dependency, avoidance, and hypochondriasis, which were initiated and maintained by a partial expression of panic disorder.

It is not clear how a psychosocial treatment would deal therapeutically with the clinical case described above, but in terms of medications, a drug such as imipramine is much more likely to treat both the depression and residual symptoms of the panic attacks than compounds such as nortriptyline, which are targeted at depression alone (Cassano & Michelini, 1995). Also, the clinician-patient relationship, the cornerstone of any treatment strategy, can be significantly improved by adopting the spectrum approach. Providing clinicians with new keys with which to interpret the patient's behavior, this approach enables an easy identification of individualized psychopathological profiles, capturing mild symptoms and details of patients' lifestyles. In such profiles, patients often recognize themselves. Receiving credible, practical, and clear interpretation of their long-lasting problems helps patients establish a positive and reassuring relationship with their therapist. With the quick establishment of preferential channels of communication, patients usually feel syntonic with the therapist and, in return, they comply more completely with the therapeutic plan.

There are diagnostic and therapeutic implications of a lifetime presence of spectrum symptoms in a patient with an Axis I disorder. Referring to the example above, missing the spectrum comorbidity means overlooking potential complications related to the concomitance of panic disorder and depression—that is, greater severity of illness (Angst & Dobler-Mikola, 1985; Pini et al., 1994), poorer prognosis (Hecth et al., 1989; Wittchen & Essau, 1989), higher rates of chronicity (Stavrakaky & Vargo, 1986), decreased patient compliance and responsiveness to treatment (Albus & Sheibe, 1993; Van Valkenburg, Akiskal, Puzantian, & Rosenthal, 1984), poorer psychosocial functioning (Reich et al., 1993), increased family loading (Clayton, 1990), higher risk for substance abuse (Clayton, 1990; Merikangas, Risch, & Weissman, 1994), and elevated odds ratios for suicide attempts (Bronish & Wittchen, 1994; King, Schmaling, Cowley, & Dunner, 1995).

From a therapeutic perspective, this patient will benefit mainly from a drug or other treatment modality acting on both the Axis I disorder *and* the spectrum symptoms. A common example is that of two patients presenting with the same severity of depressive episode. Presume that the clinician prescribes the same antidepressant (e.g., clomipramine) to both patients. After 10 to 15 days, one patient improves as expected whereas the other now evidences panic attacks as well as depression. What is needed is an instrument[3] or a clinician who probes beyond the immediate symptoms needed for a *DSM-IV* diagnosis. Without asking about the spectrum of symptoms, even those that may have occurred much earlier in the patient's lifetime, a therapist will have difficulty understanding these dramatically different outcomes. With the spectrum approach used as a magnifying lens on the patient's psychopathology, it is possible to solve the problem. The patient who improved may have chronic, mild obsessive traits, such as perfectionism, which makes clomipramine the drug of first choice. On the other hand, the patient who developed panic attacks may reveal a previous trait of separation and loss sensitivity, which explains his or her adverse reaction to the clomipramine. The patient who worsened had an overlooked panic vulnerability. When the spectrum reveals such a panic profile, the patient's hypersensitivity to antidepressants and to benzodiazepine withdrawal should be taken into account. Finally, that patient will probably need reassurance and cognitive support, as do most panic patients.

A similar example is that of a depressed, grieving patient who does not recover unless the clinician gives an antidepressant with antipanic action. An abnormal grief reaction reflects a particular vulnerability to separation, which in most cases belongs to the panic-agoraphobic spectrum. Besides, the same panic habitus is often expressed by extremely intense and tight interpersonal relationships and dependency on others, characteristics typical of panic patients.

CONCLUSION

Clinicians who seek only the diagnostic criteria for a specific disorder will probably miss a more global perspective of the entire pathology. Rigid adherence to the *DSM-IV* diagnostic criteria, and by extension, the *DSM-IV* categories, could be somewhat like looking at the world through binoculars, only backwards. Instead of a broad field, the view is very narrow, and the observer sees only part of the landscape. Such a narrow perspective is mainly justified in research, but it is unacceptable in clinical practice. The *DSM-IV* was conceived, at least in part, as a research tool, allowing common, standardized, and atheoretical communication among clinical investigators. But the *DSM-IV* is also used as a clinical manual when the practitioner is face-to-face with the client/patient. In such a nonstandardized, unstructured setting, the clinician more often than not sees the *DSM-IV* as a means to collect payment from a third party and focuses on the predominant symptom picture as the diagnosis. A more integrative approach that takes comorbidity into account not only reflects a more valid psychiatric classification, but it should improve treatment and treatment outcome.

Evidence for the dramatic intrusion of comorbidity phenomena (Axis I and spectrum comorbidity) in psychiatry has been derived from several sources, including epidemiological, pharmacological, clinical, and genetics studies. Despite this broad body of evidence, proponents of the categorical approach mostly conceive subclinical symptomatology that coexists with the disorder as background noise, overlooking the complex degree of overlap, both phenomenological and neurobiological, among the different symptoms. In fact, specific patterns of comorbidity appear to be stable, as if there were common neuronal networks that probably represent functional *loci minoris resistentiae.*

We have discussed the diagnostic improvement brought about by the punctual and refined recognition of subclinical and atypical comorbidity. Another relevant consequence involves therapeutic strategy, as comorbid syndromes often require different acute, continuation, and maintenance doses as well as a distinct timing of administration and suspension of the treatment. It is not difficult to believe that drug targets in the brain are different in different patients, for example, a patient with a pure disorder compared to a patient with the same disorder plus spectrum symptoms of panic, obsessive compulsive disorder (OCD), and related symptomatology. However, official guidelines for the therapy of depression and bipolar disorders still do not provide clinicians and researchers with any treatment-specific indications, devoting relatively little attention to the clinical importance of comorbidity, treatment strategies, and outcome (APA, 1994b; Depression Guideline Panel, 1993).

Also, the reliability of clinical trials can be questioned in the light of a more descriptive approach. Pharmacological trials are usually conducted with patients whose symptomatology fits a particular diagnosis coded by standardized criteria. The presence of soft signs and symptoms belonging to the spectrum of other disorders (observed over a lifetime) is systematically overlooked. For example, in a hypothetical trial for an antipanic medication, a panic patient, who has obsessive symptoms but lacks one symptom to fulfill the criteria for OCD, is included in the trials as well as a patient without obsessive traits. The presence of such a heterogeneous sample certainly raises doubts and questions about the reliability of such studies. Practical consequences may include poor knowledge about the spectrum of action of the treatment, difficulty in predicting response to the treatment, and/or atypical outcomes.

Diagnostic procedures should attempt to combine descriptive, categorical, and dimensional approaches, devoting more attention to the cross-sectional and longitudinal analysis of nuclear, subclinical, and atypical symptoms that may represent a pattern of full-blown and partially expressed comorbidity. Within this conceptual framework, psychopathology can be more specifically approached in clinical terms of either individualized treatment or prevention. Further, some traditional points of weakness of clinical psychiatry and psychology, such as the chronic forms of illness and the treatment-resistant disorders, may be contrasted more successfully.

NOTES

1. The United States of America and much of the world is bound by international treaty to use the *ICD-10*. However, Maser, Kaelber, and Weise (1991) demonstrated that use of the *DSM-III* and its revision was far greater than use of the *ICD* throughout the world.
2. Some diagnostic categories have been created or strengthened by virtue of their response to treatment. Examples are seasonal depression treated by light therapy and bipolar disorder treated with lithium. The observation that imipramine is successful in the treatment of both depression and panic attacks would, by this logic, weaken the argument for a categorical classification of each disorder separately and possibly strengthen the spectrum position.
3. Such an instrument, the Semi-Structured Spectrum Questionnaire, has been developed in Pisa, Italy. It has demonstrated high interrater reliability and is now being adapted for use in the United States.

REFERENCES

Akiskal, H.S., & Akiskal, K. (1992). Cyclothymic hyperthymic and depressive temperaments as subaffective variants of mood disorders. In A. Tasman & M.B. Riba (Eds.), *American Psychiatric Association Review, 15,* 632A–633A. Abstract.

Akiskal, H.S., Maser, J.D., Zeller, P.J., Endicott, J., Coryell, W., Keller, M., Warshaw, M., Clayton, P., & Goodwin, F. (1995). Switching from "unipolar" to bipolar II: An 11-year prospective study of clinical and temperamental predictors in 559 patients. *Archives of General Psychiatry, 52,* 114–123.

Albus, M., & Sheibe, G. (1993). Outcome of panic disorder with and without concomitant depression: A 2-year prospective follow-up study. *American Journal of Psychiatry, 150,* 1878–1880.

American Psychiatric Association, Committee on Nomenclature and Statistics. (1952). *Diagnostic and statistical manual: Mental disorders.* Washington, DC: American Psychiatric Association Mental Hospital Service.

American Psychiatric Association. (1968). *The diagnostic and statistical manual of mental disorders* (2nd ed.). Washington, DC: Author.

American Psychiatric Association. (1980). *The diagnostic and statistical manual of mental disorders* (3rd ed.). Washington, DC: Author.

American Psychiatric Association. (1994a). *The diagnostic and statistical manual of mental disorders* (4th ed.). Washington, DC: Author.

American Psychiatric Association. (1994b). Practice guideline for the treatment of patients with bipolar disorder. *American Journal of Psychiatry, 151*(Suppl. 1), 1–36.

Angst, J., & Dobler-Mikola, A. (1985). The Zurich study, VI: A continuum from depression to anxiety disorders? *European Archives of Psychiatry and Neurological Sciences, 235,* 178–186.

Angst, J., Vollrath, M., Merikangas, K.R., & Ernst, C. (1990). Comorbidity of anxiety and depression in the Zurich cohort study of young adults. In J.D. Maser & C.R. Cloninger (Eds.), *Comorbidity of mood and anxiety disorders* (pp. 123–137). Washington, DC: American Psychiatric Press.

Berkson, J. (1946). Limitations of the application of fourfold table analysis to hospital data. *Biometric Bulletin, 2,* 47–53.

Blashfield, R.K., McElroy, R.A., Pfohl, P., & Blum, N. (1994). Comorbidity and the prototype model. *Clinical Psychology: Science and Practice, 1*(1), 96–99.

Boyd, J.H., Burke, J.D., Jr., Gruenberg, E., Holzer, C.E., III, Rae, D.S., George, L.K., Karno, M., Stoltzman, R., McEvoy, L., & Nestadt, G. (1984). Exclusion criteria of *DSM-III. Archives of General Psychiatry, 41*(10), 983–989.

Bronish, T., & Wittchen, H.-U. (1994). Suicidal ideation and suicide attempts: Comorbidity with depression, anxiety disorders and substance abuse disorder. *European Archives of Psychiatry and Clinical Neuroscience, 244,* 93–98.

Caron, C., & Rutter, M. (1991). Comorbidity in child psychopathology: Concepts, issues and research strategies. *Journal of Child Psychology and Psychiatry, 32*(7) 1063–1080.

Cassano, G.B., Michelini, S., Shear, M.K., Coli, E., Maser, J.D., & Frank, E. (submitted). The panic-agoraphobic spectrum: A new approach to the assessment and treatment of subtle symptomatology. *American Journal of Psychiatry.*

Cassano, G.B., & Michelini, S. (1995). Pharmacological treatment of depression and comorbid anxiety disorders. In G. Gessa, W. Fratta, L. Pani, & G. Serra (Eds.), *Depression and mania: From neurobiology to treatment* (pp. 113–125). New York: Raven Press.

Cassano, G.B., & Savino, M. (1993). Symptomatology of panic disorder. An attempt to define the panic-agoraphobic spectrum phenomenology. In S. Montgomery (Ed.), *Psychopharmacology of panic* (pp. 38–57). London: Oxford University Press.

Chen, Y.W., & Dilsaver, S.C. (1995). Comorbidity of panic disorder in bipolar illness: Evidence from the Epidemiologic Catchment Area Survey. *American Journal of Psychiatry, 152,* 280–282.

Clayton, P. (1990). The comorbidity factor: Establishing the primary diagnosis in patients with mixed symptoms of anxiety and depression. *Journal of Clinical Psychiatry, 51*(Suppl.), 35–39.

Coryell, W., Endicott, J., & Winokur, G. (1992). Anxiety syndromes as epiphenomena of primary major depression: Outcome and familial psychopathology. *American Journal of Psychiatry, 149*(1), 100–107.

Depression Guideline Panel. (1993). Guideline: Depression co-occurring with other psychiatric conditions. In *Depression in primary care: Vol. 1. Detection and diagnosis* (pp. 43–54). (Publication No. 93-0550). Washington, DC: U.S. Department of Health and Human Services, Agency for Health Care Policy and Research.

Feinstein, A.R. (1970). The pre-therapeutic classification of co-morbidity in chronic disease. *Journal of Chronic Disease, 23,* 455–468.

Greenberg, W.M., Rosenfeld, D.N., & Ortega, E.A. (1995). Adjustment disorder as an admission diagnosis. *American Journal of Psychiatry, 152*(3), 459–461.

Hays, R.D., Wells, K.B., Sherbourne, C.D., Rogers, W., & Spritzer, K. (1995). Functioning and well-being outcomes of patients with a depression compared with chronic general medical illnesses. *Archives of General Psychiatry, 52,* 11–19.

Hecth, H., von Zerssen, D., Krieg, C., Possl, J. & Wittchen, H.-U. (1989). Anxiety and depression: comorbidity, psychopathology, and social functioning. *Comprehensive Psychiatry, 30,* 420–433.

Johnson, J., Weissman, M.M., & Klerman, G.L. (1990). Panic disorder, comorbidity, and suicide attempts. *Archives of General Psychiatry, 47,* 805–808.

Katz, M., Cole, J.O., & Barton, W.E. (1968). *The role of methodology of classification in psychiatry and psychopathology* (No. HSM 72-9015). Washington, DC: Department of Health, Education and Welfare.

Kendall, P.C., & Watson, D. (Eds.). (1989). *Anxiety and depression: Distinctive and overlapping features.* New York: Academic Press.

King, M.K., Schmaling, K.B., Cowley, D.S., & Dunner, D.L. (1995). Suicide attempt history in depressed patients with and without a history of panic attacks. *Comprehensive Psychiatry, 36,* 25–30.

Klein, D.N., & Riso, L.P. (1993). Psychiatric disorders: Problems of boundaries and comorbidity. In C.G. Costello (Ed.), *Basic issues in psychopathology* (pp. 19–66). New York: Guilford Press.

Klerman, G.L. (1990). Approaches to the phenomena of comorbidity. In J.D. Maser & C.R. Cloninger (Eds.), *Comorbidity of mood and anxiety disorders* (pp. 13–37). Washington, DC: American Psychiatric Press.

Klerman, G.L., Weissman, M.M., Ouellette, R., Johnson, J., & Greenwald, S. (1991). Panic attacks in the community: Social morbidity and health care utilization. *Journal of the American Medical Association, 265*(6), 742–746.

Levenson, J.L., Hamer, R.M., & Rossiter, L.F. (1990). Relation of psychopathology in general medical inpatients to use and cost of services. *American Journal of Psychiatry, 147,* 1498–1503.

Lewis, A. (1936). Prognosis in the manic-depressive psychosis. *Lancet, 2,* 997–999.

Lilienfeld, S.O., Waldman, I.D., & Isreal, A.C. (1994). A critical examination of the use of the term and concept of *comorbidity* in psychopathology research. *Clinical Psychology: Science and Practice, 1*(1), 71–83.

Maser, J.D., & Cloninger, C.R. (Eds.). (1990). *Comorbidity of mood and anxiety disorders.* Washington, D.C.: American Psychiatric Press.

Maser, J.D., Kaelber, C., & Weise, R.E. (1991). International use and attitudes toward *DSM-III* and *DSM-III-R:* Growing consensus in psychiatric classification. *Journal of Abnormal Psychology, 100*(3), 271–279.

Maser, J.D., Weise, R., & Gwirtsman, H. (1995). Depression and its boundaries with selected Axis I disorders: Implications of comorbidity. In E.E. Beckham & W.R. Leber (Eds.), *Handbook of depression* (2nd ed., pp. 86–106). New York: Guilford Press.

Merikangas, K.R., Risch, N.J., & Weissman, M.M. (1994). Comorbidity and co-transmission of alcoholism, anxiety and depression. *Psychological Medicine, 24,* 69–80.

Newcorn, J.H., & Strain, J. (1992). Adjustment disorder in children and adolescents. *Journal of the American Academy of Child and Adolescent Psychiatry, 31,* 318–327.

Nottelmann, E.D., & Jensen, P.S. (1995). Comorbidity of disorders in children and adolescents. In T.H. Ollendick & R.J. Prinz (Eds.), *Advances in Clinical Child Psychology* (Vol. 17, pp. 109–155). New York: Plenum Press.

Oldham, J.M., Skodol, A.E., Kellman, H.D., Hyler, S.E., Doidge, N., Rosnick, L., & Gallaher, P.E. (1995). Comorbidity of Axis I and Axis II disorders. *American Journal of Psychiatry, 152*(4), 571–578.

Pini, S., Goldstein, R.B., Wickramaratne, P.J., & Weissman, M.M. (1994). Phenomenology of panic disorder and major depression in a family study. *Journal of Affective Disorders, 30,* 257–272.

Regier, D.A., Farmer, M.E., Rae, D.S., Locke, B.Z., Keith, S.J., Judd, L.L., & Goodwin, F.K. (1990). Comorbidity of mental disorders with alcohol and other drug abuse: Results from the epidemiologic catchment area (ECA) study. *Journal of the American Medical Association, 264*(19), 2511–2518.

Reich, J.H., & Green, A.I. (1990). Effect of personality disorders on outcome of treatment. *Journal of Nervous and Mental Diseases, 178,* 592–600.

Reich, J.H., & Vasile, R.G. (1993). Effect of personality disorders on outcome of Axis I conditions: An update. *Journal of Nervous and Mental Diseases, 181,* 475–484.

Reich, J., Warshaw, M., Peterson, M., White, K., Keller, M., Lavori, P., & Yonkers, K.A. (1993). Comorbidity of panic and major depressive disorder. *Journal of Psychiatric Research, 27*(Suppl. 1), 23–33.

Robins, L.N. (1994). How recognizing "comorbidities" in psychopathology may lead to an improved research nosology. *Clinical Psychology: Science and Practice, 1*(1), 93–95.

Robins, L.N., & Regier, D.A. (1991). *Psychiatric disorders in America.* New York: Free Press.

Rutter, M. (1994). Comorbidity: Meanings and mechanisms. *Clinical Psychology: Science and Practice, 1*(1), 100–103.

Savino, M., Perugi, G., Simmonini, E., Soriani, A., Cassano, G.B., & Akiskal, H.S. (1993). Affective comorbidity in panic disorder: Is there a bipolar connection? *Journal of Affective Disorders, 28,* 155–163.

Spitzer, R.L. (1994). Psychiatric "co-occurrence"? I'll stick with "comorbidity." *Clinical Psychology: Science and Practice, 1*(1), 88–92.

Stavrakaky, C., & Vargo, B. (1986). The relationships of anxiety and depression: A review of literature. *British Journal of Psychiatry, 149,* 7–16.

Van Valkenburg, C., Akiskal, H.S., Puzantian, V., & Rosenthal, T. (1984). Anxious depression: Clinical family history and naturalistic outcome: Comparison with panic and major depressive disorders. *Journal of Affective Disorders, 6,* 67–82.

Widiger, T.A., & Ford-Black, M.M. (1994). Diagnoses and disorders. *Clinical Psychology: Science and Practice, 1*(1), 84–87.

Winokur, G. (1990). The concept of secondary depression and its relationship to comorbidity. *Psychiatric Clinics of North America, 13,* 567–583.

Wittchen, H.-U., & Essau, C.A. (1989). Comorbidity of anxiety disorders and depression: Does it affect course and outcome? *Psychiatry and Psychobiology, 4,* 315–323.

World Health Organization. (1990, February). *Mental and behavioral disorders: The ICD-10 classification—Diagnostic criteria for research* (Draft for field trials). Geneva, Switzerland: Author.

2

The Prevalence of Psychiatric Comorbidity

RONALD C. KESSLER

Studies of diagnostic patterns in both clinical samples (Ross, Glaser, & Germanson, 1988; Rounsaville et al., 1991; Wolf, Schubert, Patterson, Marion, & Grande, 1988) and general population samples (Boyd et al., 1984; Helzer & Pryzbeck, 1988; Kessler et al., 1994; Kessler, 1995) show that comorbidity among psychiatric disorders is highly prevalent. Over one-half of patients in psychiatric treatment typically have more than one diagnosis (Wolf et al., 1988), and three out of four patients in treatment for substance abuse or dependence also have a diagnosis of some mental disorder (Ross et al., 1988; Rounsaville et al., 1991). As many as half of all lifetime psychiatric disorders in the general population occur to people with a prior history of some other psychiatric disorder (Kessler et al., 1994; Robins & Regier, 1991).

The National Comorbidity Survey (NCS) is a collaborative epidemiologic investigation of the prevalence, causes, and consequences of psychiatric morbidity and comorbidity in the United States. The survey is supported by the National Institute of Mental Health (Grants R01 MH/DA46376 and R01 MH49098), the National Institute of Drug Abuse (through a supplement to R01 MH/DA46376) and the W. T. Grant Foundation (Grant 90135190), Ronald C. Kessler, Principal Investigator. Preparation of this report was also supported by Research Scientist Award K05 MH00507 and by Training Grant T32 MH16806. Collaborating NCS sites and investigators are the Addiction Research Foundation (Robin Room), Duke University Medical Center (Dan Blazer, Marvin Swartz), Harvard University (Richard Frank, Ronald Kessler), the Johns Hopkins University (James Anthony, William Eaton, Philip Leaf), the Max Planck Institute of Psychiatry (Hans-Ulrich Wittchen), the Medical College of Virginia (Kenneth Kendler), the University of Michigan (Lloyd Johnston), New York University (Patrick Shrout), State University of New York (SUNY) at Stony Brook (Evelyn Bromet),

Most of the published research on psychiatric comorbidity, including the work reviewed in this volume, comes from treatment samples. Such work attempts to identify common patterns of comorbidity and to determine whether patients with comorbid disorders respond to treatment differently from those with pure disorders. Treatment samples are less well suited, though, to the more basic epidemiologic questions about the prevalence of comorbidity considered in this chapter. The reason is that the patterns of comorbidity found in treatment settings do not reflect the patterns in the community as a whole. This is so because comorbidity is associated with professional help seeking (Helzer & Pryzbeck, 1988; Regier et al., 1990; Rounsaville, Dolinsky, Babor, & Meyer, 1987; Woodruff, Guze, Clayton, & Carr, 1973). As a result, it is necessary to turn to community samples for accurate information about the distribution of comorbidity. Such studies are rare. Only two major general population epidemiologic surveys have been used to study psychiatric comorbidity in the United States. The first is the Epidemiologic Catchment Area (ECA) study (Robins & Regier, 1991), a landmark survey of over 20,000 respondents carried out in the early 1980s in five U.S. communities. It documented for the first time that comorbidity among psychiatric cases is quite common in the general population. The second is the National Comorbidity Survey (NCS; Kessler et al., 1994). Carried out in the early 1990s, this was a nationally representative survey of over 8,000 respondents with the explicit aim of obtaining more detailed information about psychiatric comorbidity than that collected in the ECA study. This chapter reviews the results obtained to date from the NCS.

STUDY DESIGN

The respondents in the NCS were selected, using probability methods, from a stratified sample of small areas in 172 counties in 34 states throughout the United States. These individuals, who were all between 15 and 54 years of

the University of Toronto (R. Jay Turner), and Washington University School of Medicine (Linda Cottler). A complete list of NCS publications can be obtained from the NCS Study Coordinator, Room 1006, Institute for Social Research, University of Michigan, Box 1248, Ann Arbor, MI 48106-1248. The text of this and other NCS publications, working papers, and instruments can be obtained from the Internet by typing "141.211.207.206"; NAME = anonymous; PASSWORD = (your Internet e-mail address). Read the INSTRUCTIONS to download NCS documents. A public access NCS data file can be obtained from the Internet by typing "ftp.icpsr.umich.edu"; NAME = anonymous; PASSWORD = (your Internet e-mail address). The author appreciates the assistance with data analysis of Jinyun Liu, Christopher Nelson, Kate McGonagle, and Shanyang Zhao as well as the helpful comments of Evelyn Bromet, Fred Osher, and Hans-Ulrich Wittchen.

age, were interviewed in their homes between September 1990 and February 1992. The survey was administered by the staff of the Survey Research Center at the University of Michigan. The response rate was 82.4 percent. The data were weighted to adjust for variation in within-household probabilities of selection and systematic nonresponse and poststratified to approximate the national population distributions of major census variables. A more detailed description of the NCS sampling design is reported elsewhere (Kessler et al., 1994).

The *Diagnostic and Statistical Manual of Mental Disorders* (*DSM-III-R*) (American Psychiatric Association [APA], 1987) diagnoses were based on a modified version of the Composite International Diagnostic Interview (CIDI; World Health Organization [WHO], 1990), a fully structured diagnostic interview developed in a collaborative WHO/Alcohol, Drug, and Mental Health Services Administration (ADAMHA) project to foster epidemiologic and cross-cultural comparative research by producing diagnoses according to the definitions and criteria of both *DSM-III-R* (APA, 1987) and the *Diagnostic Criteria for Research of the International Classification of Diseases* (*ICD-10*) (WHO, 1993). The CIDI uses the same basic architecture as the Diagnostic Interview Schedule (Robins, Helzer, Cottler, & Goldring, 1988). Diagnoses reported here are based on *DSM-III-R* criteria and include mood disorders (major depression, dysthymia, mania), anxiety disorders (panic disorder, generalized anxiety disorder, phobia, posttraumatic stress disorder), substance use disorders (alcohol abuse, alcohol dependence, illicit drug abuse, illicit drug dependence), and other disorders (conduct disorder, adult antisocial behavior, schizophrenia, other nonaffective psychoses). Good reliability and validity of the CIDI diagnoses have been documented in a series of international studies conducted largely as part of the WHO field trials of the CIDI (Wittchen, 1993) as well as in reliability and validity studies carried out as part of the National Comorbidity Survey (Wittchen, Kessler, Zhao, & Abelson, 1995). An exception to this statement is the diagnosis of nonaffective psychosis (NAP), including schizophrenia, which was found to have low validity in the ECA study (Anthony et al., 1985) and was consequently assessed using a two-stage clinical reappraisal approach in the NCS (Kendler, Gallagher, Abelson, & Kessler, in press).

Twelve-month and lifetime prevalences of specific NCS/*DSM-III-R* disorders have been reported previously (Kessler et al., 1994). The diagnoses considered in this chapter differ from those reported earlier in several ways. First, posttraumatic stress disorder (PTSD) has now been added to the anxiety disorders, based on evidence from recent analyses that it is a highly prevalent disorder (Kessler, Sonnega, Bromet, Hughes, & Nelson, 1995). This diagnosis was not included in earlier reports because PTSD was a Part III NCS diagnosis. Second, we have now expanded the assessment of symptoms associated with antisocial personality disorder to distinguish between conduct disorder (CD; three or more types of antisocial behavior that occurred prior to the age of 15) and adult antisocial behavior (AAB; four or more types of antisocial behavior that occurred after the age of 18). Although both CD and AAB are required for a diagnosis of antisocial personality disorder (APA, 1987), the present analysis considers CD and AAB separately because of evidence documented in recent NCS analyses that a substantial number of respondents, women in particular, report AAB in the absence of CD (Cottler, Kessler, & Nelson, submitted). Third, there is a change in the definitions of alcohol dependence and drug dependence. In earlier reports we used the CIDI convention of defining respondents as having 12-month substance dependence when they met lifetime criteria for the disorder and had one or more 12-month dependence symptoms. This has now been changed to require a minimum of three 12-month dependence symptoms, which is the minimum specified in *DSM-III-R* as fulfilling the requirement of Criterion A for a diagnosis of dependence.

As the data were obtained from a stratified multistage sample with weights, estimates of standard errors based on the usual assumptions of equal-probability simple random sampling are biased. Therefore, more complex analysis methods were used to obtain appropriate significance tests. Estimates of standard errors of prevalences reported in this chapter were obtained using the Taylor series linearization method (Woodruff & Causey, 1976). The PSRATIO program in the OSIRIS software package (University of Michigan, 1981) was used to make these calculations. Estimates of confidence intervals of odds ratios were obtained using the method of Jackknife Repeated Replications (JRR; Kish & Frankel, 1970). The LOGISTIC program in the SAS software package (SAS Institute, 1988) was used to estimate the odds ratios (ORs). An SAS macro was used to replicate these estimates in subsamples, to compute estimates of the standard errors of the logits from the distribution of the coefficients across these replications, and to use this design-based estimate of the standard errors to compute confidence intervals of the odds ratios. The JRR estimates take into account clustering and weighting without the linearization constraint required in the Taylor series method, yielding somewhat less biased estimates of standard errors in nonlinear models such as logistic regression (Kish & Frankel, 1970; Woodruff & Causey, 1976).

LIFETIME PSYCHIATRIC COMORBIDITY

General Patterns

As noted above, the ECA investigators were the first to document that co-morbidity is widespread in the general population. Over 54 percent of re-spondents in the five local ECA sites with a lifetime history of at least one *DSM-III* psychiatric disorder were found to have a second diagnosis as well. Fifty-two percent of lifetime alcohol abusers had a second diagnosis, and 75 percent of lifetime drug abusers had a second diagnosis (Robins, Locke, & Regier, 1991). Respondents with a lifetime history of at least one mental disorder had a relative odds of 2.3 of having a lifetime history of alcohol abuse or dependence and a relative odds of 4.5 of some other drug use dis-order compared to respondents with no mental disorder (Regier et al., 1990).

Similar results have more recently been found in the National Comor-bidity Survey. Fifty-six percent of the respondents with a lifetime history of at least one *DSM-III-R* disorder also had one or more other disorders (Kessler, 1995). Fifty-two percent of respondents with lifetime alcohol abuse or dependence also had a lifetime mental disorder, whereas 36 percent had a lifetime illicit drug use disorder. Fifty-nine percent of the respondents with a lifetime history of illicit drug abuse or dependence also had a lifetime men-tal disorder and 71 percent had a lifetime alcohol use disorder.

Comorbidities of Specific Disorders

The results in Table 2-1 show the lifetime prevalences of the 16 core NCS/*DSM-III-R* disorders along with the proportions of people having these disorders who are comorbid in the sense of reporting at least one other life-time NCS/*DSM-III-R* disorder. As shown there, 19.6 percent of the popula-tion in the age range of the NCS are estimated to have had a mood disorder at some time in their lives, 28.7 percent to have had a lifetime anxiety disorder, 26.7 percent to have had a lifetime substance use disorder, and 52.5 percent to have had one or more of the NCS disorders. Lifetime comorbidity is the norm for these cases, with proportions ranging from a low of 62.1 percent for alcohol abuse to a high of 99.4 percent for mania. Seven of the 16 disor-ders have lifetime comorbidities in excess of 90 percent and the average pro-portion of comorbidity across disorders is 8.6 percent. These high comor-bidities should not be interpreted as suggesting that 86.6 percent of people with a lifetime psychiatric disorder are comorbid, as those with comorbidity are counted multiple times in the table. Instead, as shown at the end of the third numeric column of the table, 59.8 percent of the people who have ever had one of the disorders considered here have a history of multiple disorders.

TABLE 2-1
Lifetime Prevalences of National Comorbidity Survey/*DSM-III-R*
Disorders and Proportions with Lifetime Comorbidity[1]

	Lifetime Prevalence		Proportion with Lifetime Comorbidity among Those Having the Disorder	
	%	se	%	se
I. Mood Disorders				
MDE	17.2	(0.6)	83.1	(2.2)
DD	1.7	(0.3)	91.3	(1.8)
BPI	6.7	(0.4)	99.4	(0.6)
Any	19.6	(0.6)	82.2	(2.1)
II. Anxiety Disorders				
GAD	5.2	(0.4)	91.3	(1.5)
PD	3.6	(0.3)	92.2	(1.9)
SoP	13.3	(0.7)	81.0	(1.5)
SiP	11.3	(0.6)	83.4	(1.5)
AG	6.8	(0.3)	87.3	(2.9)
PTSD	7.6	(0.5)	81.0	(3.3)
Any	28.7	(1.0)	74.1	(1.5)
III. Substance Use Disorder				
AA	9.4	(0.5)	62.1	(2.6)
AD	14.2	(0.7)	80.6	(2.4)
DA	4.4	(0.4)	89.0	(2.6)
DD	7.7	(0.5)	95.7	(2.0)
Any	26.7	(1.1)	73.3	(1.3)
IV. Other Disorders				
CD	13.0	(0.7)	78.9	(2.6)
AAB	5.2	(0.3)	96.2	(1.0)
NAP	0.7	(0.1)	93.0	(4.4)
V. Any Disorders				
1+	52.5	(1.3)	59.8	(1.2)
1	21.1	(0.9)	—	—
2+	31.4	(0.1)	—	—

[1]All disorders are operationalized using *DSM-III-R* criteria ignoring diagnostic hierarchy rules. MDE = major depressive episode; DD = dysthymic disorder; BPI = bipolar I disorder; GAD = generalized anxiety disorder; PD = panic disorder; SoP = social phobia; SiP = simple phobia; AG = agoraphobia; PTSD = posttraumatic stress disorder; AA = alcohol abuse; AD = alcohol dependence; DA = illicit drug abuse; DD = illicit drug dependence; CD = conduct disorder; AAB = adult antisocial behavior (defined only for NCS respondents ages 19+ and absent, by definition, for younger respondents); NAP = nonaffective psychosis (schizophrenia, schizophreniform disorder, schizoaffective disorder, delusional disorder, atypical psychosis, psychosis not otherwise specified).

Bivariate Comorbidities

Data on lifetime (LT) comorbidities of specific pairs of disorders in the NCS are presented in Table 2-2. Results are shown in the form of odds ratios (ORs). Diagnostic hierarchy rules were not used in constructing this table so as to avoid artificially deflating estimates of comorbidity. The exceptions are substance abuse and dependence; these were defined in such a way as to be mutually exclusive even though the vast majority of people who meet criteria for dependence also meet criteria for abuse. The most striking result is that all but four of the 118 ORs shown in the table are greater than 1.0. This means that there is a positive association between the lifetime occurrences of almost every pair of NCS/*DSM-III-R* disorders.

However, there is considerable variation in the size of the ORs. It is conceivable that this variation is due to random error. To determine whether this is the case, a comparison was made between the ORs presented here and comparable ORs obtained by reanalyzing data from the Epidemiologic Catchment Area study. This comparison showed a rank-order correlation between the ORs in the two surveys of .79 (Kessler, 1995), which documents the variation in the ORs as systematic rather than random.

Several patterns related to this variation are worthy of note. First, one would expect the relative sizes of the ORs to show that disorders of a single type are more strongly related to each other than to disorders of another type. This is generally true. However, the strength of pairwise associations within the mood disorders is generally greater than within the anxiety disorders, with an average OR of 13.5 for affective disorders and 6.2 for anxiety disorders.

Second, mood disorders and anxiety disorders are strongly comorbid. In fact, pairwise associations between a mood disorder and an anxiety disorder (an average OR of 6.6) are generally stronger than between two anxiety disorders.

Third, despite a substantial clinical literature pointing to the importance of comorbidity between mood disorders and substance use disorders (Allen & Frances, 1986; DeMilio, 1989; Hasin, Grant, & Endicott, 1988; Hesselbrock, Meyer, & Keener, 1985; Keeler, Taylor, & Miller, 1979; Penick, Powell, Jackson, & Liskow, 1988; Ross et al., 1988) and between anxiety disorders and substance use disorders (Chambless, Cherney, Caputo, & Rheinstein, 1987; Hasin et al., 1988; Hesselbrock et al., 1985; Penick et al., 1988; Mullaney & Trippett, 1979; Roy, DeJong, Lamparski, Adinoff, et al., 1991; Roy, DeJong, Lamparski, George, & Linnoila, 1991; Weiss & Rosenberg, 1985), these are among the weakest comorbidities shown in the

TABLE 2-2
Lifetime Comorbidities (Odds Ratios) between Pairs of National Comorbidity Survey/DSM-III-R Disorders[1]

	Mood Disorders			Anxiety Disorders						Substance Use Disorders				Other Disorders	
	MDE	DD	BPI	GAD	PD	SoP	SiP	AG	PTSD	AA	AD	DA	DD	CD	AAB
I. Mood Disorders															
DD	14.4*														
BPI	18.0*	8.2*													
II. Anxiety Disorders															
GAD	9.7*	13.6*	10.4*												
PD	7.0*	5.2*	11.0*	12.3*											
SoP	3.6*	3.2*	4.6*	3.8*	4.8*										
SiP	4.5*	3.4*	10.1*	4.9*	7.9*	7.8*									
AG	4.8*	3.1*	7.9*	5.8*	11.9*	7.1*	8.7*								
PTSD	5.3*	5.1*	6.4*	3.9*	3.9*	2.8*	3.8*	4.2*							
III. Substance Use Disorders															
AA	0.9	0.9	0.9	0.8	1.0	1.2	1.3*	1.0	0.7*						
AD	2.7*	3.0*	7.0*	2.7*	2.0*	2.2*	2.1*	1.7*	2.6*	5.8*					
DA	1.7*	1.4	1.1	1.5	1.6	1.2	1.1	0.9	1.6*	5.8*	3.8*				
DD	2.8*	3.0*	7.2*	3.8*	3.8*	2.6*	2.5*	2.9*	4.0*	2.3*	11.9*	—			
IV. Other Disorders															
CD	1.9*	2.0*	5.8*	1.8*	1.6*	2.1*	1.8*	1.9*	2.2*	2.0*	5.6*	2.6*	5.3*		
AAB	2.4*	3.0*	7.3*	3.6*	2.2*	2.9*	2.5*	2.6*	3.5*	1.8*	10.7*	2.8*	13.7*	13.9*	
NAP	7.0*	4.2*	12.3*	6.1*	7.0*	3.0*	2.5*	4.0*	5.1*	1.1	3.3*	1.2	5.4*	2.6*	9.3*

*OR significant at the .05 level, two-tailed test

[1] All disorders are operationalized using DSM-III-R criteria ignoring diagnostic hierarchy rules. MDE = major depressive episode; DD = dysthymic disorder; BPI = bipolar I disorder; GAD = generalized anxiety disorder; PD = panic disorder; SoP = social phobia; SiP = simple phobia; AG = agoraphobia; PTSD = posttraumatic stress disorder; AA = alcohol abuse; AD = alcohol dependence; DA = illicit drug abuse; DD = illicit drug dependence; CD = conduct disorder; AAB = adult antisocial behavior (defined only for NCS respondents ages 19+ and absent, by definition, for younger respondents); NAP = nonaffective psychosis (schizophrenia, schizophreniform disorder, schizoaffective disorder, delusional disorder, atypical psychosis, psychosis not otherwise specified).

table (average ORs of 2.7 for mood-substance pairs and 2.0 for anxiety-substance pairs).

One of the main purposes of investigating comorbid disorders is to help refine definitions of syndromes and diagnoses. With this in mind, it is important to recognize that some of the strongest ORs in Table 2-2 are associated with clusters that are generally recognized as disorders in their own right. For example, the largest OR in Table 2-2 is between major depression and mania. This conjunction, of course, reflects the fact that people with bipolar disorder usually experience not only mania but also depressive episodes (Andreasen, Grove, Coryell, Endicott, & Clayton, 1988; Kessler, Rubinow, Holmes, Abelson, & Zhao, submitted; Wolf et al., 1988). Another example is the strong comorbidity between mania and nonaffective psychosis (OR = 12.3), a conjunction that is part of the definition of schizoaffective disorder (APA, 1987).

Also in Table 2-2 are a number of strong ORs associated with comorbidities that have been discussed in the clinical literature as possibly indicating the existence of a heretofore unrecognized disorder. For example, the suggestion has been made that comorbidity between major depression and panic is due to a phasic "panic-depressive illness" characterized by panic, depressive, and mixed anxious-depressive phases (Akiskal, 1986, 1990). This possibility is consistent with the finding in Table 2-2 of a pronounced association between panic and depression (OR = 7.0).

Temporally Primary and Secondary Disorders

The results in the first column of Table 2-3 show that there is considerable variation across disorders in the probability of being their temporally primary—that is, of being the lifetime NCS/*DSM-III-R* disorder with the earliest age of onset for a particular respondent. (In cases where two or more disorders were reported to have started at the same age and before any other disorders, both are coded as primary.) Simple phobia, social phobia, alcohol abuse, and conduct disorder are the only four core disorders for which the majority of lifetime cases are temporally primary. In general, anxiety disorders are more likely than others to be temporally primary; 82.8 percent of respondents having one or more lifetime anxiety disorders reported that one of these was their first disorder compared to 71.1 percent of respondents with conduct disorder, 43.8 percent of those with a mood disorder, and 48.1 percent of those with a substance use disorder.

The results in the third column of Table 2-3 show the percentage of NCS respondents who reported that each disorder was temporally primary. As a group, anxiety disorders are more likely to be temporally primary (45.3

TABLE 2-3
Percentage of Disorders That Are Temporally Primary and Distribution
of Temporally Primary National Comorbidity Survey/*DSM-III-R* Disorders[1]

	Percentage Temporally Primary Among Those Having the Disorder		Distribution of Temporally Primary Disorder	
	%	se	%	se
I. Mood Disorders				
MDE	41.1	(2.7)	13.4	(0.9)
DD	37.7	(3.1)	4.8	(0.5)
BPI	20.2	(6.0)	0.7	(0.2)
Any	43.8	(2.4)	16.4	(0.9)
II. Anxiety Disorders				
GAD	37.0	(2.9)	3.6	(0.4)
PD	23.3	(3.2)	1.6	(0.2)
SoP	63.1	(2.0)	16.0	(0.9)
SiP	67.6	(2.7)	14.5	(1.0)
AG	45.2	(4.0)	5.9	(0.7)
PTSD	52.1	(3.0)	7.5	(0.7)
Any	82.8	(1.3)	45.3	(1.4)
III. Substance Use Disorder				
AA	57.0	(2.3)	10.2	(0.6)
AD	36.8	(3.1)	9.9	(0.6)
DA	39.7	(3.0)	3.4	(0.3)
DD	20.8	(2.5)	3.0	(0.3)
Any	48.1	(1.6)	24.5	(1.0)
IV. Other Disorders				
CD	71.1	(2.0)	17.7	(1.0)
AAB	14.0	(1.8)	1.4	(0.2)
NAP	28.8	(5.6)	0.4	(0.1)

[1]All disorders are operationalized using *DSM-III-R* criteria ignoring diagnostic hierarchy rules. MDE = major depressive episode; DD = dysthymic disorder; BPI = bipolar I disorder; GAD = generalized anxiety disorder; PD = panic disorder; SoP = social phobia; SiP = simple phobia; AG = agoraphobia; PTSD = posttraumatic stress disorder; AA = alcohol abuse; AD = alcohol dependence; DA = illicit drug abuse; DD = illicit drug dependence; CD = conduct disorder; AAB = adult antisocial behavior (defined only for NCS respondents ages 19+ and absent, by definition, for younger respondents); NAP = nonaffective psychosis (schizophrenia, schizophreniform disorder, schizoaffective disorder, delusional disorder, atypical psychosis, psychosis not otherwise specified).

percent of all lifetime NCS cases reported that an anxiety disorder was their first disorder) than either mood disorders (16.4 percent), substance use disorders (24.5 percent), or other disorders (19.5 percent). Four types of disorder account for 81.7 percent of all temporally primary cases: alcohol abuse or dependence (20.1 percent), conduct disorder (17.7 percent), simple or social phobia (30.5 percent), and major depression (13.4 percent).

Predictively Primary and Secondary Disorders

It is a mistake to think of temporal priority as equivalent to causal priority, as it is possible to have comorbid disorders in which the disorder with the earlier age of onset does not significantly predict the subsequent onset of the second disorder (Kessler & Price, 1993). A more useful way to begin examining the possibility of causal priority is to investigate predictive priority—whether one disorder is significantly associated with the subsequent onset of another disorder. This was done in the NCS by using retrospective age of onset reports for each disorder to estimate a series of bivariate survival models in which onset of that disorder was treated as a time-varying predictor of the other disorders (Efron, 1988). (Nonaffective psychosis [NAP] was not included in the analysis because of low prevalence.) These models constrained the effects of earlier disorders to be constant across age of onset, time since onset, and age of onset of the outcome disorder. Despite these unrealistic simplifying assumptions, the results provide useful first approximations of the average effects of earlier disorders in predicting the onset of later disorders.

Results are reported in Table 2-4. One hundred sixty-six of the 201 co-efficients in the table are statistically significant, all of them with ORs greater than 1.0. This means that most NCS/*DSM-III-R* disorders both significantly predict the subsequent onset of other disorders and are significantly predicted by prior disorders. Thirteen of the 15 disorders considered here are pervasive predictors; that is, they significantly predict the vast majority (between 10 and 14) of the other disorders. The exceptions are alcohol abuse (AA), which predicts only three other disorders, and illicit drug abuse (DA), which predicts only seven. Twelve of the disorders are also pervasively predicted (by between 11 and 14 of the other disorders). The exceptions are AA, which is predicted by only four other disorders; drug abuse, which is predicted by nine other disorders; and conduct disorder, which is predicted by six other disorders.

A number of significant asymmetries occur in the ORs. Mood disorders generally predict anxiety disorders (average OR = 6.4), substance use disorders (average OR = 3.5), and conduct disorder/adult antisocial behavior

TABLE 2-4
The Associations (Odds Ratios) between Lifetime History of One National Comorbidity Survey/DSM-III-R Disorder (Rows) and Subsequent First Onset of Other Disorders (Columns)[1]

	Mood Disorders			Anxiety Disorders						Substance Use Disorders				Other Disorders	
	MDE	DD	BPI	GAD	PD	SoP	SiP	AG	PTSD	AA	AD	DA	DD	CD	AAB
I. Mood Disorders															
MDE	—	3.5*	7.7*	3.4*	5.1*	2.9*	3.1*	3.4*	6.7*	1.3	3.3*	2.9*	4.3*	3.3*	4.2*
DD	5.2*	—	5.9*	5.4*	3.6*	2.8*	3.1*	2.5*	6.9*	0.9	3.6*	2.1*	3.1*	2.3	3.3*
BPI	8.7**	7.3*	—	12.8*	10.8*	5.3*	16.8*	12.4*	8.2*	0.8	9.0*	2.1	9.1*	215.4*	8.5*
II. Anxiety Disorders															
GAD	4.0*	7.1*	4.9*	—	6.9*	5.9*	3.8*	4.3*	4.9*	1.1	2.9*	2.4*	4.7*	0.9	4.6*
PD	3.5*	5.1*	13.7*	5.7*	—	1.6	2.2*	2.5*	4.9*	0.7	3.2*	1.4	5.2*	3.7*	5.5*
SoP	2.9*	3.0*	2.4*	2.4*	4.3*	—	4.5*	3.8*	2.4*	1.5*	2.2*	1.6*	2.8*	2.0*	2.9*
SiP	2.9*	3.3*	0.9	2.0*	2.7*	3.4*	—	2.9*	1.8*	1.4*	2.1*	1.1	3.0*	1.1	2.6*
AG	3.4*	2.3*	2.8*	2.9*	5.0*	3.4*	4.3*	—	4.5*	1.3	2.1*	1.1	3.3*	2.4*	3.7*
PTSD	2.7*	3.7*	2.7*	2.2*	2.2*	1.9*	2.8*	2.4*	—	0.7	2.4*	1.7*	4.0*	1.9*	3.0*
III. Substance Use Disorders															
AA	1.0	1.0	1.1	0.9	1.5	0.7	1.1	1.0	0.6	—	—[2]	4.5*	3.2*	—[3]	2.6*
AD	2.0*	2.0*	5.4*	2.3*	1.6*	2.2*	1.4	1.6*	2.6*	—[2]	—	3.0*	8.2*	—[3]	17.0*
DA	1.4*	1.3	0.9	1.2	2.3*	0.7	1.8*	1.0	1.8*	2.5*	3.4*	—	—[2]	—[3]	3.2*
DD	2.0*	3.0*	6.3*	2.9*	3.6*	2.4*	1.2	2.6*	2.9*	1.0	5.6*	—[2]	—	—[3]	17.0*
IV. Other Disorders															
CD	2.0*	2.3*	5.6*	2.1*	1.6*	1.9*	2.0*	1.7*	2.2*	2.0*	5.2*	2.66*	5.3*	—	14.5*
AAB	2.1*	3.5*	6.4*	3.5*	2.0*	2.9*	2.8*	2.1*	4.3*	1.1	5.2*	2.1*	8.5*	—[4]	—

*OR significant at the .05 level, two-tailed test

[1] All disorders are operationalized using DSM-III-R criteria ignoring diagnostic hierarchy rules. MDE = major depressive episode; DD = dysthymic disorder; BPI = bipolar I disorder; GAD = generalized anxiety disorder; PD = panic disorder; SoP = social phobia; SiP = simple phobia; AG = agoraphobia; PTSD = posttraumatic stress disorder; AA = alcohol abuse; AD = alcohol dependence; DA = illicit drug abuse; DD = illicit drug dependence; CD = conduct disorder; AAB = adult antisocial behavior (defined only for NCS respondents ages 19+ and absent, by definition, for younger respondents); NAP = nonaffective psychosis (schizophrenia, schizophreniform disorder, schizoaffective disorder, delusional psychosis, atypical psychosis, psychosis not otherwise specified).

[2] Substance abuse and dependence do not overlap by definition.

[3] Age of onset of CD was not assessed in the NCS and is arbitrarily set at 10 for purposes of the analyses reported in this table. The ORs in the CD column consequently describe the associations between having other disorders prior to age 10 and having CD. The ORs for substance use disorders could not be computed because of the small numbers of respondents who reported the onset of these disorders prior to age 10.

[4] AAB does not predict CD by definition.

(CD/AAB) (average OR = 4.3) more strongly than these three predict mood disorders (average ORs of 4.0, 2.3, and 3.6, respectively). Anxiety disorders generally predict alcohol and drug dependence (average OR = 2.9) more strongly than these two predict anxiety (average OR = 2.3). And substance use disorders generally predict CD/AAB (average OR = 7.4) more strongly than CD/AAB predict substance use disorders (average OR = 5.3).

Multivariate Disorder Clusters

The odds ratios in Table 2-2 vary greatly in size. Many of the largest ORs seem to form multivariate clusters. For example, CD, AAB, alcohol dependence, and drug dependence are much more powerful predictors of each other than of other disorders. To provide some descriptive information about the extent to which such clusters exist, researchers analyzed the NCS data by means of latent class analysis (LCA; Lazarsfeld & Henry, 1968; McCutcheon, 1987). Latent class analysis postulates the existence of a discrete latent variable defining multivariate disorder clusters that account for observed patterns of comorbidity. When this model holds, the observed cell probabilities in the cross-classification among lifetime disorders will be equal to the product of the within-class marginal disorder prevalences multiplied by the class prevalences and summed across classes of the latent variable. As described in this chapter, the model contains 15 parameters for disorder prevalences within each of k classes of the latent variable in addition to k parameters for class prevalences.

The latent class model was fitted for values of k between one and nine using the iterative-fitting NAG FORTRAN library routine E04UCF (Nag, 1990) and the method of maximum likelihood (Eaves et al., 1993). The fit of LCA models with successively higher values of k was assessed by evaluating differences in the likelihood-ratio chi-squares for pairs of models with 16 degrees of freedom (15 conditional symptom probabilities and one class prevalence) to determine whether a small number of classes underlie the observed patterns of comorbidity among the NCS disorders. Results showed that this is the case and that an eight-class model is the best solution for explaining the observed distribution of disorder profiles for the 5,877 Part II NCS respondents in the 32,768 (2^{15}) logically possible symptom profiles formed by the cross-classification of the 15 disorders (1,015 of which were observed).

The results in Table 2-5 show the conditional symptom prevalences, sample proportions, and average number of disorders in each class of the eight-class model. Class 1 is the largest of the eight, with 56.6 percent of the sample. Included here are the 47.0 percent of respondents having no lifetime

TABLE 2-5
Within-Class Prevalences of Lifetime National Comorbidity Survey/*DSM-III-R*
Disorders for the Eight-Class Latent Class Analysis Model[1]

	LCA Class							
	C1	*C2*	*C3*	*C4*	*C5*	*C6*	*C7*	*C8*
I. Mood Disorders								
MDE	0.0	11.2	69.7	20.1	12.5	94.7	70.6	100.0
DD	0.0	3.3	28.8	4.3	4.2	33.6	32.9	18.8
BPI	0.0	0.5	3.4	3.4	1.0	9.2	26.0	2.9
Any	0.0	14.1	78.1	27.2	16.1	96.2	80.7	100.0
II. Anxiety Disorders								
GAD	0.0	2.2	17.5	7.9	1.7	48.3	35.6	63.2
PD	0.0	0.0	0.0	38.8	0.0	71.0	25.7	24.3
SoP	4.3	13.6	33.0	19.1	12.7	70.0	50.0	9.1
SiP	3.1	10.2	29.1	22.8	4.8	72.2	56.9	52.7
AG	1.4	4.8	18.5	20.3	0.8	56.1	35.9	5.9
PT	0.0	0.4	0.0	100.0	0.0	100.0	52.7	31.5
PTSD	2.6	2.7	18.8	8.8	9.4	26.8	42.3	25.5
Any	11.3	25.5	66.8	100.0	26.7	100.0	96.4	85.3
III. Substance Use Disorders								
AA	0.0	100.0	2.0	15.3	0.0	5.5	0.0	100.0
AD	0.0	0.0	8.5	6.4	81.4	4.9	100.0	0.0
DA	0.8	17.0	3.8	8.3	11.9	3.9	7.1	0.0
DD	0.0	13.0	2.7	7.9	31.0	10.0	63.8	100.0
Any	0.8	100.0	16.2	30.8	91.9	21.7	100.0	100.0
IV. Other Disorders								
CD	4.9	22.3	11.9	5.3	38.0	11.3	59.4	42.4
AAB	0.0	7.3	3.1	1.5	20.9	1.8	47.4	100.0
V. Any Disorders Mean Number								
of Disorders	0.2	2.1	2.5	2.9	2.3	6.2	7.1	6.8
(% of Sample)	(56.6)	(8.3)	(14.4)	(3.9)	(11.9)	(1.8)	(2.9)	(0.2)
(*n*)	(3329)	(486)	(844)	(231)	(701)	(106)	(170)	(10)

[1]All disorders are operationalized using *DSM-III-R* criteria ignoring diagnostic hierarchy rules. MDE = major depressive episode; DD = dysthymic disorder; BPI = bipolar I disorder; GAD = generalized anxiety disorder; PD = panic disorder; SoP = social phobia; SiP = simple phobia; AG = agoraphobia; PTSD = posttraumatic stress disorder; AA = alcohol abuse; AD = alcohol dependence; DA = illicit drug abuse; DD = illicit drug dependence; CD = conduct disorder; AAB = adult antisocial behavior (defined only for NCS respondents ages 19+ and absent, by definition, for younger respondents).

disorder and the 9.4 percent with pure disorders that are not strongly related to any comorbid profile (CD, phobia, PTSD, and drug abuse).

The other seven classes consist of the most common comorbid disorder profiles. Each of Classes 2 through 5 are defined by a single core disorder and a small number of other comorbid disorders (averages ranging between 1.1 and 1.9). The core disorder in Class 2 is alcohol abuse and the most common comorbid disorders are conduct disorder and drug abuse. The core disorder in Class 3 is major depression and the most common comorbid disorders are social phobia, simple phobia, and dysthymia. The core syndrome in Class 4 is panic and the most common comorbid disorders are phobias and major depression. The core disorder in Class 5 is alcohol dependence and the most common comorbid disorders are conduct disorder, adult antisocial behavior, and drug dependence. A total of 38.5 percent of respondents are in one of these low-comorbidity classes.

Each of Classes 6 through 8, in comparison, is defined by a much larger number of disorders (averages ranging between 6.2 and 7.1) with multiple core disorders (4.9 percent of the sample). The core disorders in Class 6 are major depression and panic and the most common secondary disorders are dysthymia and the anxiety disorders other than panic. The core disorders in Class 7 are major depression and alcohol dependence and the most common secondary disorders are drug dependence, CD, AAB, and all the anxiety disorders. Finally, the core disorders in Class 8 are major depression, AAB, alcohol abuse, and drug dependence, whereas the most common secondary disorders are generalized anxiety disorder, simple phobia, and CD.

TWELVE-MONTH PSYCHIATRIC COMORBIDITY

General Patterns

The evidence reviewed so far has concerned the lifetime comorbidity of multiple disorders. Of greater clinical interest is the joint occurrence of multiple disorders in the same person over a recent interval of time. The results in the first column of Table 2-6 show the 12-month prevalences of the 14 core *DSM-III-R* disorders assessed for recent prevalence in the National Comorbidity Survey. Conduct disorder and adult antisocial behavior, which were included in the lifetime analyses, are not reported here because they were assessed on a lifetime basis only. The results displayed in the remainder of the table are the proportions of the remaining disorders that are lifetime pure (i.e., no other lifetime NCS/*DSM-III-R* disorder), lifetime comorbid but 12-month pure (i.e., at least one other lifetime NCS/*DSM-III-R* disorder but no other 12-month disorder), and 12-month comorbid.

TABLE 2-6
Twelve-Month Prevalences of National Comorbidity Survey/DSM-III-R Disorders and Proportions with Lifetime and 12-Month Comorbidity[1]

	12-Month Prevalence		Proportions among 12-Month Disorders					
			That Are Pure in Both 12 Months and Lifetime		That Are Pure in 12 Months But Comorbid in Lifetime		That Are Comorbid in Both 12 Months and Lifetime	
	%	se	%	se	%	se	%	se
I. Mood Disorders								
MDE	10.2	(0.66)	15.6	(1.8)	14.4	(1.8)	69.9	(2.5)
DD	2.7	(0.3)	9.6	(3.4)	2.4	(1.0)	88.0	(2.8)
BPI	1.4	(0.3)	0.0	(—)	1.9	(1.4)	98.1	(1.4)
Any	11.4	(0.6)	16.3	(1.8)	13.8	(1.7)	69.9	(2.2)
II. Anxiety Disorders								
GAD	3.2	(0.3)	7.8	(2.2)	9.6	(3.6)	82.6	(4.0)
PD	2.3	(0.3)	3.8	(2.1)	8.1	(2.6)	88.1	(3.2)
SoP	7.8	(0.4)	17.4	(1.7)	14.4	(1.8)	68.1	(2.2)
SiP	8.8	(0.5)	15.9	(1.7)	15.9	(1.9)	68.3	(2.3)
AG	3.9	(0.4)	9.4	(3.1)	8.4	(2.7)	82.2	(4.2)
PTSD	3.9	(0.4)	17.8	(4.4)	12.6	(2.9)	69.5	(5.5)
Any	19.3	(0.8)	21.5	(1.6)	19.9	(1.4)	58.6	(2.0)
III. Substance Use Disorders								
AA	2.5	(0.2)	43.9	(5.4)	9.1	(2.9)	47.1	(5.7)
AD	7.3	(0.5)	28.7	(2.7)	19.4	(1.9)	52.0	(3.0)
DA	0.8	(0.2)	13.0	(9.3)	19.1	(9.7)	67.9	(1.2)
DD	2.9	(0.3)	5.2	(1.5)	11.6	(3.2)	83.3	(3.2)
Any	11.5	(0.5)	30.2	(2.4)	18.6	(1.7)	51.3	(2.4)
IV. Other Disorders								
NAP	0.3	(0.1)	14.2	(9.0)	22.4	(8.6)	63.4	(15.5)
V. Any Disorders								
1+	30.9	(0.6)	30.8	(1.6)	24.5	(1.5)	44.7	(2.0)
1	17.1	(0.5)	55.6	(2.5)	44.4	(2.5)	—	(—)
2+	13.8	(0.5)	—	(—)	—		100	(—)

[1]All disorders are operationalized using *DSM-III-R* criteria ignoring diagnostic hierarchy rules. MDE = major depressive episode; DD = dysthymic disorder; BPI = bipolar I disorder; GAD = generalized anxiety disorder; PD = panic disorder; SoP = social phobia; SiP = simple phobia; AG = agoraphobia; PTSD = posttraumatic stress disorder; AA = alcohol abuse; AD = alcohol dependence; DA = illicit drug abuse; DD = illicit drug dependence; CD = conduct disorder; AAB = adult antisocial behavior (defined only for NCS respondents ages 19+ and absent, by definition, for younger respondents); NAP = nonaffective psychosis (schizophrenia, schizophreniform disorder, schizoaffective disorder, delusional disorder, atypical psychosis, psychosis not otherwise specified).

As shown in Table 2-6, 11.4 percent of the population in the age range of the NCS is estimated to have had a mood disorder at some time in the 12 months prior to the interview, 19.3 percent to have had a 12-month anxiety disorder, 11.5 percent to have had a 12-month substance use disorder, and 30.9 percent to have had one or more of the 12-month disorders assessed in the NCS. Twelve-month comorbidity is the norm for each of these disorders, with proportions ranging from a low of 47.1 percent for alcohol abuse to a high of 88.1 percent for panic disorder. The average proportion of comorbidity across the disorders is 73.4 percent and 44.7 percent of those with a 12-month disorder carry multiple diagnoses.

Bivariate Comorbidities

Data on 12-month comorbidities of specific pairs of disorders are presented in Table 2-7. The format is the same as in Table 2-2, except that the odds ratios now refer to 12-month prevalence rather than to lifetime prevalence. As in Table 2-2, the vast majority of the 89 coefficients in Table 2-7 are greater than 1.0 (92 percent) and statistically significant (79 percent). This means that there is a positive association between the 12-month occurrences of almost every pair of NCS/*DSM-III-R* disorders. And, as in Table 2-2, the major exceptions are for alcohol and drug abuse. In fact, there is a very strong consistency in the relative sizes of the ORs in Table 2-7 compared to those in Table 2-2. The rank-order correlation between the odds ratios for lifetime and 12-month comorbidity is .89.

Despite these consistencies, three-fourths of the ORs in Table 2-7 are larger than those in Table 2-2. In fact, the average Table 2-7 OR (6.8) is 55 percent larger than the average Table 2-2 OR (4.4). This tendency is least apparent for the relationships of mood and anxiety disorders with substance use disorders (ORs averaging 2.8 and 2.1, respectively, in Table 2-8 compared to 2.7 and 2.0 in Table 2-2). This finding is consistent with evidence from the treatment literature that individuals often use alcohol and drugs to self-medicate depression and anxiety and that this can be effective over short periods of time (thus the comparatively low ratio of 12-month to lifetime odds ratios) even though prolonged self-medication of this sort leads to an exacerbation of the mood and anxiety disorders (Khantzian, Gawin, Kleber, & Riordan, 1984).

Comorbidity and Severity

As earlier reported, the vast majority of NCS respondents who meet the criteria established by a National Institute of Mental Health (NIMH) task force (National Advisory Mental Health Council, 1993) for 12-month severe and

TABLE 2-7
Twelve-Month Comorbidities (Odds Ratios) between Pairs of National Comorbidity Survey/DSM-III-R Disorders[1]

	Mood Disorders			Anxiety Disorders						Substance Use Disorders			
	MDE	DD	BPI	GAD	PD	SoP	SiP	AG	PTSD	AA	AD	DA	DD
I. Mood Disorders													
DD	28.3*												
BPI	27.9*	17.4*											
II. Anxiety Disorders													
GAD	14.8*	28.2*	14.0*										
PD	9.6*	10.6*	19.6*	17.7*									
SoP	4.7*	3.8*	6.2*	4.2*	6.0*								
SiP	6.0*	4.8*	13.4*	5.7*	11.4*	8.6*							
AG	7.9*	5.9*	14.9*	9.5*	23.1*	9.2*	11.4*						
PTSD	7.8*	7.8*	8.7*	5.2*	6.2*	3.7*	3.5*	4.4*					
III. Substance Use Disorders													
AA	1.1	0.9	1.0	0.5	0.5	2.3*	1.2	1.1	1.5				
AD	2.9*	1.2	6.7*	3.4*	1.4	2.2*	2.3*	1.8*	1.5	12.2*			
DA	1.5	3.4*	2.6*	1.7	0.2	1.7	0.7	0.1	2.2*	5.5*	5.2*		
DD	4.3*	2.8*	6.4*	5.4*	3.6*	3.4*	2.5*	4.2*	3.0*	—	13.6*	—	
IV. Other Disorders													
NAP	13.0*	6.2*	9.5*	12.5*	11.1*	4.5*	4.9*	7.6*	8.5*	0.9	3.7*	0.8	8.8*

*OR significant at the .05 level, two-tailed test

[1] All disorders are operationalized using *DSM-III-R* criteria ignoring diagnostic hierarchy rules. MDE = major depressive episode; DD = dysthymic disorder; BPI = bipolar I disorder; GAD = generalized anxiety disorder; PD = panic disorder; SoP = social phobia; SiP = simple phobia; AG = agoraphobia; PTSD = posttraumatic stress disorder; AA = alcohol abuse; AD = alcohol dependence; DA = illicit drug abuse; DD = illicit drug dependence; CD = conduct disorder; AAB = adult antisocial behavior (defined only for NCS respondents ages 19+ and absent, by definition, for younger respondents); NAP = nonaffective psychosis (schizophrenia, schizophreniform disorder, schizoaffective disorder, delusional disorder, atypical psychosis, psychosis not otherwise specified).

persistent mental illness have a lifetime history of three or more NCS/*DSM-III-R* disorders (Kessler et al., 1994). The results in Table 2-8 extend this to consider the criteria established by the Substance Abuse and Mental Health Services Administration (SAMHSA, 1993) for disorders that are sufficiently serious to qualify for treatment under State Block Grant funds. As shown in Table 2-8, there is a strong relationship between comorbidity and prevalence of this serious mental illness (SMI; Kessler, Berglund et al., 1995). Among respondents having a 12-month mood disorder, 48.3 percent of those with 12-month comorbidity met criteria for SMI compared to fewer than half as many of those with a lifetime pure disorder (22.6 percent, z = 4.4, p < .05) and fewer than two-thirds as many of those with a 12-month pure disorder and lifetime comorbidity (31.3 percent, z = 2.7, p < .05). Among respondents having a 12-month anxiety disorder, 37.7 percent of those with 12-month co-morbidity met criteria for a serious mental illness compared to only one-third as many of those with a lifetime pure disorder (11.4 percent, z = 7.0, p < .05) and one-fourth as many of those with a 12-month pure disorder and lifetime comorbidity (9.6 percent, z = 7.1, p < .05).

The results in Table 2-9 provide a somewhat different perspective on the relationship between comorbidity and severity by showing the relationships of lifetime comorbidity, defined in terms of the eight latent class analysis classes, with various 12-month disorders. As shown there, 12-month preva-lences of all disorders are quite low in Class 1. Twelve-month prevalences of core disorders are in the range of 30 percent to 60 percent in Classes 2 through 5 and in the range of 56 percent to 87 percent in Classes 6 through 8. The highest prevalences of 12-month SMI (45.4 percent to 67.5 percent) are found in the classes characterized by high lifetime comorbidity (Classes 6 through 8). Intermediate prevalences of SMI (14.7 percent to 18.1 per-cent) are found in the classes characterized by comorbid anxiety-depres-sion (Class 3) and comorbid panic (Class 4). Much lower prevalences of SMI (3.2 percent to 4.2 percent) are found in the classes characterized by core diagnoses of alcohol abuse (Class 2) and alcohol dependence (Class 5) with low anxiety-depression comorbidity.

DISCUSSION

It is important to acknowledge several limitations in the above results. First, they are based on diagnoses generated from fully structured interviews ad-ministered by interviewers who are not clinicians. Although good reliabil-ity and validity of these interviews has been documented in controlled stud-ies (Wittchen, 1993), most of the interviews were carried out in patient

TABLE 2-8
Prevalence of 12-Month Serious Mental Illness (SMI) among Respondents with Various Pure and Comorbid National Comorbidity Survey/DSM-III-R Disorder[1]

	Lifetime Pure		12-Month Pure Lifetime Comorbid		12-Month Comorbid	
	%	se	%	se	%	se
I. Mood Disorders						
MDE	21.0	(5.5)	31.6	(5.6)	45.6	(3.4)
DD	32.3	(14.2)	0.0	(—)	51.6	(5.2)
BPI	—	(—)	100	(—)[2]	100	(—)[2]
Any	22.6	(5.0)	31.3	(5.5)	48.3	(3.1)
II. Anxiety Disorders						
GAD	17.2	(9.9)	19.2	(12.8)	54.5	(5.6)
PD	0.0	(—)	11.4	(9.6)	56.5	(4.3)
SoP	9.2	(3.3)	8.6	(2.8)	35.7	(2.9)
SiP	5.6	(4.3)	9.9	(5.3)	33.6	(3.2)
AG	9.3	(7.9)	2.7	(2.2)	44.8	(4.5)
PTSD	20.5	(11.0)	9.2	(6.1)	50.9	(3.9)
Any	11.4	(2.8)	9.6	(2.8)	37.7	(2.5)
III. Substance Use Disorders						
AA	0.0[3]	(—)	0.0[3]	(—)	16.1	(4.8)
AD	0.0[3]	(—)	0.0[3]	(—)	32.3	(3.1)
DA	0.0[3]	(—)	0.0[3]	(—)	10.0	(4.9)
DD	0.0[3]	(—)	0.0[3]	(—)	31.0	(4.5)
Any	0.0[3]	(—)	0.0[3]	(—)	29.9	(2.9)
IV. Other Disorders						
NAP	100[2]	(—)	100[2]	(—)	100[2]	(—)
V. Any Disorders						
1	9.9	(4.7)	12.5	(3.9)	—	(—)
2+	—	(—)	—	(—)	33.7	(2.8)

[1] All disorders are operationalized using *DSM-III-R* criteria ignoring diagnostic hierarchy rules. MDE = major depressive episode; DD = dysthymic disorder; BPI = bipolar I disorder; GAD = generalized anxiety disorder; PD = panic disorder; SoP = social phobia; SiP = simple phobia; AG = agoraphobia; PTSD = posttraumatic stress disorder; AA = alcohol abuse; AD = alcohol dependence; DA = illicit drug abuse; DD = illicit drug dependence; CD = conduct disorder; AAB = adult antisocial behavior (defined only for NCS respondents ages 19+ and absent, by definition, for younger respondents); NAP = nonaffective psychosis (schizophrenia, schizophreniform disorder, schizoaffective disorder, delusional disorder, atypical psychosis, psychosis not otherwise specified).

[2] SMI is present by definition among people with BPI and NAP.

[3] SMI is absent by definition among people with pure substance use disorders.

TABLE 2-9
Conditional Prevalences of 12-Month National Comorbidity
Survey/*DSM-III-R* Disorders within Subsamples Defined by the
Eight Lifetime Latent Class Analysis (LCA) Classes

	LCA Class							
	C1	*C2*	*C3*	*C4*	*C5*	*C6*	*C7*	*C8*
I. Any Mood Disorder								
%	0.0	6.2	44.3	16.1	7.9	66.1	55.6	80.6
(se)	(0.0)	(1.3)	(2.6)	(3.1)	(1.3)	(4.8)	(4.7)	(13.7)
II. Any Anxiety Disorder								
%	5.8	17.9	49.4	62.9	13.2	87.3	82.0	78.2
(se)	(0.6)	(1.7)	(2.2)	(4.3)	(1.2)	(4.4)	(3.3)	(13.6)
III. Any Substance Use Disorder								
%	0.2	30.4	6.0	7.6	43.2	7.0	57.8	80.7
(se)	(0.1)	(2.5)	(1.0)	(1.8)	(2.4)	(2.1)	(5.1)	(13.5)
IV. Serious Mental Illness (SMI)								
%	0.8	4.2	18.1	14.7	3.2	49.3	45.4	67.5
(se)	(0.2)	(1.0)	(1.7)	(3.4)	(0.5)	(6.1)	(4.7)	(15.4)

samples. Little is known about the magnitude of classification errors when fully structured diagnostic interviews are used in general population samples. Errors of this sort could lead to systematic bias in estimates of comorbidity. For example, Horwath, Johnson, and Hornig (1993) documented that structured interviews like those used in the National Comorbidity Survey can systematically misclassify simple phobics as agoraphobics, leading to an underestimate of the comorbidity between panic and agoraphobia. We do not know the extent to which biases of this sort affected the results found here concerning prevalence and patterns of comorbidity.

Second, the results concerning temporal priority and prediction are all based on retrospective age of onset reports. Although special efforts were made to improve the accuracy of these reports in the National Comorbidity Survey (Kessler, Mroczek, & Belli, in press), recall bias could have distorted recall and, with it, the accuracy of results concerning primary-secondary disorder patterns.

Third, the results have been reported in summary form with no attention to the likelihood that comorbidity varies depending on such things as the age and sex of the respondent, or their age at onset of the disorder. This is a serious limitation, as clinical evidence shows a number of clear specifications of this sort. For example, comorbid alcoholism is much more often found in patient samples to be primary and associated with Antisocial Personality Disorder (ASPD) among men and secondary and associated with mood disorders and anxiety disorders among women (Hesselbrock et al., 1986; Roy, DeJong, Lamparski, George, et al., 1991). Furthermore, strong and consistent evidence has been found that depressed patients with an early onset have a stronger family history of both depression and alcoholism than those with a late onset (e.g., Mendlewicz & Baron, 1981). These and other specifications are being examined in ongoing analyses of the NCS data, but our current understanding of them is too incomplete to include in this report.

Despite these limitations, the results reported above show clearly that psychiatric comorbidity is highly prevalent. Indeed, the majority of people who suffer from any one psychiatric disorder also have a history of at least one other. It is hard to imagine that correction of measurement or design problems would lead to a modification of this conclusion. The NCS results also suggest that comorbid disorders are, in general, more severe than pure disorders (Kessler, 1995). In fact, the major societal burden of psychiatric disorder is found to fall on people with comorbidity, with nearly 90 percent of NCS respondents having a severe 12-month psychiatric impairment reporting a lifetime history of three or more comorbid psychiatric disorders (Kessler et al., 1994).

What causes such a high rate of comorbidity among psychiatric disorders is not clear. Common causes of either a biological or environmental sort, effects of one disorder on the subsequent onset of other disorders, and diagnostic confusion are probably all at work to some degree. Analysis of temporal relationships does little to help clarify this picture, as most disorders are found to be significant predictors of the subsequent onset of other disorders. There is some variation in this regard, such as the finding that substance abuse is both less strongly predictive and less strongly predicted than the other disorders considered here, and the finding that mania is much more strongly predictive than the other disorders. However, the main impression one gets from the NCS results is that most disorders are related to most other disorders in ways that are very difficult to sort out.

An initial attempt to make some progress in this sorting operation showed that seven broadly defined comorbidity profiles can be detected in the multivariate cross-classification of the National Comorbidity Survey disorders. The most prevalent of these profiles (Class 3, 14.4 percent of the sample) is characterized by high prevalences of both mood disorders (78 percent) and anxiety disorders (67 percent), but low prevalences of other disorders (3 percent to 12 percent). The second most prevalent profile (Class 5, 11.9 percent of the sample) is characterized by a high prevalence of substance use (mostly dependence) disorders (92 percent) and comorbid conduct disorders and adult antisocial behavior (46 percent), with lower prevalences of mood (16 percent) and anxiety (27 percent) disorders. The third most prevalent profile (Class 2, 8.3 percent of the sample) is characterized by 100 percent prevalence of alcohol abuse and moderately high prevalences of mood disorders (14 percent), anxiety disorders (26 percent), and CD/AAB (25 percent). These three profiles describe 80 percent of all lifetime comorbidity in the NCS respondents. The other 20 percent is made up of four less common profiles, two of which have a core of panic and the other two of which are characterized by high prevalences of mood disorders (81 percent to 100 percent), anxiety disorders (85 percent to 96 percent), substance dependence (100 percent), and CD/AAB (74 percent to 100 percent).

The isolation of these profiles provides a good beginning for more detailed analysis. It might be that one or more of these profiles will prove to be useful in advancing our understanding of the pathophysiology of psychiatric disorder and possibly even in improving our ability to offer effective treatments. To justify the laboratory, treatment, and longitudinal studies that would be required to show whether this is the case, preliminary epidemiologic evidence is needed to demonstrate that respondents with these combinations of disorders are distinct from those with pure disorders in terms of family history, age of onset, risk factors, and clinical course. These issues are being explored in ongoing analysis of the NCS data. Cross-national collaborations are also being developed to determine whether these results can be replicated in epidemiologic studies in other parts of the world.

REFERENCES

Akiskal, H.S. (1986). Mood disturbances. In G. Winokur & P. Clayton (Eds.), *The medical basis of psychiatry*. Philadelphia: Saunders.

Akiskal, H.S. (1990). Toward a clinical understanding of the relationship of anxiety and depressive disorders. In J.D. Maser & C.R. Cloninger (Eds.), *Comorbidity of mood and anxiety disorders* (pp. 597–610). Washington, DC: American Psychiatric Press.

Allen, M.H., & Frances, R.J. (1986). Varieties of psychopathology found in patients with addictive disorders: A review. In R.E. Meyer (Ed.), *Psychopathology and addictive disorders*. New York: Guilford Press.

American Psychiatric Association. (1987). *Diagnostic and statistical manual of mental disorders (3rd ed., rev.)*. Washington, DC: Author.

Andreasen, N.C., Grove, W.M., Coryell, W.H., Endicott, J., & Clayton, P.J. (1988). Bipolar versus unipolar and primary versus secondary affective disorder: Which diagnosis takes precedence? *Journal of Affective Disorders, 15*, 69–80.

Anthony, J.C., Folstein, M., Romanoski, A.J., VonKorff, M.R., Nestadt, G.R., Chahal, R., Merchant, A., Brown, C.H., Shapiro, S., Kramer, M., & Gruenberg, E.M. (1985). Comparison of the lay Diagnostic Interview Schedule and a standardized psychiatric diagnosis. Experience in eastern Baltimore. *Archives of General Psychiatry, 42*, 667–675.

Boyd, J.H., Burke, J.D., Jr., Gruenberg, E., Holzer, C.E., Rae, D.S., George, L.K., Karno, M., Stoltzman, R., McEvoy, L., & Nestadt, G. (1984). Exclusion criteria of *DSM-III:* A study of co-occurrence of hierarchy-free syndromes. *Archives of General Psychiatry, 41*, 983–989.

Chambless, D.L., Cherney, J., Caputo, G.D., & Rheinstein, B.J. (1987). Anxiety disorders and alcoholism. *Journal of Anxiety Disorders, 1*, 24–40.

Cottler, L.B., Kessler, R.C., & Nelson, C.B. (submitted). Antisocial personality disorder in the National Comorbidity Survey.

DeMilio, L. (1989). Psychiatric syndromes in adolescent substance abusers. *American Journal of Psychiatry, 146*, 1212–1214.

Eaves, L.J., Silberg, J.L., Hewitt, J.K., Rutter, M., Meyer, J.M., Neale, M.C., & Pickles, A. (1993). Analyzing twin resemblance in multisymptom data: Genetic applications of a latent class model for symptoms of conduct disorder in juvenile boys. *Behavior Genetics, 23*, 5–19.

Efron, B. (1988). Logistic regression, survival analysis and the Kaplan-Meier Curve. *Journal of the American Statistical Association, 83*, 414–425.

Hasin, D., Grant, B., & Endicott, J. (1988). Treated and untreated suicide attempts in substance abuse patients. *Journal of Nervous Mental Diseases, 176*, 289–294.

Helzer, J.E., & Pryzbeck, T.R. (1988). The co-occurrence of alcoholism with other psychiatric disorders in the general population and its impact on treatment. *Journal of Studies on Alcohol, 49*, 219–224.

Hesselbrock, V.M, Hesselbrock, M.N., & Workman-Daniels, K.L. (1986). Effect of major depression and antisocial personality on alcoholism: Course and motivation patterns. *Journal of Studies in Alcohol, 47*, 207–212.

Hesselbrock, M.N., Meyer, R.E., & Keener, J.J. (1985). Psychopathology in hospitalized alcoholics. *Archives of General Psychiatry, 42*, 1050–1055.

Horwath, E., Johnson, J., & Hornig, C.D. (1993). Epidemiology of panic disorder in African-Americans. *American Journal of Psychiatry, 150*, 465–469.

Keeler, M.H., Taylor, C.I., & Miller, W.C. (1979). Are all recently detoxified alcoholics depressed? *American Journal of Psychiatry, 136*, 586–588.

Kendler, K.S., Gallagher, T.J., Abelson, J.M., & Kessler, R.C. (in press). Lifetime prevalence, demographic risk factors and diagnostic validity of nonaffective psychosis as assessed in a U.S. community sample: The National Comorbidity Survey. *Archives of General Psychiatry.*

Kessler, R.C. (1995). The epidemiology of psychiatric comorbidity. In M. Tsuang, M. Tohen, & G. Zahner (Eds.), *Textbook of psychiatric epidemiology* (pp. 179–198). New York: Wiley.

Kessler, R.C., Berglund, P.A., Leaf, P.J., Kouzis, A.C., Bruce, M.L., Friedman, R.M., Grosser, R.C., Kennedy, C., Kuehnel, T.G., Laska, E.M., Manderscheid, R.W., Narrow, B., Rosenbeck, R.A., Santoni, T.W., & Schneier, M. (1995). *Estimation of the 12-month prevalence of Serious Mental Illness (SMI).* NCS

Working Paper #8. Ann Arbor: University of Michigan, Institute for Social Research.

Kessler, R.C., McGonagle, K.A., Zhao, S., Nelson, C.B., Hughes, M., Eshleman, S., Wittchen, H.-U., & Kendler, K.S. (1994). Lifetime and 12-month prevalence of *DSM-III-R* psychiatric disorders in the United States: Results from the National Comorbidity Survey. *Archives of General Psychiatry, 51,* 8–19.

Kessler, R.C., Mroczek, D.K., & Belli, R.F. (in press). Retrospective adult assessment of childhood psychopathology. In D. Shaffer & J. Richters (Eds.), *Assessment in child psychopathology.* New York: Guilford Press.

Kessler, R.C., & Price, R.H. (1993). Primary prevention of secondary disorders: A proposal and agenda. *American Journal of Community Psychology, 21,* 607–634.

Kessler, R.C., Rubinow, D.R., Holmes, C., Abelson, J.M., & Zhao, S. (submitted). *DSM-III-R* bipolar disorder in a general population survey.

Kessler, R.C., Sonnega, A., Bromet, E., Hughes, M., & Nelson, C.B. (1995). Posttraumatic stress disorder in the National Comorbidity Survey. *Archives of General Psychiatry, 52,* 1048–1060.

Khantzian, E.J., Gawin, F.H., Kleber, H.D., & Riordan, C.E. (1984). Methylphenidate treatment of cocaine dependence: A preliminary report. *Journal of Substance Abuse Issues, 1,* 107–112.

Kish, L., & Frankel, M.R. (1970). Balanced repeated replications for standard errors. *Journal of the American Statistical Association, 65,* 1071–1094.

Lazarsfeld, P.R., & Henry, N.W. (1968). *Latent structure analysis.* Boston: Houghton Mifflin.

McCutcheon, A.L. (1987). *Latent class analysis.* Newbury Park, CA: Sage.

Mendlewicz, J., & Baron, M. (1981). Morbidity risks in subtypes of unipolar depressive illness: Differences between early and late onset forms. *British Journal of Psychiatry, 139,* 463–466.

Mullaney, J.A., & Trippett, C.J. (1979). Alcohol dependence and phobias: Clinical description and relevance. *British Journal of Psychiatry, 135,* 565–573.

Nag. (1990). *Nag FORTRAN Library Introductory Guide.* Downers Grove, IL: Author.

National Advisory Mental Health Council. (1993). Health care reform for Americans with severe mental illnesses. *American Journal of Psychiatry, 150,* 1447–1476.

National Institute of Mental Health. (1993). *The prevention of mental disorders: A national research agenda.* Rockville, MD: Author.

Penick, E.C., Powell, B.J., Jackson, J.O., & Liskow, B.I. (1988). The stability of coexisting psychiatric syndromes in alcoholic men after one year. *Journal of Studies on Alcohol, 49,* 395–405.

Regier, D.A., Farmer, M.E., Rae, D.S., Locke, B.Z., Keith, B.J., Judd, L.L., & Goodwin, F.K. (1990). Comorbidity of mental health disorders with alcohol and other drug abuse. *Journal of the American Medical Association, 264,* 2511–2518.

Robins, L.N., & Regier, D.A. (Eds.). (1991). *Psychiatric disorders in America.* New York: Free Press.

Robins, L.N., Helzer, J.E., Cottler, L.B., & Goldring, E. (1988). *The Diagnostic Interview Schedule, Version III-R.* St. Louis, MO: Washington University School of Medicine.

Robins, L.N., Locke, B.Z., & Regier, D.A. (1991). Overview: Psychiatric disorders in America. In L.N. Robins & D.A. Regier (Eds.), *Psychiatric disorders in America* (pp. 328–366). New York: Free Press.

Ross, H.E., Glaser, F.B., & Germanson, T. (1988). The prevalence of psychiatric disorders in patients with alcohol and other drug problems. *Archives of General Psychiatry, 45,* 1023–1031.

Rounsaville, B.J., Anton, S.F., Carroll, K., Budde, D., Prusoff, B.A., & Gawin, R. (1991). Psychiatric diagnosis of treatment-seeking cocaine abusers. *Archives of General Psychiatry, 48,* 43–51.

Rounsaville, B.J., Dolinsky, Z.S., Babor, T.F., & Meyer, R.E. (1987). Psychopathology as a predictor of treatment outcome in alcoholics. *Archives of General Psychiatry, 44,* 505–513.

Roy, A., DeJong, J., Lamparski, D., Adinoff, B., George, T., Moore, V., Garnett, D., Kerich, M., & Linnoila, M. (1991). Mental disorders among alcoholics: Relationship to age of onset and cerebrospinal fluid neuropeptides. *Archives of General Psychiatry, 48,* 423–427.

Roy, A., DeJong, J., Lamparski, D., George, T., & Linnoila, M. (1991). Depression among alcoholics: Relationship to clinical and cerebrospinal fluid variables. *Archives of General Psychiatry, 48,* 428–432.

SAS Institute. (1988). *SAS 6.05.* Cary, NC: Author.

Substance Abuse and Mental Health Services Administration (SAMHSA). (1993). Final notice establishing definitions for (1) children with a serious emotional disturbance, and (2) adults with a serious mental illness. *Federal Register, 58,* 29422–29425.

University of Michigan. (1981). *OSIRIS VII.* Ann Arbor: University of Michigan, Institute for Social Research.

Weiss, K.J., & Rosenberg, D.J. (1985). Prevalence of anxiety disorder among alcoholics. *Journal of Clinical Psychiatry, 46,* 3–5.

Wittchen, H.-U. (1993). Reliability and validity studies of the WHO-Composite International Diagnostic Interview (CIDI): A critical review. *Journal of Psychiatric Research, 28,* 57–84.

Wittchen, H.-U., Kessler, R.C., Zhao, S., & Abelson, J. (1995). Reliability and clinical validity of UM-CIDI *DSM-III-R* generalized anxiety disorder. *Journal of Psychiatric Research, 29,* 95–110.

Wolf, A.W., Schubert, D.S.P., Patterson, M.B., Marion, B., & Grande, T.P. (1988). Associations among major psychiatric diagnoses. *Journal of Consulting Clinical Psychology, 56,* 292–294.

Woodruff, R.S., & Causey, B.D. (1976). Computerized method for approximating the variance of a complicated estimate. *Journal of the American Statistical Association, 71,* 315–321.

Woodruff, R.A., Jr., Guze, S.B., Clayton, P.J., & Carr, D. (1973). Alcoholism and depression. *Archives of General Psychiatry, 28,* 97–100.

World Health Organization. (1990). *Composite International Diagnostic Interview* (Version 1.0). Geneva, Switzerland: Author.

World Health Organization. (1993). *The ICD-10 classification of mental and behavioral disorders: Diagnostic criteria for research.* Geneva, Switzerland: Author.

3

Assessment of Comorbidity

TOVA FERRO
DANIEL N. KLEIN

The term *comorbidity* was introduced into the medical literature by Feinstein (1970) to refer to patients with two co-occurring diseases. In the past decade, numerous studies have documented extensive comorbidity among psychiatric disorders (Biederman, Newcorn, & Sprich, 1991; Boyd et al., 1984; Brady & Kendall, 1992; Caron & Rutter, 1991; Gunderson & Phillips, 1991; Maser & Cloninger, 1990). Comorbidity has a number of important clinical implications. First, it plays a significant role in the treatment of psychiatric disorders. For example, Kupfer and Carpenter (1990) compared treatment outcome of individuals with major depression and comorbid alcoholism to the outcome of those with major depression without lifetime diagnoses of most Axis I disorders or antisocial personality disorder. They found that the pure major depressive group responded to treatment and remitted more rapidly than did those with comorbid alcoholism. Furthermore, in a review of the literature, Reich and colleagues (Reich & Green, 1991; Reich & Vasile, 1993) reported that patients with comorbid Axis II pathology exhibited a poorer response to treatment of Axis I disorders than did patients with Axis I pathology alone. Second, comorbid pathology also appears to influence the course of disorders. Pfohl, Coryell,

Preparation of this chapter was supported by National Institute of Mental Health grants F31-MH10459 (Dr. Ferro) and R01-MH45757 (Dr. Klein).

Zimmerman, and Stangl (1987) found that depressed inpatients with a greater degree of personality pathology were approximately one half as likely to improve at both discharge and six-month follow-up as were patients with a lesser degree of personality pathology. Likewise, Keller, Lavori, Endicott, Coryell, and Klerman (1983) found that patients who had comorbid major depression and dysthymia were more likely to experience a relapse of major depression than those with major depression alone. Third, observing patterns of comorbidity can provide clues about causal relationships between disorders. Finally, data on comorbidity can point to problems in the classification system and suggest refinements and revisions.

In light of its impact on the areas discussed above, the assessment of comorbidity is a critical part of any diagnostic evaluation, regardless of whether it is conducted for research or clinical purposes. In this chapter, the authors outline some of the major factors that affect the assessment of comorbidity, discuss some strategies by which to distinguish between the various explanations of comorbidity, and describe the major assessment methods and instruments for assessing comorbidity.

FACTORS AFFECTING THE ASSESSMENT OF COMORBIDITY

Comorbidity can result from a number of factors including base rates, classification system, assessment methods, and the establishment of boundaries in the wrong place. Understanding the nature of comorbidity can have important etiological, prognostic, and treatment implications.

Effects of Base Rates

Chance

The base rates of disorders within the population affect comorbidity by determining the chance co-occurrence of disorders (Finn, 1982; Meehl, 1973). For example, of two disorders with high prevalence rates, a significant number of individuals will experience both disorders simply on the basis of chance. An awareness of the base rates of disorders is important because it can inform diagnosticians as to what rates of comorbidity they can reasonably expect and therefore can assist them in evaluating the relationship between disorders. The likelihood that comorbidity will occur by chance can be readily calculated by multiplying the base rate (or prevalence) of each of the relevant disorders.

Sampling

Certain samples tend to exhibit elevated rates of comorbidity. Berkson (1946), for example, noted that clinical populations yield high rates of co-morbidity for the following reason: The likelihood of seeking treatment is higher for individuals with multiple disorders than for individuals with only one disorder because treatment seeking is a function of the combined like-lihood of referral for each disorder. As a result, rates of comorbidity in clin-ical samples are likely to be higher than in the general population.

Clinical samples may also have higher rates of comorbidity because the probability that an individual will seek treatment for a particular disorder may increase as a result of a second comorbid disorder (Galbaud du Fort, Newman, & Bland, 1993). For example, Galbaud du Fort and colleagues (1993) found a higher rate of treatment seeking for alcoholism among in-dividuals who also experienced a comorbid depression than for those with alcoholism alone.

Finally, clinical samples tend to have higher rates of comorbidity than the general population because the patients who are the hardest to treat (e.g., due to comorbidity) tend to stay the longest in the mental health sys-tem. These characteristics can lead to the clinician's illusion that comor-bidity is more common than it actually is in the general population or among consecutive admissions of patients to treatment settings (Cohen & Cohen, 1984).

Population Stratification

Population stratification can influence diagnosis of comorbidity when the risk factors associated with two disorders have an increased prevalence in the same stratum of the population. Within these strata, the likelihood that the disorders will co-occur is no greater than chance. However, because of the increased prevalence of risk factors for both disorders within the same subgroup, the rate of comorbidity is higher than that expected by chance for the population as a whole. Unless population stratification is taken into account, the two disorders will appear to co-occur at a greater than chance frequency. For example, a strong association has frequently been reported for alcoholism and depression. However, due to assortative mating between individuals with depression and those with alcoholism, risk factors for both disorders may be higher within many of these families than among the gen-eral population (Klein & Riso, 1993; Merikangas, 1982; Merikangas, Leck-man, Prusoff, Pauls, & Weissman, 1985). Rather than indicating true comorbidity, the relationship found between depression and alcoholism in families may simply indicate that high base rates of both disorders exist within a particular stratum of the population. Likewise, many disorders are associated with low socioeconomic status (SES; Kessler et al., 1994; Robins, Locke, & Regier, 1991). High comorbidity in a low SES sample may simply reflect chance co-occurrence that is elevated due to population stratification. Assessments of comorbidity should routinely consider the risk factors associated with the population stratum from which a sample is drawn.

Classification System Factors

Breadth of the Classification System

The coverage of a classification system affects the assessment of comorbidity. When the number of diagnostic categories included in the nomenclature is increased, an individual is more likely to fall into multiple categories (Frances, Widiger, & Fyer, 1990). For example, the inclusion of caffeine- and nicotine-related disorders in the *Diagnostic and Statistical Manual* (*DSM-IV*) (American Psychiatric Association [APA], 1994) has presumably led to an increase in the percentage of the general population who meet the criteria for several *DSM* diagnoses. Therefore, it is important for clinicians to be aware of the scope of the diagnostic system in assessing comorbidity.

Hierarchical Exclusion Criteria

Hierarchical exclusion criteria also have a great impact on the assessment of comorbidity. In some classification systems, diagnostic hierarchies are clearly specified; this is the case with the *DSM-IV,* which stipulates, for instance, that generalized anxiety disorder is ruled out if a current mood disorder exists.

Although the two most recent editions of the *DSM*—the *DSM-III-R* (APA, 1987) and the *DSM-IV* (APA, 1994)—have eliminated many of the diagnostic hierarchies imposed by earlier editions, they have retained two general hierarchical principles. First, the presence of an organic etiology that can account for symptom expression overrides the diagnosis of another disorder. For example, if panic attacks occur within the context of hyper- or hypothyroidism, a diagnosis of organic anxiety syndrome in *DSM-III-R,* or anxiety disorder due to a general medical condition in *DSM-IV,* would override that of panic disorder. Second, the more recent versions of the *DSM* still indicate that some pervasive disorders, such as schizophrenia, override a diagnosis of a less pervasive disorder even if core features of the less pervasive disorder are present. In this regard, it would not be possible to make a diagnosis of both schizophrenia and dysthymia.

Another hierarchical approach to diagnosis found in the *DSM*s, including the *DSM-IV,* is the stipulation of a principal diagnosis. The principal diagnosis is defined as the disorder responsible for the patient's treatment seeking, which is usually the focus of treatment (APA, 1994, p. 3). The determination of a principal diagnosis can often be somewhat arbitrary when the patient presents with more than one diagnosis, and it can lead to the neglect of other comorbid disorders or even the disregard of comorbidity altogether.

Diagnostic Thresholds

A classification system further influences the assessment of comorbidity through its specification of diagnostic thresholds. This issue has been raised in relation to the *DSM-III-R* in which several disorders, such as major depression, simple phobia, substance abuse, and personality disorders, have relatively low thresholds (Frances et al., 1990). The existence of such low thresholds raises the potential for comorbidity because meeting criteria for numerous individual diagnoses becomes easier, thus increasing the likelihood that the patient will meet criteria for more than one disorder. An appreciation of the effect of diagnostic thresholds on comorbidity will inform its assessment.

Criterion Overlap

Another classification-related problem for the assessment of comorbidity is the problem of criterion overlap. When similar symptoms are included in the criteria sets for several different disorders, inflated rates of comorbidity result (Klein & Riso, 1993; Widiger, 1989). For instance, higher rates of comorbidity may result from the difficulty in distinguishing major depression from borderline personality disorder in light of shared affective symptomatology. Likewise, higher rates of comorbidity between social phobia and avoidant personality disorder may result from common symptoms of social avoidance. However, close attention to the phenomenology and context of symptoms can provide clues to differential diagnosis that go beyond the *DSM* criteria. For example, Weston and associates (1992) reported success in differentiating borderline personality disorder from major depression through a phenomenological examination of the affective symptoms of the two disorders. They found that affective dysregulation in subjects with borderline personality disorder, as opposed to those with major depression, was less episodic, had an interpersonal focus, and was related to poor impulse control. Of particular note was the finding that depression severity was unrelated to these distinctions.

Similarly, Benjamin (1993) describes an approach for making distinctions at the symptom level. For example, inappropriate anger is a criterion for borderline, narcissistic, histrionic, and antisocial personality disorders. Benjamin demonstrates how, through an examination of their interpersonal context, different manifestations of anger can be distinguished from one another and clearly placed in the appropriate diagnostic category. She describes the unique circumstances that are likely to trigger an angry reaction, the nature of the angry response, and the ends to which the response is directed. For example, a panicky anger, in response to perceived abandonment with the intention of inspiring nurturance, is exhibited in cases of borderline personality disorder; a cold anger, designed to maintain control without regard or care for its consequences, occurs in cases of antisocial personality disorder. In contrast, with histrionic personality disorder, anger expressed through temper tantrums functions to elicit praise, admiration, and nurturance from others. Finally, narcissistic personality disordered patients feel deserving of special treatment and express anger when their expectations are not met. Taken together, these reports suggest that a qualitative examination of the overlapping symptoms of two disorders may facilitate differential diagnosis.

Although the criteria may be faithfully applied, determining whether the comorbidity is real or is simply an artifact of double counting certain features can have important implications. Thus, treatments are likely to differ for a patient diagnosed as having borderline personality disorder, major depression, or both conditions. The same is true of the patient whose anger is treated as a criterion of two or more personality disorders as opposed to one.

The degree of bias produced by overlapping criteria may also vary as a function of severity. More severely disturbed patients tend to exhibit a greater number of symptoms, including nonspecific symptoms that are shared by several disorders, than do less severely disturbed patients. As a result, the more severe group also exhibits greater comorbidity (Caron & Rutter, 1991).

In addition to the qualitative approaches described by Weston and colleagues (1992) and Benjamin (1993), one can determine whether the patient continues to meet criteria for both diagnoses if the overlapping criteria are disregarded (Widiger, 1989). This is a common approach in evaluating depression in medical patients, when symptoms like fatigue as well as changes in sleep and weight can be due to a physical condition. In such cases, clinicians often focus more on the cognitive and affective symptoms of depression to determine whether a diagnosis is warranted. This strategy must be used cautiously for several reasons. First, the deletion of criteria changes the original diagnostic construct (Widiger, 1989). For example, the construct of borderline personality disorder is clearly altered when its affective components are excluded. In addition, this strategy makes meeting criteria for the disorder more difficult because there are fewer criteria. Of course, one could also reduce the number of criteria required or substitute new nonoverlapping criteria, but this would alter the construct even further. However, if the patient continues to meet criteria for both disorders after the deletion of the overlapping features, it would be a powerful argument in favor of the existence of real comorbidity.

Assessment Factors

Halo Effects

Halo effects affect the assessment of comorbidity when a rating instrument, diagnostician, or patient assumes that two disorders either cannot or must be associated with one another (Frances et al., 1990). Halo effects can cause diagnosticians to underestimate comorbidity if they assume that a certain disorder precludes the diagnosis of other disorders. If a diagnostician believes that a diagnosis of obsessive compulsive disorder (OCD) cannot coexist with a diagnosis of borderline personality disorder, the presence of OCD will lead the diagnostician to overlook the latter. Halo effects can also cause overestimates of comorbidity when the presence of one disorder biases the diagnostician (or patient) toward endorsing the criteria for a second disorder. If a diagnostician believes that a strong association exists between OCD and obsessive compulsive personality disorder (OCPD), the presence of OCD will predispose the diagnostician to make a diagnosis of OCPD as well.

Moreover, halo effects may cause the diagnostician's attention to be caught by a particularly salient feature of a disorder and thus be misdirected. When this happens, the diagnostician's attention becomes focused on a tangential area and the initial avenue of inquiry is prematurely closed. Kendell (1968) describes an example of such a problem in his report of the effect of rater biases on diagnosis of depression. He found that raters with strong opinions regarding the diagnostic distinction between psychotic and neurotic depression were more likely to direct their attention to, and exaggerate, the predominant psychotic or neurotic symptoms exhibited by patients and cease their inquiry into the opposing set of features (Kendell, 1968).

Response Set

The patient's response set, or tendency to answer routinely in a fixed way, can also influence comorbidity. The most commonly studied response sets include socially desirable, acquiescent, and deviant response sets (Paulhus, 1991; Wiggins, 1973). Individuals with a socially desirable response set have a tendency to give answers that present them in a favorable light. An acquiescent response set occurs in individuals who demonstrate a tendency to agree with all statements and questions that are put to them. Those with a deviant response set tend to answer questions in a statistically deviant manner as compared to either the general, or a particular (e.g., clinical), population.

The use of gate questions and skipouts in many commonly employed, structured diagnostic interviews may cause them to be particularly vulnerable to the effects of response sets. In the course of such interviews, patients may learn that if they answer "no," the assessment will be shortened. For example, Kessler and others (1994) hypothesized that subjects in the Epidemiologic Catchment Area (ECA) study learned that by saying "no" to the gate questions on the Diagnostic Interview Schedule (DIS; Robins, Helzer, Croughan, & Ratcliff, 1981), they could greatly shorten the diagnostic assessment because the interviewer would skip the rest of the section; the result was lower than expected rates of certain disorders (e.g., major depression). To alleviate this problem, the researchers redesigned a subsequent version of the instrument (the Composite International Diagnostic Interview [CIDI]; World Health Organization [WHO], 1990) placing all gate questions at the beginning of the interview (Kessler et al., 1994). This approach has since been adopted by the *DSM-IV* version of the Structured Clinical Interview for *DSM-III-R* (SCID; Spitzer, Williams, Gibbon, & First, 1992).

Time Frame

Finally, the time frame employed in making diagnostic assessments will also have a great effect on the assessment of comorbidity. If, for example, a patient's lifetime is under consideration, he or she is more likely to receive multiple diagnoses than if only his or her current state is being assessed.

Establishing Boundaries in the Wrong Places

Distinguishing Comorbid Conditions from Associated Features

A major problem for the assessment of comorbidity is the determination of whether a symptom (or set of symptoms) is indicative of a comorbid condition or is simply an associated feature of the disorder in question. This problem is one of the toughest challenges for differential diagnosis, especially for inexperienced diagnosticians. The *DSM* handles the problem with exclusion criteria, such as "not due to . . ." or "not better accounted for by . . . ," but these criteria are not always easy to apply. For example, the presence of somatic complaints during a major depressive episode may give rise to comorbid diagnoses of major depression and somatoform disorder (e.g., hypochondriasis). However, with a careful assessment, it may become clear that the full somatoform syndrome is not met and that, in fact, the patient's somatic complaints are simply an associated feature of the major depressive episode as described in the *DSM-IV* (APA, 1994, p. 323).

Perhaps a graver problem (related to the misdirection of a rater's attention and the resulting premature closure that was discussed earlier) would be to focus so narrowly on the existence of somatic complaints that a diagnosis of major depression is overlooked in favor of a somatoform disorder. The key to making a differential diagnosis under uncertain circumstances is to evaluate thoroughly the existence of the full second syndrome as well as the associated features, typical and atypical, of the original disorder. In this way, a rater is less likely to be misled by a particularly salient feature. Furthermore, the diagnostician also needs a thorough understanding of the core concept of the disorder that the criteria are intended to draw upon.

An important issue arising from the problem described above is when and/or whether an associated feature should be diagnosed in addition to a full syndrome. Widiger and Trull (1991) have suggested that when an associated feature necessitates additional treatment or causes additional impairment, it, too, should be diagnosed. As an example, Widiger and Trull state that a social phobia resulting from anorexia or stuttering, which would not be diagnosable in the *DSM-IV,* can be as debilitating as any diagnosable phobia. At the current time, the presence of an associated feature, even if it causes major impairment in and of itself, is not considered as comorbidity. However, both clinicians and researchers should bear the significance of such associated features in mind.

Multiformity

Multiformity is another major problem for the assessment of comorbidity. It refers to the fact that disorders can often assume phenomenologically heterogeneous forms, including symptoms that are typically associated with other disorders (Klein & Riso, 1993). Possible examples of multiformity include the relationship between somatization and antisocial personality disorder (Cloninger, 1978; Lilienfeld, 1992), and between Gilles de la

Tourette's syndrome and obsessive compulsive disorder (Pauls, Towbin, Leckman, Zahner, & Cohen, 1986). In some cases of multiformity, the comorbid condition may be a more severe form of one of the pure disorders. For example, albeit controversial (Weissman et al., 1993), some studies have suggested that major depression with concurrent panic attacks may represent a more severe form of mood disorder than major depression without panic attacks (Coryell et al., 1988; Leckman, Weissman, Merikangas, Pauls, & Prusoff, 1983; Van Valkenburg, Akiskal, Puzantian, & Rosenthal, 1984; Weissman et al., 1986). If this is true, assessment is made more difficult because the diagnostician must determine when or if depression with panic indicates the existence of two separate disorders, and when or if it is simply a multiform expression of one of the pure disorders. Coryell and colleagues (1988) reported that patients who experienced panic attacks during major depressive episodes exhibited a greater number of depressive symptoms and a more chronic course than did patients with major depression without panic attacks, although the two groups did not differ in family history of mood and anxiety disorders. It is interesting that both groups had lower rates of anxiety disorders in relatives than did patients with panic disorder and secondary depression. Coryell and associates concluded that patients with concurrent major depression and panic attacks have a single multiform disorder. Moreover, the variant of major depression that included concurrent panic attacks appeared to be more severe than major depression without panic attacks.

CLINICAL AND ASSESSMENT STRATEGIES

An assessment of comorbidity offers an opportunity to examine the causal relationship between the index and comorbid disorders. For example, if during a thorough assessment of comorbidity, one disorder is determined to have an earlier onset than another, this finding may contribute to the establishment of causality. There are several strategies that can be used to help determine the nature of the relationship between two comorbid conditions.

Longitudinal Course

A longitudinal strategy is the major method of attempting to understand the nature of comorbidity in the individual patient. Generally, longitudinal course is examined retrospectively through history taking. However, if a patient is seen in treatment over a long period of time, a prospective approach may be possible. For example, if the clinician would like to understand the relationship between major depression and panic disorder, an examination of the course of both disorders during a retrospective period of time would be made. The nature of the relationship between the two disorders during this period may indicate whether they are truly comorbid. For example, at the earliest point at which a retrospective assessment is made, a patient is found to have a major depressive disorder. Subsequently, the patient experiences recurrent episodes of major depression and at a later time also meets criteria for panic attacks, with panic attacks occurring both during and between depressive episodes. In this scenario, the patient would be diagnosed with comorbid major depressive disorder and panic disorder. Conversely, if a patient meets criteria for major depressive disorder subsequent to and only during the course of panic disorder, this situation would raise the possibility that the depression is a complication of panic disorder rather than an independent condition.

Family History

Gathering family history information from a patient in a clinical setting is one of the most useful means of assessing and understanding the nature of comorbidity. The presence or absence of disorders in family members will help to give an indication of whether true comorbidity exists. For example, if the patient has three first-degree relatives diagnosed with major depressive disorder and another two with panic disorder, the presence of both disorders in the patient can more clearly be interpreted as true comorbidity than if the family were positive for only one disorder or the other. In the latter case, it would be impossible to rule out the existence of multiformity as opposed to comorbidity.

Treatment Response

A final approach to assessing comorbidity is the treatment response strategy. Thus, treatment outcome can help explicate the nature of the relationship between the two disorders in question. For example, if a short-term, time-limited, cognitive-behavioral treatment of major depression is carried out with a patient who also has features of borderline personality disorder and both disorders resolve, it would appear that the features of borderline personality disorder were simply associated features of major depression. However, if borderline features persist after resolution of the major depressive episode, it would suggest that the patient has two distinct disorders.

The treatment response strategy can also be used to illuminate Widiger and Trull's (1991) question of when an associated feature might deserve the status of a comorbid disorder. For example, if a patient does not meet diagnostic criteria for a social phobia because it exists within the context of an eating disorder, but a particular treatment is successful only with regard to the eating disorder, this situation would suggest that social phobia should be considered as a true comorbid condition (Widiger & Trull, 1991).

SPECIAL PROBLEMS FOR THE ASSESSMENT OF COMORBIDITY

Substance-Related Disorders

In the presence of heavy substance use, a clinician often has difficulty determining whether a disorder is substance induced and should therefore be ruled out diagnostically or is an independent comorbid condition. Recently, *DSM-IV* delineated criteria for making such a determination. Using the new *DSM* criteria, and depression and alcohol use as an example, one must determine the following: Has the depression preceded the alcohol use by at least one month? Has the depression persisted for at least one month after alcohol use or withdrawal has ceased? Is the depression excessive given the amount and duration of alcohol use? Does other evidence exist suggesting that the depression is not causally related to alcohol use (e.g., previous episodes of nonsubstance related depression) (APA, 1994, p. 374)? If any of the above can be established and the criteria for both major depression and alcohol abuse are met, then both diagnoses are made. If none of the above can be established and the depression began within one month of alcohol use, then a diagnosis of alcohol-induced mood disorder with depressive features is made, and onset is specified as occurring during either intoxication or withdrawal. Finally, if a diagnosis of major depression is not warranted (i.e., the depression is not excessive and does not require clinical attention in and of itself), then only a diagnosis of alcohol use is made.

State versus Trait Distinction in the Diagnosis of a Comorbid Personality Disorder

A common problem in the assessment of Axis II comorbidity involves making the distinction between state and trait. Axis I disorders, which frequently co-occur with personality disorders, can affect assessments of Axis II because of mood-state biases and the difficulty that patients may have in distinguishing premorbid traits from current symptoms (Hirschfeld et al., 1983; Reich, Noyes, Coryell, & O'Gorman, 1986).

This problem can be alleviated through several means. First, the *DSM* definition of personality disorders stipulates that they must be "enduring patterns of perceiving, relating to, and thinking about the environment and oneself that are exhibited in a wide range of social and personal contexts" (APA, 1994, p. 630). In this way, the diagnostician must firmly establish the personality disorder criteria in question to have been present both before and after an episodic disorder, such as major depression.

The method by which personality disorders are assessed will also help to make the distinction between state and trait. For example, semistructured interviews that are designed for use by experienced clinicians will be more successful in making this distinction than either self-report measures or structured interviews designed for lay interviewers because they have the flexibility that allows for clarification. They also incorporate the use of the interviewer's observations and often require convincing examples for a positive rating to be made. Finally, albeit controversial (O'Boyle & Self, 1990; Stuart, Simons, Thase, & Pilkonis, 1992), there is some evidence suggesting that state biases may be found less often with the use of direct interviews given by clinical interviewers than with self-report inventories (Loranger et al., 1991). Assessment methods are discussed in more depth in the following section.

Because of the interpersonal and socially undesirable nature of personality disorders, several researchers have advocated the use of informants and multiple sources of information for making assessments of personality disorders (Ferro & Klein, in press; Tyrer et al, 1979; Zimmerman, 1994). There has been some recent support for the usefulness of informant interviews. For example, Ferro and Klein (in press) found that concordance on Axis II disorders between two informants was higher than between subjects and informants, lending support to the idea that, in addition to reporting on some of the same aspects of personality pathology, informants have access to unique information about patients. Furthermore, Lara, Ferro, and Klein (in press) found that even when Axis I psychopathology was controlled statistically, informants' reports of personality disorders were significantly correlated with nondiagnostic indices of personality dysfunction (e.g., social adjustment) reported by subjects. These findings held even in subjects who denied diagnosable Axis II psychopathology in direct interviews, suggesting that informants can provide important information on personality disorders that may not be available from assessments with patients themselves. Finally, even though patients and informants often provide contradictory reports, two studies have shown that clinicians can integrate this information and arrive at diagnoses with high reliability (Klein, Ouimette, Kelly, Ferro, & Riso, 1994; Zimmerman, Pfohl, Stangl, & Corenthal, 1986).

ASSESSMENT METHODS AND INSTRUMENTS

Clinical versus Structured Interviews

Diagnostic evaluations, and thus assessments of comorbidity, can be made through the use of unstructured clinical interviews or structured interview schedules administered by either lay or clinical interviewers. One advantage of the unstructured clinical interview is that the interview is more flexible and inquiry is driven by the interviewer's clinical knowledge and experience. In this way, the clinical interview includes all aspects of a patient's history, including information that might not be found in a standard structured interview. For example, in a clinical interview, it is routine to inquire about developmental history and social functioning, two important areas that are not included in most structured interviews. Flexibility and clinical knowledge also make it easier for the interviewer to be aware of and respond to patient response sets so that they do not interfere with an accurate assessment of comorbidity.

Conversely, structured interviews draw less on clinical judgment and are therefore less prone to halo effects. Because of the interview's structured nature, including the use of strictly delineated criteria and ordering of questions, interviewers are less likely to fall prey to their own biases. Employment of structured interviews also allows for the use of lay interviewers, a practice that minimizes clinician time and expenses in research or busy clinical settings.

In actuality, many structured interviews are semistructured (e.g., the SCID and Personality Disorder Examination [PDE]; Loranger, 1988) and combine the advantages of the structured format with the clinical experience and knowledge that clinicians bring to bear during an assessment of diagnostic comorbidity. For this reason, we recommend that, whenever possible, semistructured interview methods be employed.

Interview versus Self-Report Measures

Categorical-Dimensional Distinctions

One distinction between interview and self-report assessment methods is that interview methods tend to be categorical and self-report methods dimensional. Although the covariation of dimensions within a dimensional system can be examined, comorbidity is only truly relevant in a categorical system in which clearly delineated entities exist. Many dimensional systems, however, impose a categorical format on their continuous scales. For example, the Millon Clinical Multiaxial Inventory (MCMI; Millon, 1983) and the Beck Depression Inventory (BDI; Beck, Rush, Shaw, & Emery, 1979) both impose cutoff scores that indicate the presence or absence of disorder and thus become categorical instruments. Some fundamentally categorical instruments—the PDE, for example—also give dimensional profiles in addition to categorical diagnoses.

Prevalence Rates

The use of self-report measures as opposed to interview measures has been found to result in higher prevalence rates of disorder and thus, comorbidity. Although interview measures are assumed to be more valid, in part because of the seemingly excessive rates of disorder found when self-report measures are used, the authors are not aware of any studies of differential validity for Axis I diagnoses. One study has examined the differential validity of interview and self-report measures for Axis II disorders. Pfohl and colleagues (1987) found that Axis II assessments made with both the Structured Interview for *DSM-III* Personality Disorders (SIDP; Pfohl, Stangl, Zimmerman, Bowers, & Corenthal, 1983) and the Personality Diagnostic Questionnaire (PDQ; Hyler et al., 1988) were related to differences in treatment outcome at discharge and at six-month follow-up, although the SIDP was more strongly related to outcome at discharge.

Widiger and Frances (1987) have suggested that the increase in self-report-diagnosed personality disorders as compared to interview diagnoses may be due to the combination of two factors: on the one hand, patients may overstate the presence of personality pathology because they fail to distinguish between state and trait or because the nature of many personality disorders is to exaggerate or acquiesce; on the other hand, clinical interviewers may minimize the existence of further personality pathology once they have determined the existence of several disorders because they find it difficult to conceptualize the existence of multiple disorders.

Specificity

Self-report measures also tend to be less specific than interviews. For example, many self-report measures of depression assess anxiety symptoms as well (Di Nardo & Barlow, 1990; Fechner-Bates, Coyne, & Schwenk, 1994). For example, Fechner-Bates and associates (1994) found that the Center for Epidemiologic Studies Depression Scale (CES-D; Radloff, 1977) was as good at detecting cases of anxiety disorder on the SCID as it was in identifying instances of depression. Furthermore, most subjects with high scores on the CES-D were not depressed on the basis of *DSM* criteria, and a substantial group of subjects with low scores on the CES-D met criteria for depression.

Flexibility

Interviews allow for more flexibility of assessment and, thus, are better able to tease apart the various explanations of comorbidity discussed earlier. For example, an interview allows the interviewer to take patient behavior into account during an assessment and offers the opportunity to clarify the patient's responses, identify inconsistencies, and assess temporal and contextual factors. As a result, an interviewer can assess the chronology of two disorders accurately and determine whether they overlapped in time or if one of them occurred prior to the other. Furthermore, there is some evidence that subjects are often confused by questions on self-reports, in part as a result of reverse-scored items (Zimmerman, 1994). On the other hand, self-report measures often incorporate the inclusion of scales for the assessment of response styles (Widiger & Frances, 1987) that can be helpful in evaluating comorbidity.

Time and Financial Constraints

Self-report measures are much cheaper to administer than interviews and usually require much less time to complete.

Which Method to Use

In part the decision between use of interview and self-report measures should be based on the purpose of the evaluation and the staff and resources available. Keep in mind, however, that it is possible to examine symptomatology within a primarily categorical approach and to derive categories from a dimensional approach. One interview, the Structured Clinical Interview for *DSM-III-R* Personality Disorders (SCID-II; Spitzer, Williams, & Gibbon, 1987), incorporates aspects of both the self-report and interview methods. First, a self-report screen is administered to the patient and then the areas the patient has indicated as problems are further followed up with an interview assessment.

Coverage

Diagnostic coverage varies from instrument to instrument and a diagnostician should give serious consideration to its influence when assessing comorbidity. For example, some assessment instruments were developed for very specific areas of inquiry such as Gunderson and associates' Diagnostic Interview for Borderlines (1981) and Diagnostic Interview for Narcissism (1990). Likewise, the Anxiety Disorders Interview Schedule (1983) of Di Nardo and associates is very comprehensive in the domain of anxiety disorders but somewhat less so for other Axis I disorders. These contrast with instruments such as the SCID and PDE that were designed for comprehensive assessments of Axis I and Axis II disorders, respectively. Also, some instruments focus only on the present (e.g., the Present State Exam [PSE]; Wing, Cooper, & Sartorius, 1974) rather than on the lifetime history of illness, as others do. This emphasis can have a large impact on comorbidity assessment, as patients are more likely to have met criteria for a diagnosis of two or more disorders during a lifetime assessment than during a cross-sectional assessment.

The more focused an assessment instrument is, the less suited it is for assessing comorbidity. This focus should be taken into careful consideration when a diagnostician chooses an instrument, or modifies it because of time or economic constraints. The effect that a decrease in scope will have on revealing comorbidity should, likewise, be acknowledged when he or she interprets the assessment that results.

Use of Skipouts

Skipouts have an effect on the assessment of comorbidity, as discussed earlier, and differ from instrument to instrument. An instrument's skipouts usually mirror the inclusion and exclusion criteria of the classification system for which it was designed. Some instruments, however, have incorporated extra skipouts. For example, the *DSM-III-R* SCID excludes a diagnosis of dysthymia if the patient has been in a depressive episode for more than half the time during the two years preceding the assessment, effectively ruling out many instances of current double depression.

Assessment instruments vary greatly in their use of skipouts. For example, the PSE has no skipouts. Likewise, the PDE inquires about all *DSM* personality disorder criteria. The net effect of this design is that it allows comorbidity to be more thoroughly and flexibly assessed and it decreases the pull for clinician biases and patient response sets. In contrast, the Schedule for Schizophrenia and Affective Disorders-Lifetime Version (SADS-L; Spitzer & Endicott, 1977) and SCID have numerous skipouts. Although use of these saves time, their employment can lead to a less comprehensive assessment and is vulnerable to various biases. As noted earlier, Kessler and others (1994) reorganized the CIDI to address this problem, placing all the gate questions together at the beginning of the instrument. In summary, diagnosticians should be aware of the influence that individual instruments can have on the assessment of comorbidity through the use of skipouts.

Clinical versus Lay Interviewers

Assessment instruments have been designed for use by both clinical and lay interviewers. For example, the DIS and CIDI were designed for Axis I assessments by lay interviewers, in contrast to the SADS and SCID. For Axis II assessments, the PDE, SIDP, and the SCID-II were designed for use by clinical interviewers whereas the Personality Interview Questions (Widiger, 1985) was developed for lay interviewers.

There are advantages and disadvantages inherent to using both clinical and lay interviewers. Lay interviewers cost less to use but do not have the flexibility of clinical interviewers to clarify patients' reports and elicit examples; they are also less aware of patient response sets. For example, the DIS employs only forced choice questions, in which a symptom is described and the patient answers either yes or no. In contrast, the SCID incorporates many open-ended questions and allows the interviewer to ask additional questions not included in the interview format and to challenge patient responses that present conflicting information (Spitzer, 1983). The SCID also allows for the incorporation of other information, such as data from a clinical chart or family member, in making diagnoses. Clinical interviewers, on the other hand, may have preconceptions that leave them susceptible to premature closure and halo effects, as suggested by Kendell (1968). Little research has examined the validity of lay versus clinical interviewers. In the one relevant study of which we are aware, the predictive validity of lay versus psychiatrist diagnoses were compared using the DIS in an epidemiological setting, and virtually no significant differences were found between the two methods (Helzer, Spitznagel, & McEvoy, 1987).

For clinical assessments, the question of lay versus clinical interviewers is generally irrelevant, as evaluations are conducted by clinicians. However, the issue is more salient for researchers, who must base their decision to use lay or clinical interviews on the nature of the study and the resources available.

CONCLUSION

In summary, a diagnosis of comorbidity can be the result of a number of factors including base rates, classification system, assessment methods, and the places where boundaries are drawn. This chapter has described some of the major factors to consider in an assessment of comorbidity in addition to several specific assessment strategies and methods. Finally, when comorbidity is evaluated in a knowledgeable manner and its nature understood, the implications for etiology, prognosis, and treatment are significant.

REFERENCES

American Psychiatric Association. (1987). *Diagnostic and statistical manual of mental disorders* (3rd ed., rev.). Washington, DC: Author.

American Psychiatric Association. (1994). *Diagnostic and statistical manual of mental disorders* (4th ed.). Washington, DC: Author.

Beck, A. T., Rush, A. J., Shaw, B. F., & Emery, G. (1979). *Cognitive therapy for depression.* New York: Guilford Press.

Benjamin, L. S. (1993). *Interpersonal diagnosis and treatment of personality disorders.* New York: Guilford Press.

Berkson, J. (1946). Limitations of the application of fourfold table analysis to hospital data. *Biometrics, 2,* 47–53.

Biederman, J., Newcorn, J., & Sprich, S. (1991). Comorbidity of attention deficit hyperactivity disorder with conduct, depressive, anxiety, and other disorders. *American Journal of Psychiatry, 148,* 564–577.

Boyd, J. H., Burke, J. D., Gruenberg, E., Holzer, C. E., Rae, D. S., George, L. K., Karno, M., Stoltzman, R., McEvoy, L., & Nestadt, G. (1984). Exclusion criteria of *DSM-III. Archives of General Psychiatry, 41,* 983–989.

Brady, E. U., & Kendall, P. C. (1992). Comorbidity of anxiety and depression in children and adolescents. *Psychological Bulletin, 111,* 244–255.

Caron, C., & Rutter, M. (1991). Comorbidity in child psychopathology: Concepts, issues, and research strategies. *Journal of Child Psychology and Psychiatry, 32,* 1063–1080.

Cloninger, C. R. (1978). The link between hysteria and sociopathy: An integrative model of pathogenesis based on clinical, genetic, and neurophysiological observations. In H. S. Akiskal & W. L. Webb (Eds.), *Psychiatric diagnosis: Exploration of biologic predictors* (pp. 189–218). New York: Spectrum.

Cohen, P., & Cohen, J. (1984). The clinician's illusion. *Archives of General Psychiatry, 41,* 1178–1182.

Coryell, W., Endicott, J., Andreasen, N. C., Keller, M. B., Clayton, P. J., Hirschfeld, R. M. A., Scheftner, W. A., & Winokur, G. (1988). Depression and panic attacks: The significance of overlap as reflected in follow-up and family study data. *American Journal of Psychiatry, 145,* 293–300.

Di Nardo, P. A., & Barlow, D. H. (1990). Syndrome and symptom co-occurrence in the anxiety disorders. In J. D. Maser & C. R. Cloninger (Eds.), *Comorbidity of mood and anxiety disorders* (pp. 205–230). Washington, DC: American Psychiatric Press.

Di Nardo, P. A., O'Brien, G. T., Barlow, D. H., Waddell, M. T., & Blanchard, E. B. (1983). Reliability of *DSM-III* anxiety disorder categories using a new structured interview. *Archives of General Psychiatry, 40,* 1070–1074.

Fechner-Bates, S., Coyne, J. C., & Schwenk, T. L. (1994). The relationship of self-reported distress to depressive disorders and other psychopathology. *Journal of Consulting and Clinical Psychology, 62,* 550–559.

Feinstein, A. R. (1970). The pre-therapeutic classification of co-morbidity in chronic disease. *Journal of Chronic Disease, 23,* 455–468.

Ferro, T., & Klein, D. N. (in press). Family history assessment of personality disorders: Concordance with direct interview and between pairs of informants. *Journal of Personality Disorders.*

Finn, S. E. (1982). Base rates, utilities, and *DSM-III:* Shortcomings of fixed-rule systems of psychodiagnosis. *Journal of Abnormal Psychology, 91,* 294–302.

Frances, A., Widiger, T., & Fyer, M. R. (1990). The influence of classification methods on comorbidity. In J. D. Maser & C. R. Cloninger (Eds.), *Comorbidity of mood and anxiety disorders* (pp. 41–59). Washington, D.C.: American Psychiatric Press.

Galbaud du Fort, G., Newman, S. C., & Bland, R. C. (1993). Psychiatric comorbidity and treatment seeking: Sources of selection bias in the study of clinical populations. *Journal of Nervous and Mental Disease, 181,* 467–474.

Gunderson, J., Kolb, J., & Austin, V. (1981). The diagnostic interview for borderline patients. *American Journal of Psychiatry, 138,* 896–903.

Gunderson, J. G., & Phillips, K. A. (1991). A current view of the interface between borderline personality disorder and depression. *American Journal of Psychiatry, 148,* 967–975.

Gunderson, J. G., Ronningstam, E., & Bodkin, A. (1990). The diagnostic interview for narcissistic patients. *Archives of General Psychiatry, 47,* 676–680.

Helzer, J. E., Spitznagel, E. L., & McEvoy, L. (1987). The predictive validity of lay Diagnostic Interview Schedule diagnoses in the general population. *Archives of General Psychiatry, 44,* 1069–1077.

Hirschfeld, R. M. A., Klerman, G. L., Clayton, P. J., Keller, M. B., McDonald-Scott, P., & Larkin, B. H. (1983). Assessing personality: Effects of the depressive state on trait measurement. *American Journal of Psychiatry, 140,* 695–699.

Hyler, S. E., Rieder, R. D., Williams, J. B. W., Spitzer, R. L., Hendler, J., & Lyons, M. (1988). The Personality Diagnostic Questionnaire: Development and preliminary results. *Journal of Personality Disorders, 2,* 229–237.

Keller, M. B., Lavori, P. W., Endicott, J., Coryell, W., & Klerman, G. L. (1983). "Double depression": Two year follow-up. *American Journal of Psychiatry, 140,* 689–694.

Kendell, R. E. (1968). An important source of bias affecting ratings made by psychiatrists. *Journal of Psychiatric Research, 6,* 135–141.

Kessler, R. C., McGonagle, K. A., Zhao, S., Nelson, C. B., Hughes, M., Eshleman, S., Wittchen, H.-U., & Kendler, K. S. (1994). Lifetime and 12-month prevalence of *DSM-III-R* psychiatric disorders in the United States. *Archives of General Psychiatry, 51,* 8–19.

Klein, D. N., Ouimette, P. C., Kelly, H. S., Ferro, T., & Riso, L. P. (1994). Test-retest reliability of team consensus best-estimate diagnoses of Axis I and II disorders in a family study. *American Journal of Psychiatry, 151,* 1043–1047.

Klein, D. N., & Riso, L. P. (1993). Psychiatric disorders: Problems of boundaries and comorbidity. In C. G. Costello (Ed.), *Basic issues in psychopathology* (pp. 19–66). New York: Guilford Press.

Kupfer, D. J., & Carpenter, L. L. (1990). Clinical evidence of comorbidity: A critique of treated samples and longitudinal studies. In J. D. Maser & C. R. Cloninger (Eds.), *Comorbidity of mood and anxiety disorders* (pp. 231–238). Washington, DC: American Psychiatric Press.

Lara, M. E., Ferro, T., & Klein, D. N. (in press). Informants' reports of Axis II disorders in relatives: Construct validity of the family history interview for personality disorders. *Journal of Personality Disorders.*

Leckman, J. F., Weissman, M. M., Merikangas, K. R., Pauls, D. L., & Prusoff, B. A. (1983). Panic disorder and major depression: Increased risk of depression, alcoholism, panic, and phobic disorders in families of depressed probands with panic disorder. *Archives of General Psychiatry, 40,* 1055–1060.

Lilienfeld, S. O. (1992). The association between antisocial personality and somatization disorder: A review and integration of theoretical models. *Clinical Psychology Review, 12,* 641–662.

Loranger, A. W. (1988). *Personality Disorder Examination manual.* Yonkers, NY: DV Communications.

Loranger, A. W., Lenzenweger, M. F., Gartner, A. F., Susman, V. L., Herzig, J., Zammit, G. K., Gartner, J. D., Abrams, R. C., & Young, R. C. (1991). Trait-state artifacts and the diagnosis of personality disorders. *Archives of General Psychiatry, 48,* 720–728.

Maser, J. D., & Cloninger, C. R. (Eds.). (1990). *Comorbidity of mood and anxiety disorders.* Washington, DC: American Psychiatric Press.

Meehl, P. E. (1973). *Psychodiagnosis: Selected papers.* Minneapolis: University of Minnesota Press.

Merikangas, K. R. (1982). Assortative mating for psychiatric disorders and psychological traits. *Archives of General Psychiatry, 39,* 1173–1180.

Merikangas, K. R., Leckman, J. F., Prusoff, B. A., Pauls, D. L., & Weissman, M. M. (1985). Familial transmission of depression and alcoholism. *Archives of General Psychiatry, 42,* 367–372.

Millon, T. (1983). *Millon Clinical Multiaxial Inventory manual* (3rd ed.). Minneapolis, MN: National Computer Services.

O'Boyle, M., & Self, D. (1990). A comparison of two interviews for *DSM-III-R* personality disorders. *Psychiatry Research, 32,* 85–92.

Paulhus, D. L. (1991). Measurement and control of research bias. In P. R. Shaver & L. Wrightsman (Eds.), *Measures of personality and social psychological attitudes* (pp. 17–59). San Diego: Academic Press.

Pauls, D. L., Towbin, K. E., Leckman, J. F., Zahner, G. E. P., & Cohen, D. J. (1986). Gilles de la Tourette's syndrome and obsessive compulsive disorder: Evidence supporting a genetic relationship. *Archives of General Psychiatry, 43,* 1180–1182.

Pfohl, B., Coryell, W., Zimmerman, M., & Stangl, D. (1987). Prognostic validity of self-report and interview measures of personality disorder in depressed inpatients. *Journal of Clinical Psychiatry, 48,* 468–472.

Pfohl, B., Stangl, D. A., Zimmerman, M., Bowers, W., & Corenthal, C. (1983). *Structured Clinical Interview for* DSM-III *Personality Disorders (SIDP).* Iowa City: Department of Psychiatry, University of Iowa.

Radloff, L. S. (1977). The CES-D scale: A self-report depression scale for research in the general population. *Applied Psychological Measurement, 1,* 385–401.

Reich, J. H., & Green, A. I. (1991). Effect of personality disorders on outcome of treatment. *Journal of Nervous and Mental Disease, 179,* 74–82.

Reich, J., Noyes, R., Jr., Coryell, W., & O'Gorman, T. W. (1986). The effect of state anxiety on personality assessment. *American Journal of Psychiatry, 143,* 760–763.

Reich, J. J., & Vasile, R. G. (1993). Effect of personality disorders on the treatment outcome of Axis I conditions: An update. *Journal of Nervous and Mental Disease, 181,* 475–484.

Robins, L. N., Helzer, J. E., Croughan, J. L., & Ratcliff, K. S. (1981). National Institute of Mental Health Diagnostic Interview Schedule: Its history, characteristics and validity. *Archives of General Psychiatry, 38,* 381–389.

Robins, L. N., Locke, B. Z., & Regier, D. A. (1991). An overview of psychiatric disorders in America. In L. N. Robins & D. A. Regier (Eds.), *Psychiatric disorders in America* (pp. 328–366). New York: Free Press.

Spitzer, R. L. (1983). Psychiatric diagnosis: Are clinicians still necessary? *Comprehensive Psychiatry, 24,* 399–411.

Spitzer, R. L., & Endicott, J. (1977). *Schedule for Affective Disorders and Schizophrenia (SADS)* (3rd ed.). New York: New York State Psychiatric Institute, Biometrics Research.

Spitzer, R. L., Williams, J. B. W., & Gibbon, M. (1987). *Structured Clinical Interview for* DSM-III-R *Personality Disorders (SCID-II).* New York: New York State Psychiatric Institute, Biometrics Research.

Spitzer, R. L., Williams, J. B. W., Gibbon, M., & First, M. B. (1992). The Structured Clinical Interview for *DSM-III-R* (SCID), I: History, rationale, and description. *Archives of General Psychiatry, 49,* 624–629.

Stuart, S., Simons, A. D., Thase, M. E., & Pilkonis, P. (1992). Are personality disorder assessments valid in acute major depression? *Journal of Affective Disorders, 24,* 281–289.

Tyrer, P., Alexander, M. S., Cicchetti, D., Cohen, M. S., & Remington, M. (1979). Reliability of a schedule for rating personality disorders. *British Journal of Psychiatry, 135,* 168–174.

Van Valkenburg, C., Akiskal, H. S., Puzantian, V., & Rosenthal, T. (1984). Anxious depressions: Clinical, family history, and naturalistic outcome-comparisons with panic and major depressive disorders. *Journal of Affective Disorders, 6,* 67–82.

Weissman, M. M., Merikangas, K. R., Wickramaratne, P., Kidd, K. K., Prusoff, B. A., Leckman, J. F., & Pauls, D. L. (1986). Understanding the clinical heterogeneity of major depression using family data. *Archives of General Psychiatry, 43,* 430–434.

Weissman, M. M., Wickramaratne, P., Adams, P. B., Lish, J. D., Horwath, E., Charney, D., Woods, S. W., Leeman, E., & Frosch, E. (1993). The relationship between panic disorder and major depression: A new family study. *Archives of General Psychiatry, 50,* 767–780.

Weston, D., Moses, M. J., Silk, K. R., Lohr, N. E., Cohen, R., & Segal, H. (1992). Quality of depressive experience in borderline personality disorder and major depression: When depression is not just depression. *Journal of Personality Disorders, 6,* 382–393.

Widiger, T. (1985). *Personality Interview Questions.* Unpublished manuscript. Lexington: University of Kentucky.

Widiger, T. A. (1989). The categorical distinction between personality and affective disorders. *Journal of Personality Disorders, 3,* 77–91.

Widiger, T. A., & Frances, A. (1987). Interviews and inventories for the measurement of personality disorders. *Clinical Psychology Review, 7,* 49–75.

Widiger, T. A., & Trull, T. J. (1991). Diagnosis and clinical assessment. *Annual Review of Psychology, 42,* 109–133.

Wiggins, J. S. (Ed.). (1973). *Personality and prediction: Principles of personality assessment.* Reading, MA: Addison-Wesley.

Wing, J. K., Cooper, J. E., & Sartorius, N. (1974). *Description and classification of psychiatric symptoms.* Cambridge, England: Cambridge University Press.

World Health Organization. (1990). *Composite International Diagnostic Interview (CIDI),* version 1.0. Geneva, Switzerland: Author.

Zimmerman, M. (1994). Diagnosing personality disorders: A review of issues and research methods. *Archives of General Psychiatry, 51,* 225–245.

Zimmerman, M., Pfohl, B., Stangl, D., & Corenthal, C. (1986). Assessment of *DSM-III* personality disorders: The importance of interviewing an informant. *Journal of Clinical Psychiatry, 47,* 261–263.

PART II
Treatment Strategies

4

Psychological Treatment of Anxiety Disorder Patients with Comorbidity

WILLIAM C. SANDERSON
LATA K. McGINN

More often than not, patients with a principal diagnosis of an anxiety disorder suffer from additional comorbid psychiatric disorders as well, especially mood, anxiety, and personality disorders. Thus, the practice of diagnosing a patient with one disorder is inadequate to convey the patient's overall level of psychopathology. Although the several versions of the *Diagnostic and Statistical Manual of Mental Disorders,* third edition, revised; and fourth edition (*DSM-III-R* and *DSM-IV*) (American Psychiatric Association [APA], 1987, 1994), allow for the assignment of multiple diagnoses, the use of this categorical diagnostic system may provide the clinician with a false sense of patient homogeneity (i.e., all patients with a particular diagnosis are the same). In addition, when a clinician's focus is the diagnosis of syndromes, the presence of comorbid symptoms that may not be severe enough to warrant a diagnosis for a specific disorder may be missed or downplayed, leading to inadequate treatment planning and implementation. This chapter presents an approach to the assessment and psychotherapeutic treatment of anxiety disorder patients that is *symptom focused* rather than disorder based. Unlike the disorder-based approaches, symptom-focused treatment

75

provides a framework that allows clinicians to tailor their treatment to address the specific symptom configuration of each patient, maximizing treatment efficiency.

PREVALENCE AND SIGNIFICANCE OF COMORBIDITY

Patients with a principal anxiety disorder diagnosis have been shown to suffer frequently from an additional co-occurring Axis I disorder (i.e., *syndrome comorbidity*). Several large studies using *DSM-III-R* (APA, 1987) criteria found that 50 percent to 70 percent of patients with anxiety disorders are diagnosed with at least one comorbid disorder (deRuiter, Ruken, Garssen, van Schaik, & Kraaimaat, 1989; Sanderson, Di Nardo, Rapee, & Barlow, 1990). The rate of comorbidity among patients with a principal anxiety disorder diagnosis is quite variable. For the most part, patients with generalized anxiety disorder (GAD) and panic disorder with agoraphobia (PD) have the highest rate of comorbidity, whereas those with specific phobia have the lowest. For patients presenting with comorbidity, the most frequently assigned comorbid diagnoses are specific phobia, social phobia, and dysthymia.

High rates of comorbidity are not limited to patients with anxiety disorders and are frequently encountered among patients with a principal diagnosis of commonly occurring mood disorders as well. Nearly two thirds of patients with dysthymia and major depression are assigned at least one comorbid diagnosis (see, e.g., Sanderson, Beck, & Beck, 1990). Approximately one half of these patients are diagnosed with a comorbid anxiety disorder, most frequently social phobia and generalized anxiety disorder.

The diagnosis of actual syndromes (disorders) is the most conservative approach to examining comorbidity and overlap between disorders. However, the more common occurrence is for patients to present with *symptom comorbidity*. In these instances, patients with a principal diagnosis of a specific disorder may manifest symptoms of one or more other disorders, yet not fulfill diagnostic criteria sufficiently to warrant a comorbid diagnosis. For example, independent of whether diagnostic criteria for a mood disorder are satisfied, the majority of PD patients report a moderate level of depressive symptomatology (Lesser et al., 1988). In fact, patients with one anxiety disorder invariably present with *symptoms* of other anxiety and mood disorders as well. Features such as panic attacks, social evaluative fears, worry, phobias, obsessive compulsive thoughts or behavior, and depression, which are the identifying characteristics of panic disorder, social phobia, generalized anxiety disorder, specific phobia, obsessive compulsive disorder, and major depression/dysthymia, respectively, are often present to some degree in patients suffering from any one specific anxiety disorder (cf. Di Nardo & Barlow, 1990; Rathus & Sanderson, in press).

Thus far, we have focused on comorbid Axis I disorders and symptoms. However, several recent studies found high rates of Axis II personality disorders among patients with anxiety disorders as well (Friedman, Shear, & Frances, 1987; Green & Curtis, 1988; Reich & Noyes, 1987; Sanderson, Wetzler, Beck, & Betz, 1994; Turner, 1987). These studies indicate that as many as two thirds of patients with certain anxiety disorders are diagnosed with a personality disorder, although there is a significant range in the rates of comorbidity across anxiety disorder categories, with social phobia and generalized anxiety typically having the highest rate and specific phobia the lowest.

In summary, most patients with a principal diagnosis of an anxiety disorder present with comorbid symptoms and syndromes. There is considerable overlap between patients, especially with regard to features of depressive, anxiety, and personality disorders. Thus, rather than a focus on one disorder, a thorough evaluation consists of an assessment of a patient's entire symptom configuration.

TREATMENT IMPLICATIONS OF COMORBIDITY

Perhaps the most important indicator of the usefulness of a classification system is the extent to which the diagnostic information guides the selection of optimal treatment. Clearly, from a descriptive standpoint, comorbidity must be taken into account to capture adequately the patient's presenting symptomatology. But does the presence of these additional symptoms and disorders have any bearing on treatment outcome? Although to date, there are very few studies examining the impact of comorbidity on treatment outcome (traditionally, most studies have focused only on the principal disorder), the available data suggest that anxiety disorder patients with comorbid Axis I and Axis II psychiatric disorders display more severe symptoms than patients without comorbidity (Coryell et al., 1988; Lesser et al., 1988; Sanderson, Friedman, Asnis, & Wetzler, 1992), are less responsive to treatment (Noyes et al., 1990; Rathus, Sanderson, Miller, & Wetzler, 1995; Reich, 1988; Sanderson, Beck, & McGinn, 1994; Turner, 1987), and are more likely to require additional treatment (Brown, Antony, & Barlow, 1995). These findings are certainly corroborated by clinicians.

Considering the emerging data on the extent and significance of comorbidity, comprehensive treatment requires an intervention that addresses the patient's full range of symptoms. Treatment carried out in clinical research effectiveness trials must be limited and highly controlled so that the effect of a treatment on one particular disorder can be evaluated. In actual clinical practice, however, patient response would be maximized if the treatment were broadened to address each patient's entire symptom presentation (Sanderson, Raue, & Wetzler, 1995; Wolfe, 1994).

DIMENSIONAL MODEL OF PSYCHOPATHOLOGY: ASSESSMENT AND TREATMENT IMPLICATIONS

Categories versus Dimensions

Clearly, from the clinician's standpoint, the identification of co-occurring syndromes offers important information. Treating a patient with PD and major depression (MD) requires a different approach from treating a patient with PD alone, whether the treatment modality be psychotherapy, pharmacotherapy, or a combination. However, as detailed earlier, the clinician cannot rely on comorbid disorders alone to capture important clinical information. For example, although 73 percent of patients with generalized anxiety disorder (GAD) reported experiencing panic attacks, only 27 percent met the *DSM-III-R* criteria for panic disorder (Sanderson & Barlow, 1990). It may be that the presence of panic attacks will require treatment attention even among those patients not meeting criteria sufficiently to warrant the diagnosis of PD.

The current classification system (*DSM-IV*), which is based on a categorical model, provides the clinician with a false sense of patient homogeneity (i.e., all patients with a principal diagnosis of X are alike). By definition, categorical models of classification assume the existence of homogenous groups with little overlap (Blashfield, 1990). Considering the comorbidity data discussed above, overlap is more the rule than the exception. Patients within a particular diagnostic group can be quite heterogenous, largely influenced by their comorbid symptoms.

Yet because of the dominance of categorical classification models, almost all treatment outcome studies investigate the efficacy of a treatment within a group of patients with a specific diagnosis, either excluding or ignoring comorbidity. For example, many treatment studies on patients with anxiety disorders exclude patients with a comorbid depressive disorder. Under this condition, the treatment being tested may be one that applies to only a specific subset of all patients with that disorder, as patients with comorbid depression are common. Likewise, by ignoring comorbidity as a factor, clinicians may be losing important information. Perhaps among the patients who did not respond to treatment, a common comorbid symptom may be identified, and consequently, treatment may be modified to address this symptom.

Symptom-Focused Treatment

For optimum treatment planning, the authors endorse a dimensional approach to classification. In this format, assessment involves ascertaining the presence and severity of various symptoms. Consistent with the proposals of several other researchers (e.g., Blashfield, 1990; Di Nardo & Barlow, 1990), the approach advocated here is the use of the essential features of the *DSM-IV* anxiety and depression diagnostic categories as dimensional symptoms (see Figure 4-1), wherein there is considerable overlap and co-occurrence. Thus, from here on, *symptom* refers to the essential features of a *DSM* anxiety or depressive disorder.

The proposal made here is that, following a symptomatic assessment of the patient, treatment be conducted in a *symptom-focused* fashion (Sanderson, in press). In this model, treatment strategies are selected to relieve specific symptoms in a sequential fashion based on severity. In some cases, the less severe symptoms will clear as the clinician treats the more severe symptoms. However, in other cases, the next most severe symptom will need to be addressed, and so on.

This conceptual scheme is absolutely essential in the current health care climate. As noted by Clarkin and Kendall (1992), just as clinical researchers are documenting the prevalence and significance of comorbidity, the clinician is being pressured to offer decreasing services. As a result, clinicians are now presumably in the position in which they understand the clinical importance of providing comprehensive treatment that addresses comorbid symptoms, yet they are required to treat patients with fewer sessions. Hence, more efficient treatment models that aggressively target the patient's complete symptomatology are necessary to provide optimal care and prevent relapse (McGinn, Young, & Sanderson, 1995).

GENERAL APPROACH OF PSYCHOLOGICAL TREATMENT

Psychological treatment interventions based on cognitive behavioral therapy (CBT) are the most widely studied psychotherapeutic interventions for patients with anxiety disorders (Chambless et al., in press). Cognitive behavioral

SYMPTOM SEVERITY
consider functional impairment resulting from that symptom
with regard to occupational, educational, and interpersonal
functioning

check if present	SYMPTOM	mild	moderate	severe	very severe
	WORRY persistent apprehensive expectation focused on a variety of life situations (e.g., family, finances, work)				
	CHRONIC AROUSAL restlessness, difficulty concentrating, edginess, muscle tension, disturbed sleep				
	PHOBIA marked and persistent fear of a specific object or situation. Includes AGORAPHOBIA anxiety about being in places or situations from which escape might be difficult or in which help may not be available. The situaton may be avoided as in a phobia.				
	SOCIAL EVALUATIVE ANXIETY marked and persistent fear of social or performance situations				
	OBSESSIVE THOUGHTS recurrent and persistent thoughts, impulses, images, or ideas that are intrusive and inappropriate and are accompanied by significant anxiety .				
	COMPULSIVE BEHAVIORS AND THOUGHTS repetitive behaviors (e.g., hand washing, checking) or mental acts (e.g., counting, repeating words silently) aimed at preventing some dreaded event or situation (e.g., checking the stove to make sure it is off to prevent a fire). However, the compulsive behavior is either (1) not connected in a realistic way to prevent the event or (2) is excessive.				
	PANIC ATTACKS bouts of fear or a feeling of impending doom, accompanied by accelerated autonomic nervous system activity				
	POST-TRAUMATIC MEMORIES anxiety and other characteristic somatic symptoms (e.g., intrusive recollections of the event, autonomic arousal, persistent avoidance of stimuli associated with the traumatic event) following exposure to a traumatic event in which actual or threatened death, or serious injury occurred				
	DEPRESSION depressed mood, loss of interest or pleasure in nearly all activities, feeling of worthlessness, hopelessness, thoughts of death and suicide.				

Figure 4-1 Symptom evaluation form.

therapy has been shown to be an effective treatment for each of the anxiety disorders (cf. Barlow, 1988; Brown, Hertz, & Barlow, 1992). As described later, the specific details of treatment vary from disorder to disorder; in general, however, each of these therapies directly addresses the specific cognitive, behavioral, and emotional psychopathology of the patient.

Essentially, anxiety as an emotional disorder arises when individuals consistently overestimate the danger of a situation and/or underestimate their ability to cope with the demands of a threatening situation. In either case, there is an exaggerated perception of the threat or danger and the subsequent generation of anxiety or panic. To alleviate their anxiety/panic, anxiety-disordered individuals come up with maneuvers, such as avoidance, that paradoxically maintain the anxiety/panic in the long run through the mechanism of negative reinforcement. Depending on the disorder, various stimuli provoke anxiety, whether it be a social situation for the social phobic patient, heart palpitations for the panic disorder patient, or germs for the obsessive compulsive disorder patient (Rapee, Sanderson, McCauley, & Di Nardo, 1992).

The primary aim of CBT is to extinguish the association between the stimulus and the anxiety/panic response and to extinguish the association between ineffective avoidance behaviors and the temporary relief of anxiety. Cognitive behavioral therapy attempts to remediate the exaggerated threat/appraisal of the patient by (1) increasing the accuracy of the patient's appraisal and (2) increasing the patient's ability to cope with the demands of a stressful situation or conditions.

Cognitive Restructuring

Central to the cognitive model of anxiety (Beck & Emery, 1985) is the notion that the thinking of anxiety-disordered individuals is characterized by faulty information processing styles. As noted above, patients with anxiety disorders consistently overestimate the danger of situations and/or underestimate their ability to cope with such threats, thereby generating anxiety. The individual anticipates threats to self and family, and such threats may be either physical (e.g., life threatening, as in danger associated with flying) or psychological (e.g., threat to self-esteem, as in fear of looking foolish during public speaking). Hence, cognitive restructuring is a strategy employed to reduce patient anxiety by correcting this faulty appraisal style, which presumably generates the anxiety. In other words, when individuals prone to pathological levels of anxiety learn to perceive both the actual danger and their ability to cope with such situations more accurately, their anxiety will decrease.

Specifically, cognitive restructuring focuses on reducing a patient's anxiety by (1) identifying the erroneous beliefs and perceptions of threat that generate anxiety, and (2) challenging and modifying the fearful thoughts by guiding the patient to access information incompatible with the anxiety response (corrective information). The therapist first works with the patient to uncover fear-related cognitions (automatic thoughts) during periods of increased anxiety or panic using a thought monitoring form (Figure 4-2). Because the information processed during these episodes is automatic and extremely rapid, patients may have significant difficulty identifying these cognitions in the beginning. Once this identification is accomplished, patients then learn to challenge the accuracy of their threat appraisal of the stimulus through a process of guided discovery (learning to search for accurate information with the therapist's assistance). Because patients with anxiety disorders typically exaggerate the threat in their respective anxiety-provoking situations, they can be taught to reappraise situations consciously by using various structured exercises, ultimately decreasing their anxiety and panic response. (For a full discussion of cognitive therapy, see Beck, 1995.)

Exposure

The goal of exposure is (1) to break or disconnect the associations between sensations of fear or anxiety and the phobic but objectively safe stimuli (extinction), and (2) to break or disconnect the associations between the *reduction* of anxiety and the escape or avoidance of the phobic stimulus. In systematic exposure, individuals confront the phobic stimuli that trigger their anxiety and panic attacks for a prolonged period of time until their anxiety reaction decreases. Eventually, because the phobic stimulus is not followed by the feared consequence, the association between the phobic stimulus (conditioned stimulus) and the anxiety response (conditioned response) is weakened and a new association develops with the previously feared stimulus (no anxiety).

Because exposure is done in a systematic, hierarchical fashion, patients learn to tolerate manageable levels of anxiety as they confront low-grade phobic situations. Methods such as cognitive restructuring, relaxation, and breathing exercises are often used to decrease the patient's arousal when he or she confronts the phobic stimulus. By tolerating the anxiety caused by the phobic stimulus rather than escaping it, the patient will experience increased efficacy in coping with higher-level phobic situations. Hence, exposure provides a "corrective" experience allowing the patient to disconfirm the threatening appraisal by facing progressively more threatening experiences and enhancing the patient's attention to the absence of the feared consequences.

In vivo exposure involves actual confrontation with the phobic stimulus both in and out of therapy sessions. To accomplish this confrontation, phobic stimuli that create anxiety are initially identified and arranged hierarchically according to the amount of anxiety they evoke. Because the patient is typically not able to confront the stimulus (e.g., petting a dog), the hierarchy also involves the presentation of different levels of the stimulus (e.g., pictures of dogs, watching a movie about dogs, observing a dog from a distance). Exposure is then initiated with those items producing the least

THOUGHT RECORD

Name_____ Date_____

I. Describe the situation: _____

II. Specify feelings/emotion(s) and rate the intensity of each from 1 (just present) to 100 (very intense) (for example: 20 may equal mild, 50 may equal moderate).

1. Emotion _____ Rating= _____ 2. Emotion _____ Rating= _____

3. Emotion _____ Rating= _____ 4. Emotion _____ Rating= _____

III. Complete the 3 columns

AUTOMATIC THOUGHTS write each and rate your belief in each from 1 (do not believe) to 100 (completely believe)	COGNITIVE DISTORTION (S)	RATIONAL RESPONSES substitute more realistic thoughts

IV. Outcome: Describe how you feel after completing the above (e.g., better, not better, etc). _____

Figure 4-2 Thought record.

amount of anxiety and continued on to those items producing increasing levels of anxiety. Anxiety levels are periodically monitored (every five to ten minutes) during exposure sessions so that patients can directly observe the decrease in their anxiety that occurs over time. Exposure to a particular item may be omitted when it evokes minimal or no anxiety for two or three successive sessions. Although the optimal length of exposure may vary across disorders and individual patients, a rule of thumb is to ensure that exposure sessions are not terminated until the patient's anxiety is lessened. There is also some evidence that exposure sessions of short duration may actually increase the patient's anxiety level (Rachman, 1969). In fact, this is the very process that facilitates the development of the phobia.

Imaginal exposure involves visualizing the phobic stimuli in imagination. Imaginal exposure may be used in conjunction with or in lieu of in vivo exposure. When possible, imaginal exposure should precede exposure in vivo so as to prime the patient's coping response. In this way, imaginal exposure can serve to inoculate the patient against the higher levels of anxiety experienced during in vivo exercises. Finally, at times, in vivo exposure may not be feasible, and thus confrontation with the phobic stimulus can be accomplished only by imaginal exposure (e.g., when exposing a rape victim to the traumatic memory).

To implement imaginal exposure, several scenes of gradually increasing levels of anxiety are prepared in advance of sessions. Specifically, each scene should create a graphic, imaginal picture for the patient with equal emphasis placed on descriptions of external situations (e.g., traveling on a train) and internal fear cues (thoughts, images, physiological responses). Scenes are hierarchically arranged according to both the level of the stimulus (looking at a dog versus petting it) and the amount of detail presented (imagining petting a dog, then increasing cues such as the feel of the dog). Homework sessions involve listening to the audiotape of the imaginal exposure conducted in the session.

Relaxation Procedures

Progressive Muscle Relaxation

Progressive muscle relaxation (PMR) is used to reduce the physiological components of anxiety. The PMR exercise described here is based on the Jacobsonian technique of alternating muscle contraction and relaxation (Bernstein & Borkovec, 1973; Brown, O'Leary, & Barlow, 1993). Patients are initially trained to discriminate between muscle tension and relaxation in each of 16 muscle groups distributed throughout the body (e.g., biceps, triceps). The goal of discrimination training is to facilitate rapid relaxation to individual muscle groups by enabling patients to detect sources and early signs of muscle tension and substitute the learned relaxation response. Relaxation-deepening exercises such as deep, diaphragmatic breathing (see complete description in next section) are also employed to facilitate total body relaxation. Sessions may take up to 30 minutes to conduct and are usually taped so that patients may practice the exercises at home.

Once the patient has mastered PMR using all muscle groups (typically over a span of two weeks), the number exercised is gradually reduced to only four muscle groups, specifically focusing on the patient's problematic areas. Reducing the number allows patients the time and flexibility to conduct the exercises as and when needed. During the next phase, relaxation by recall is introduced; in this phase the patient is required to release the tension in each of the four targeted areas by recalling the release of tension experienced during the PMR exercises (as opposed to alternating tension and relaxation). Finally, when the patient has mastered relaxation by recall, cue-controlled relaxation is introduced; in this step, the patient learns to relax all muscle groups by pairing the relaxation with cues such as deep, diaphragmatic breathing (e.g., learning to relax muscle groups when exhaling and saying the word "relax").

Initially, patients are advised to practice PMR exercises twice a day at home. However, as the relaxation exercises are shortened and conducted through the process of recall and cue control, patients are also instructed to use them as and when needed, particularly in high-stress situations. To ensure continued success of relaxation by recall and cue-controlled relaxation, patients are instructed to practice periodically the full 16-muscle-group PMR exercises.

Breathing Retraining

Like PMR, breathing retraining is used to reduce the somatic component of anxiety. Specifically, patients learn diaphragmatic breathing to counteract the shallow, irregular, and rapid breathing patterns often exhibited by individuals experiencing anxiety or stress. This breathing is characterized by the use of chest muscles (thoracic breathing) and is associated with an increase in respiration rate (hyperventilation). Opinions vary on whether anxiety symptoms develop as a result of hyperventilation or whether hyperventilation develops after the anxiety has already begun (cf. McGinn & Sanderson, 1995, for a review). In either case, breathing retraining is believed to prevent hyperventilation and cause changes in autonomic functioning, thereby leading to overall relaxation (Clark, Salkovskis, & Chalkley, 1985).

In abdominal or diaphragmatic breathing, the process of breathing is even and nonconstricting; the inhaled air (oxygen) is drawn deep into the lungs and exhaled (carbon dioxide) as the diaphragm constricts and expands. This type of breathing involves movement in and out of the abdominal rather than the chest muscles, and it allows for the most efficient exchange of oxygen and carbon dioxide with the least effort (see Schwartz, 1987, for a complete description).

Patients initially learn to practice breathing with their abdominal muscles at their regular rate (i.e., approximately 15 breaths per minute). Often, this is difficult as most people tend to breathe with their chest or shoulder muscles. Once diaphragmatic breathing is mastered, the meditative component is introduced in which patients are instructed to focus only on their breathing, covertly counting numbers when they inhale and repeating the word "relax" or "calm" when they exhale (e.g., "1," "relax," "2," "relax"). When patients are able to focus on their breathing *and* keep its rate normal, the final phase of breathing retraining is introduced in which patients learn to slow their breathing to 10 or fewer breaths per minute.

Patients are instructed to practice deep, diaphragmatic breathing outside the session. Initially, as they learn all the different components of breathing retraining, patients are advised to practice the exercise for 10 consecutive minutes twice a day. As they master the technique and learn to control their breathing quickly, they are advised to use the method in many different situations as and when needed (e.g., when they face phobic stimuli).

Symptom-Focused Treatment Strategies

Because of the frequency of comorbidity, effective psychotherapeutic treatment of patients with anxiety disorders involves evaluating their entire symptom configurations, rather than diagnosing disorders alone, and selecting therapeutic strategies to target those symptoms. The primary symptom-focused treatment strategies are presented below.

Chronic Worry

Worry is best defined as persistent apprehensive expectation focused on a variety of life situations (such as family, finances, or health). Worry itself can be a functional activity in that it allows one to problem solve and prepare for future threats. As an example, if a person worries sufficiently about what his or her financial status will be during retirement, he or she may be motivated to establish a retirement savings account that will provide adequate retirement income, thus terminating the negative emotional state.

However, most individuals suffering from chronic worry lose the functional aspect of their worry. Perhaps driven by an increased sense of vulnerability, worriers tend to catastrophize—focus on the worst possible outcome—and overestimate probabilities—convince themselves that the worst possible outcome will occur. As a result of the anxious arousal generated by such thinking, chronic worriers typically become overwhelmed and, consequently, are not able to engage in effective problem solving.

Cognitive Restructuring. Cognitive restructuring is a well-studied, effective strategy used to diminish worry (Beck & Emery, 1985). In cognitive restructuring, the patient identifies specific thoughts or predictions that trigger anxiety, then subjects each thought to logical analysis, as described above. Patients are taught to circumvent their process of anxious apprehension by switching to a model of accurate information processing and problem solving, as shown in the following example. James, a patient suffering from chronic worry has a meeting scheduled by his boss. He begins to feel extremely anxious, thinking that he is going to be fired, that he will never be able to find another job, and that he will become financially bankrupt. The anxiety and worry spiral. Step one is to have the patient list the content of his worry.

1. I will be fired during the meeting.
2. I will never be able to find another job and will become bankrupt.

The next step is to have the patient evaluate the accuracy of each thought. Clinicians often begin by considering the evidence on which each one is based. With regard to the first thought, is there any evidence that this is likely to happen—has James recently received a negative job performance evaluation? Is there any evidence to the contrary—for example, has he always received positive evaluations or recently been promoted? Another line of questioning focuses on generating alternative explanations that may be equally likely or more likely to be accurate. For example, are there any reasons, other than to fire James, that his boss would have called the meeting? Decatastrophizing is another important cognitive strategy. Decatastrophizing involves having the patient imagine what the impact of the negative event would be. By considering the actual impact of the negative event, the patient can engage in problem solving and implement coping techniques. In the above example, James would evaluate the actual impact of being fired, with the goal of developing ways to cope with being unemployed.

When this strategy is used, the patient can often see the negative event as being more manageable than it previously appeared.

Chronic Somatic Arousal

Almost all patients with anxiety disorders manifest chronic somatic arousal, the most likely exception being those with very specific anxiety-eliciting stimuli, such as specific phobias. Common, tension-related central nervous system symptoms include restlessness, edginess, fatigue, irritability, muscle tension, or sleep disturbance. Progressive muscle relaxation appears to be the best psychotherapeutic strategy for diminishing chronic somatic arousal, or anxiety. Patients are encouraged to use progressive muscle relaxation, detailed above, preferably two times each day, to lower their baseline arousal level.

Phobia

Phobia is defined as a marked and persistent fear of a specific object or situation. In a specific phobia, the object or situation invariably provokes anxiety. A variation of specific phobia is agoraphobia, typically developed as a secondary response in someone experiencing panic attacks. Agoraphobia is defined as anxiety about being in places or situations from which escape might be difficult or in which help may not be available. Patients with agoraphobia typically worry that if they have a panic attack in a situation and cannot escape or get help, a catastrophe may result. Thus, they may avoid agoraphobic situations just as people with specific phobias avoid the circumstances that cause their fears. The important distinction is that in the case of specific phobia, the person is afraid of the stimulus or object itself (e.g., fear of flying because the plane may crash). In contrast, patients with agoraphobia fear the onset of a panic attack in that situation (e.g., fear of flying because the person will be unable to get off the plane if a panic attack occurs)—not the situation itself.

Situational Exposure. The best treatment strategy for phobias is a combination of *imaginal* and *in vivo exposure*. The first step is to develop an individualized fear and avoidance hierarchy. The goal is to have the patient visualize the agoraphobic situation prior to actually confronting it. By confronting such anxiety-provoking situations mentally, patients learn how to cope before they confront the situations in actuality. In time, patients are asked to visualize effective coping techniques and responses. In this way, visualization serves as an inoculation: If patients can handle small amounts of manufactured anxiety, they will be better prepared to handle anxiety in a naturalistic setting. A typical format is to use imaginal exposure in session, then have patients actually confront the situations outside the session.

Social Anxiety

The hallmark feature of social anxiety is excessive anxiety, or panic attacks, in situations in which the person is subject to scrutiny by others while performing a specific task—speaking in public, eating in a restaurant, urinating in public restrooms, for example. Individuals generally fear that they will show anxiety symptoms or act in a way that will be humiliating or embarrassing. The feared social or performance situation is either endured with anxiety or avoided altogether.

Although social anxiety is the predominant feature of social phobia, some degree of social anxiety is experienced by many individuals in the general population (Heimberg, Dodge, & Becker, 1987) and is perhaps the most common comorbid symptom experienced by patients with other anxiety disorders (Rapee, Sanderson, & Barlow, 1988). Hence, treatment strategies designed to treat symptoms of social anxiety may be applicable for socially anxious patients with or without a diagnosis of social phobia.

Treatment outcome data indicate that cognitive behavioral therapies are effective in treating social anxiety (see Hope, Holt, & Heimberg, 1993, for a complete review). The goal of cognitive behavioral strategies is to alleviate the anxiety and avoidance behaviors associated with the social or performance situations. When possible, group treatment is the format of choice for patients with social anxiety because it gives participants the opportunity to learn vicariously, see others with similar problems, and make a public commitment to change (Heimberg, 1991; Sank & Shaffer, 1984). Group treatment also provides the opportunity for multiple role-play partners and allows all group members to help one another challenge distorted thoughts (Heimberg, 1991; Sank & Shaffer, 1984).

Simulated exposure consists of five- to ten-minute role-plays of anxiety-provoking situations during treatment sessions. Anxiety-provoking situations are based on fear and avoidance hierarchies of rank-ordered situations rated for fear, avoidance, and fear of negative evaluation by others. They can range from initiating a conversation with a stranger to giving a presentation at a staff meeting. Nonperfectionistic, behavioral goals should be set for the simulated exposure tasks; these may require some negotiation as patients with social anxiety tend to have unrealistic or unmeasurable goals (e.g., "I should feel no anxiety" or "I should be responsible for filling in all the pauses in a conversation") (Heimberg, 1991). During a role-play, patients' anxiety levels and automatic thoughts are monitored periodically and the exposure task is continued until the anxiety decreases or plateaus and goals have been met. Patients' performance and anxiety levels, as well as the automatic thoughts and rational responses used during the role-play, are then discussed, with the goal of identifying self-statements that increase patient anxiety and those that decrease it to facilitate future performance.

In a group format, other group members serve as role-play partners in addition to the therapist. Outsiders may also be brought in to serve as role-play partners in both individual and group formats. Props may be used to make the simulated exposures as realistic as possible. For example, a patient may be required to stand at a podium while giving a talk; food may be brought in if a patient has a fear of eating in public.

Although in vivo exposure is described as the treatment of choice for the anxiety disorders in general (Barlow & Beck, 1984), simulated exposure techniques form the bulk of treatment for social anxiety for multiple reasons (Heimberg, 1991). One reason is that in vivo exposure exercises are harder to design and implement in the treatment of social anxiety. Unlike simple exposure exercises, such as having a panic disorder patient enter a train, patients with social anxiety must perform a complex sequence of interpersonal behaviors during the phobic situation, exposing themselves to a variety of feared interpersonal consequences. In vivo exposure exercises are not only more complicated but are also less easily available to patients suffering from social anxiety who may have cut themselves off from all but necessary social contact. Because social situations are inherently unpredictable, it is also harder to design in vivo exercises in advance, and harder to ensure that patients repeat the same social situation or expose themselves to easier situations before difficult ones. Finally, the success of in vivo exposure usually comes from prolonged exposure to the feared situation, which is believed to lead to habituation of anxiety. Because several social or performance situations often involve only a brief exchange, patients with anxiety may not remain in them until their anxiety peaks and then diminishes. However, to facilitate transfer-of-training to real-life social or performance situations, clinicians generally assign in vivo exposure exercises to patients during each session. Specific homework assignments are negotiated with patients and are coordinated with simulated exposure tasks conducted during sessions.

Cognitive Restructuring. Typically, cognitive restructuring is used in conjunction with exposure exercises in the treatment of social anxiety. Automatic thoughts regarding feared and avoided situations are elicited, cognitive distortions are identified, and rational responses are developed before individuals engage in simulated or actual in vivo exercises. Then, individuals are instructed to use cognitive restructuring techniques before, during, and after each exposure exercise to facilitate exposure tasks.

Cognitive restructuring may be particularly useful for patients who do not exhibit behavioral avoidance of feared situations. Such individuals may use cognitive maneuvers to avoid anxiety—for example, to distract themselves or to withdraw into themselves—thus preventing the experience of full-blown anxiety during social or performance tasks. Others may distort social or performance encounters—see them as unsuccessful despite objective evidence to the contrary.

It is not clear whether exposure plus cognitive therapy is more effective than exposure alone (Hope et al., 1993). However, because the fear of negative evaluation, the hallmark of social phobia, is essentially a cognitive construct, several researchers believe that cognitive interventions may play a more important role in the treatment of social phobia than in other anxiety disorders (Butler, 1989). Further, studies have shown that exposure alone has no substantial impact on fear of negative evaluation (Butler, Cullington, Munby, Amies, & Gelder, 1984) and that fear of negative evaluation has a strong relationship to treatment outcome (Mattick & Peters, 1988; Mattick, Peters, & Clarke, 1989). These findings suggest that altering distorted thoughts related to these fears may significantly affect treatment outcome.

Obsessive Thoughts

Obsessions are defined as persistent, intrusive, and inappropriate thoughts, ideas, impulses, or images that cause a person significant anxiety. To alleviate the anxiety, the person attempts to suppress or ignore the obsessions or to neutralize them with some other thought or behavior. The goal of cognitive behavioral strategies is to alleviate the anxiety associated with these obsessive thoughts, thereby reducing the frequency and persistence of the thoughts.

Exposure. An examination of the relative efficacy of behavioral techniques for the treatment of obsessive thoughts indicates that obsessive thoughts respond primarily to exposure (Foa, Steketee, Grayson, Turner, & Latimer, 1984) and that a combination of in vivo and imaginal exposure appears to be superior to other strategies in maintaining long-term gains, particularly for those patients who cognitively avoid their feared consequences (Foa, Steketee, Turner, & Fischer, 1980).

To design successful exposure sessions for patients who present with obsessive thoughts, clinicians must first thoroughly assess the nature of presenting symptoms. This assessment includes identifying the *fear/threat cues* that cause the patients anxiety (such as fearing that they will be contaminated by a toilet seat or that they will harm their loved ones) and discovering *the consequences they fear,* because many patients with obsessive thoughts are afraid that something terrible will happen if they fail to neutralize or suppress these thoughts (Riggs & Foa, 1993). Obtaining specific information about the patient's feared consequence is extremely important in deciding which parts of the treatment will be more useful.

To eliminate obsessive thinking, patients are confronted over a prolonged period of time with anxiety-evoking stimuli (the fear/threat cues), either imaginally or in vivo (Riggs & Foa, 1993). As patients tolerate prolonged confrontation with these fear/threat cues without trying to escape or neutralize the thought with some other thought or action, they learn that their feared consequences do not occur; as a result, their anxiety associated with these thoughts ultimately decreases. As they become habituated to these thoughts, patients experience a reduction in obsessive thoughts.

In vivo exposure involves direct prolonged confrontation with external fear/threat cues (such as contact with contamination) whereas imaginal exposure involves prolonged confrontation with feared disasters (such as hitting a pedestrian while driving). Often, *imaginal exposure* may be the first step before patients are directly exposed to anxiety-evoking stimuli (imagining sitting on a public toilet before actually sitting on it). In other cases, in vivo exposure may not be feasible and only imaginal exposure may be used, as for patients who fear that their loved ones may be killed in a fire. In yet other cases, in vivo exposure may be the only treatment of choice. For example, patients who do not express specific feared consequences but rather fear that the emotional distress from the obsessive thoughts will be intolerable tend to benefit only from in vivo exposure.

Cognitive Restructuring. Although behavioral techniques have been empirically validated for the treatment of obsessive thoughts and compulsive behaviors (see Foa, Steketee, & Ozarow, 1985, for a full review), preliminary evidence suggests that cognitive strategies may be effective in conjunction with exposure and response prevention (Salkovskis & Warwick, 1985). Patients with obsessive thoughts often have specific belief systems and irrational ideas that can be helped with cognitive techniques. For example, patients with obsessive thoughts have erroneous belief systems (e.g., if I have a thought about killing my mother, it is like actually killing my mother), a condition that leads to erroneous estimates of threat (e.g., I am capable of killing my mother). They also exhibit a tendency to perceive these intrusive thoughts as ego dystonic (e.g., I am a bad person for having such evil thoughts; people don't have thoughts about harming their own mothers), which leads to increased anxiety. Finally, such patients also have a tendency to devalue their own ability to deal with threat; this assessment causes anxiety (e.g., I am a weak person and I have no control over my thoughts), which leads them to neutralize their thoughts through passive avoidance or ritualized thoughts or behaviors. Cognitive restructuring involves helping patients identify the erroneous beliefs and perceptions of threat, normalize their obsessive thoughts, and challenge their tendency to devalue their own ability to deal adequately with such threat.

Compulsive Thoughts and Behaviors

Compulsions are repetitive behaviors, such as hand washing, or mental acts, such as praying silently, that the person feels compelled to perform according to rigid rules or to alleviate the anxiety created by the obsessive thoughts. Behavioral strategies attempt to block ritualized behaviors or thoughts with the goal of breaking the association between ritualized behaviors and thoughts and the patient's subsequent feelings of relief or reduced anxiety.

Response Prevention. Efficacy studies indicate that ritualized behaviors and thoughts respond primarily to response prevention (Foa et al., 1984). To maximize treatment efficacy, clinicians should obtain detailed information on how patients attempt to alleviate their anxiety. Their rituals may be mental (e.g., counting numbers) or behavioral (e.g., washing their hands, checking stove). They may be fairly explicit (e.g., washing hands) or fairly subtle (e.g., blinking, walking on alternate tiles).

Although rituals serve to alleviate anxiety, they become aversive for many patients. First, the rituals never alleviate the anxiety completely and hence they become more and more prolonged: Hand washing can occur over and over because the person is never positive that all germs have been eliminated. Second, the rituals take up so much time that they interfere with other aspects of the person's daily life: He or she may spend up to eight hours a day checking the gas stove (Riggs & Foa, 1993). Sometimes when one compulsion becomes too aversive, the patient will switch to another one. The therapist must be alert to all compulsions, even shifts in rituals during treatment, and address them as well (Riggs & Foa, 1993).

Response prevention involves the blocking of compulsions, such as helping the patient leave the kitchen without checking the stove, and begins during the first treatment session. Patients are given a rationale for response preventions, presented with specific rules for accomplishing them, and are generally assisted by family members to comply with response prevention rules. By the end of treatment, patients must be presented with guidelines for normal behavior because many do not know what normal behavior is.

Data from *DSM-IV* field trials indicate that compulsive thoughts or behaviors occur in the context of obsessive thoughts (Foa & Kozak, in press). Hence, for patients who present with ritualized thoughts or behaviors, treatment strategies used to reduce ritualized thoughts or behaviors should be used in conjunction with strategies designed to reduce obsessive thoughts.

Panic Attacks

Although almost all patients suffering from anxiety disorders experience panic attacks, the treatment strategies described in this section are to address those attacks not typically associated with any particular stimuli. When a particular stimulus is the anxiety producer, the stimulus itself is feared, as when a social phobic patient enters a party and experiences panic. Instead, the strategies in this section are for patients experiencing panic attacks that are themselves the source of fear. In these cases, the panic attack is not limited to particular stimuli, and the patient fears the panic attack itself. For a more thorough description of these techniques, see Craske and Barlow (1993).

Psychoeducation. Patients experiencing panic attacks have typically been to many different doctors without receiving a clear diagnosis and explanation of their disorder. In the absence of such information, these patients often imagine that they are going to die, go crazy, or lose control. In almost all cases, they suspect that the doctor has overlooked some life-threatening physical condition that would account for their symptomatology. Therefore, the psychoeducation phase consists of a didactic presentation about panic attacks. The primary goal is to debunk common myths about the danger of panic attacks: Panic attacks are a sign of an undetected brain tumor; palpitations cause heart attacks; hyperventilation leads to fainting. These myths seem to drive the panic process. Written materials, such as pamphlets and books, are valuable educational tools because patients may reread them as desired. Several excellent self-help books are available that offer simple, supportive information about panic attacks (Barlow & Craske, 1989; Burns, 1989).

Cognitive Restructuring. The first step is to help the patient identify how certain cognitions accentuate or provoke panic. The clinician does this by helping the patient retrospectively examine the thoughts, beliefs, and assumptions he or she experienced during a typical panic attack. The patient can vividly remember the first and most recent panic attacks, and a detailed discussion of those experiences is a useful place to begin this examination. Through a series of questions, the therapist tries to determine the patient's idiosyncratic panic sequence and to uncover unrealistic catastrophic thoughts. Under such questioning, the validity of these cognitions is implicitly and explicitly challenged.

A typical panic sequence follows this line:

1. I was sitting in a meeting at work.
2. I noticed my heart began to beat faster. (physical symptom)
3. I assumed these palpitations were the early signs of a panic attack, and that I would lose control and start to yell. Everyone would think I was crazy! (catastrophic thought)
4. I became even more anxious, worried about losing control, and started to perspire profusely. (escalation)
5. I excused myself from the meeting. (escape and avoidance)
6. I felt depressed and discouraged because I couldn't even handle an innocuous work meeting. (hopelessness)

This description of a typical panic sequence reveals the patient's interior monologue which must be made explicit because most patients are unaware of their own thinking. There is also a tendency for patients to deny that they engage in catastrophic ways of thinking because these beliefs seem so incredible once the panic attack has subsided. The therapeutic setting should promote the patient's sense of comfort and acceptance so as to facilitate patient disclosure.

Once patients become aware of the importance of their cognitions in eliciting and fueling their panic attacks, they are in a position to reevaluate the validity of these cognitions and ultimately to challenge them. In particular, clinicians should target patients' catastrophic misinterpretations of their panic-related somatic cues (Clark, 1986). Other common misinterpretations include the overestimation of the consequences of panic, such as public humiliation, losing one's job, or interpersonal rejection.

The final phase of cognitive restructuring is to *decatastrophize* the situation with the patient, especially when dealing with agoraphobic avoidance. This is easily accomplished through a series of questions: If your worst fear came true, would it really be as bad as you imagine? Consider a patient who believes he or she will have a panic attack on a plane, will scream wildly, and will try to escape. In fact, if the person's worst fears were realized and he or she did have a panic attack, the most likely outcome would be a feeling of great discomfort—not screaming, attempts to escape, and embarrassment. Decatastrophizing greatly reduces the patient's need to avoid panic-related situations.

Respiratory Control. Respiratory control helps patients regain a sense of control over the somatic features of panic and anxiety. They are taught a method of breathing that increases their relaxation and prevents hyperventilation (Clark et al., 1985). Hyperventilation initiates a cascade of somatic symptoms such as dizziness, chest pain, breathlessness, and paresthesias that culminate in panic. These symptoms instill a frightening sense that one's body is out of control.

Under stress and anxiety, respiration rate often increases; this symptom is characterized by the use of chest muscles and short, shallow breaths. To combat this tendency, the patient is taught to use diaphragmatic breathing— breathing that involves in-and-out movement of the abdomen, not the chest—at a regular rate—approximately 15 breaths per minute. This exercise is practiced outside the session in many different situations. Patients learn to control their breathing quickly and to recognize this as an effective strategy they can rely on once they notice the onset of panic.

Interoceptive Exposure. Interoceptive exposure is a technique employed to address directly the *fear of fear* often present in patients who experience panic attacks—that is, patients who are afraid of the symptoms of fear. Specifically, patients are exposed to internal somatic sensations associated with panic in order to weaken their association. Interoceptive exposure is based on the patient's individualized hierarchy of feared internal sensations, such as dizziness and palpitations. For example, a patient who fears cardiac symptoms may be exposed to one minute of increased heart rate by using an exercise bike, then two minutes, and so on. Systematic exposure to these sensations may be achieved using idiosyncratic methods, such as overbreathing, spinning, and physical exertion.

Posttraumatic Memories

Individuals who suffer from anxiety associated with a previously experienced traumatic event tend to reexperience the traumatic event persistently, exhibit a numbing of general responsiveness not present before the trauma, and avoid stimuli associated with the trauma. Often, such individuals alternate between episodes of reexperiencing and numbing or avoidance behaviors.

Reexperiencing episodes may take the form of recollections, dreams, a sense of reliving the experience, illusions, hallucinations, or dissociative (flashback) episodes. Affected individuals may experience intense psychological distress and heightened physiological reactivity on exposure to internal or external cues that symbolize or resemble an aspect of the traumatic event. Avoidance behaviors or general numbing may occur in any of the following ways: efforts to avoid thoughts, feelings, activities, places, or people associated with the trauma; inability to recall an important aspect of the trauma; a diminished interest or participation in significant activities; a feeling of detachment or estrangement from others; a restricted range of affect manifested in the inability to have loving feelings; and a sense of a foreshortened future, shown by lack of expectation of having a career, marriage, children, or a normal life span.

Although the fear and anxiety directly associated with trauma are natural, behavioral theories suggest that these emotions become associated with other stimuli present during the trauma (conditioning), generalize to other stimuli not present (stimulus generalization) and are maintained because by avoiding or escaping these stimuli, the individual does not learn that they are not inherently frightening (negative reinforcement). The goal of cognitive-behavioral treatment is to reduce the fear or anxiety (1) directly associated with the trauma and (2) indirectly associated with the trauma as a result of conditioning.

Prolonged Imaginal Exposure (to the Traumatic Event). According to Foa (Foa & Kozak, 1986; Foa, Steketee, & Rothbaum, 1989), systematic exposure to the traumatic memory in a safe environment alters the patient's feared memory, thus enabling him or her to reevaluate the threat cues and habituate to the fear. Prolonged imaginal exposure to the traumatic event is considered crucial for treatment success and requires considerable therapist expertise because emotions displayed may be extremely powerful (Foa, Rothbaum, Riggs, & Murdoch, 1991).

Specifically, the patient is asked to recall the traumatic event in detail and is helped to process the memory until it is no longer acutely distressing (habituation). Initially, patients are exposed to trauma memories that provoke a minimum anxiety level; in subsequent sessions, however, more and more detail about external cues (e.g., physical location of the rape, the smell in the room) and internal cues (thoughts, physiological responses, feared consequences) are elicited. Patient anxiety levels are monitored periodically throughout the exposure period, and sessions are terminated only when anxiety levels decrease. To facilitate habituation, exposure sessions are taped and patients are instructed to listen to the tapes regularly at home.

In Vivo Exposure to Current and Future Life Issues. In this phase, patients are exposed to stimuli in their current life that generate fear and/or avoidance but are not directly associated with the traumatic event (such as going out alone if the patient is a rape victim). These stimuli become indirectly associated with the traumatic event through conditioning; as a result, they lead to fear and avoidance.

The patient generates a hierarchical list of major stimuli that are currently feared and avoided: for a rape victim, dating men; for a burn victim, cooking. The goal is to expose patients to each feared event or stimulus on the hierarchy. Patients are initially exposed to situations that are minimally threatening to ensure that they can manage the anxiety that is triggered when they perform new behaviors. They are moved upward on the systematic exposure hierarchy when their anxiety is minimal. In vivo tasks can be conducted during the session—for the patient to wear the clothes she wore when she was raped, to go to the scene of the trauma—and outside the session—for a rape victim to go on a date.

To better prepare patients for in vivo exercises and to increase the likelihood of success outside therapy, clinicians may expose patients to each level of the hierarchy imaginally during sessions before in vivo exposure takes place. Several scenes of gradually increasing anxiety-evoking potential are prepared prior to exposure sessions, with each script creating a vivid, imaginal picture for the patient. Generally, the greater the detail of these images, the more effective they are in ultimately reducing anxiety associated with the phobic stimuli: Where is the party? What are the guests wearing? What is the weather like? Equal emphasis should be placed on descriptions of external situations and the patient's thoughts, images, and physiological responses in the feared scene: talking to men at a party, thinking of being raped by each man she talks to, experiencing heart racing and breathing difficulty.

Role-Playing. Role-playing may also be considered before in vivo exposure takes place if patients need further preparation for a situation than is provided by imaginal exposure, if they lack certain skills or behaviors, or if they perceive themselves as lacking certain skills. If indicated, patients may be referred for specialized training, such as assertiveness training.

Cognitive Restructuring. Because patients' reactions directly to the trauma are natural and not distorted, cognitive restructuring focuses only on current and future life issues. It involves modifying *distorted thoughts* that develop as a result of the trauma and that interfere with social and occupational functioning—thoughts for a rape victim as to why she was raped, or that all men are bad. Among other areas, cognitive distortions are assessed in the following areas: (1) beliefs about the world (all men are potential rapists), (2) helplessness versus controllability (I have no control over my life), (3) personal responsibility (maybe the way I dressed made him rape me), and (4) phobic situations (I can never date again). In general, cognitive restructuring attempts to change the patient's self-image from passive victim to active survivor, thus empowering the patient.

The patient's maladaptive cognitions (I caused the rape) are first identified, and their impact on the patient's current life are discussed (the patient does not date because of these thoughts). The cognitive distortions, or overgeneralizations, evident in the thoughts are then noted and more realistic, rational responses are substituted: Because one man raped me does not mean that every man is a potential rapist.

Depression

One of the best-documented treatments for depression is cognitive therapy, a therapeutic strategy that focuses directly on the disturbed information processing maintained by depressed patients (Beck, Rush, Shaw, & Emery, 1979). Specifically, as detailed in Beck's *cognitive triad of depression* (Beck et al., 1979), depressed patients typically have a negative view of *themselves,* seeing themselves as worthless, inadequate, unlovable, and deficient). They are equally negative about their *environment,* seeing it filled with obstacles and failure, and their *future,* seeing it as hopeless.

As a result of this cognitive triad, which serves as a template for processing information, depressed patients consistently distort their interpretations of events, thus maintaining the depression. A depressed patient often exaggerates failures in his or her life and underplays successes, consequently feeling like a failure as a person. Distorted information processing is a core process contributing to depressed mood. Thus, the primary goal of cognitive therapy is to "correct" this process, using the general principles of cognitive restructuring described above. The overall aim of this approach is to help patients learn to think more logically and thereby experience improvements in affect, motivation, and behavior.

In many cases, comorbid depression in patients with anxiety disorder is secondary, or a reaction to the anxiety disorder. For example, patients whose life functioning is impaired by social anxiety feel bad about themselves, their environment, and their future. As a result, the depression often clears up as the other disorder is successfully treated and does not have to be addressed directly. Thus, as a rule of thumb, unless the depression is so severe that it impedes treatment of the anxiety disorder, a useful approach seems to be to address the anxiety disorder first, then reevaluate the depression.

CONCLUSION

Patients with a principal diagnosis of an anxiety disorder commonly suffer from comorbid disorders and symptoms; thus, the practice of describing a patient with one disorder is inadequate to convey the overall level of the patient's psychopathology, leading to inadequate treatment planning and implementation. This chapter has presented an approach to the assessment and psychotherapeutic treatment of anxiety disorder patients that is symptom focused, rather than disorder based, and has provided a framework that allows clinicians to tailor their treatment to address the specific symptom configuration of each patient. The authors recommend that clinicians adopt this strategy as a primary approach to maximizing treatment efficiency for patients with anxiety disorders.

REFERENCES

American Psychiatric Association. (1987). *Diagnostic and statistical manual of mental disorders* (3rd ed., rev.). Washington, DC: Author.

American Psychiatric Association. (1994). *Diagnostic and statistical manual of mental disorders* (4th ed.). Washington, DC: Author.

Barlow, D.A., & Beck, A.T. (1984). The psychosocial treatment of anxiety disorders. In J.B.W. Williams & R.L. Spitzer (Eds.), *Psychotherapy research: Where are we and where should we go?* (pp. 29–66). New York: Guilford Press.

Barlow, D.H. (1988). *Anxiety and its disorders.* New York: Guilford Press.

Barlow, D.H., & Craske, M.G. (1989). *Mastery of your anxiety and panic.* Albany, NY: Graywind.

Beck, A.T., & Emery, G. (1985). *Anxiety disorders and phobias: A cognitive perspective.* New York: Basic Books.

Beck, A.T., Rush, A.J., Shaw, B., & Emery, G. (1979). *Cognitive therapy of depression.* New York: Guilford Press.

Beck, J. (1995). *Cognitive therapy: Basics and beyond.* New York: Guilford Press.
Bernstein, T.A., & Borkovec, T.D. (1973). *Progressive relaxation training.* Champaign, IL: Research Press.
Blashfield, R.K. (1990). Comorbidity and classification. In J.D. Maser & C.B. Cloninger (Eds.), *Comorbidity in anxiety and mood disorders* (pp. 61–82). Washington, DC: American Psychiatric Press.
Brown, T.A., Antony, M.M., & Barlow, D.H. (1995). Diagnostic comorbidity in panic disorder: Effect on treatment outcome and course of comorbid diagnoses following treatment. *Journal of Consulting and Clinical Psychology, 63,* 408–418.
Brown, T.A., Hertz, R.M., & Barlow, D.H. (1992). New developments in cognitive behavioral treatments of anxiety disorders. In A. Tasman & M.B. Riba (Eds.), *Review of psychiatry* (Vol. 11, pp. 285–306). Washington, DC: American Psychiatric Press.
Brown, T.A., O'Leary, T.A., & Barlow, D.H. (1993). Generalized anxiety disorder. In D.A. Barlow (Ed.), *Clinical handbook of psychological disorders* (pp. 137–188). New York: Guilford Press.
Burns, D.D. (1989). *The feeling good handbook: Using the new mood therapy in everyday life.* New York: Morrow.
Butler, G. (1989). Issues in the application of cognitive and behavioral strategies to the treatment of social phobia. *Clinical Psychology Review, 9,* 91–186.
Butler, G., Cullington, A., Munby, M., Amies, P., & Gelder, M. (1984). Exposure and anxiety management in the treatment of social phobia. *Journal of Consulting and Clinical Psychology, 52,* 642–650.
Chambless, D.L., Sanderson, W.C., Shoham, V., Johnson, S.B., Pope, K., Crits-Christoph, P., Baker, M., Johnson, B., Woody, S.R., Sue, S., Beutler, L., Williams, D., & McCurry, S. (in press). Empirically validated therapies: A project of the Division of Clinical Psychology, American Psychological Association, Task Force on Psychological Interventions. *The Clinical Psychologist.*
Clark, D.M. (1986). A cognitive approach to panic. *Behaviour Research and Therapy, 24,* 461–471.
Clark, D.M., Salkovskis, P.M., & Chalkley, A.J. (1985). Respiratory control as a treatment for panic attacks. *Journal of Behavior Therapy & Experimental Psychiatry, 16,* 23–30.
Clarkin, J.F., & Kendall, P.C. (1992). Comorbidity and treatment planning: Summary and future directions. *Journal of Consulting and Clinical Psychology, 60,* 904–908.
Coryell, W., Endicott, J., Andreasen, N.C., Keller, M.B., Clayton, P.J., Hirschfeld, R.M.A., Scheftner, W.A., & Winokur, G. (1988). Depression and panic attacks: The significance of overlap as reflected in follow-up and family study data. *American Journal of Psychiatry, 145,* 293–300.
Craske, M.G., & Barlow, D.H. (1993). Panic disorder and agoraphobia. In D.H. Barlow (Ed.), *Clinical handbook of psychological disorders.* New York: Guilford Press.
deRuiter, C., Ruken, H., Garssen, B., van Schaik, A., & Kraaimaat, F. (1989). Comorbidity among the anxiety disorders. *Journal of Anxiety Disorders, 3,* 57–68.

Di Nardo, P.A., & Barlow, D.H. (1990). Syndrome and symptom comorbidity in the anxiety disorders. In J.D. Maser & C.R. Cloninger (Eds.), *Comorbidity in anxiety and mood disorders* (pp. 205–230). Washington, DC: American Psychiatric Press.

Foa, E.B., & Kozak, M.J. (1986). Emotional processing of fear: Exposure to corrective information. *Psychological Bulletin, 99,* 20–35.

Foa, E.B., & Kozak, M.J. (in press). Report on the *DSM-IV* field trial for obsessive-compulsive disorder. In *DSM-IV sourcebook.* Washington, DC: American Psychiatric Association.

Foa, E.B., Rothbaum, B.O., Riggs, D.S., & Murdoch, T.B. (1991). Treatment of posttraumatic stress disorder in rape victims: A comparison between cognitive-behavioral procedures and counseling. *Journal of Consulting and Clinical Psychology, 59*(5), 715–723.

Foa, E.B., Steketee, G., Grayson, J.B., Turner, R.M., & Latimer, P. (1984). Deliberate exposure and blocking of obsessive-compulsive rituals: Immediate and long-term effects. *Behavior Therapy, 13,* 450–472.

Foa, E.B., Steketee, G., & Ozarow, B. (1985). Behavior therapy with obsessive-compulsives: From theory to treatment. In M. Mavissakalian (Ed.), *Obsessive-compulsive disorder: Psychological and pharmacological treatment* (pp. 49–129). New York: Plenum Press.

Foa, E.B., Steketee, G., & Rothbaum, B.O. (1989). Behavior/cognitive conceptualizations of post-traumatic stress disorder. *Behavior Therapy, 20,* 155–176.

Foa, E.B., Steketee, G., Turner, R.M., & Fischer, S.C. (1980). Effects of imaginal exposure to feared disasters in obsessive-compulsive checkers. *Behavior Research and Therapy, 18,* 449–455.

Friedman, C.J., Shear, M.K., & Frances, A. (1987). *DSM-III* personality disorders in panic patients. *Journal of Personality Disorders, 1,* 132–135.

Green, M.A., & Curtis, G.C. (1988). Personality disorders in panic patients: Response to elimination of medication. *Journal of Personality Disorders, 2,* 303–314.

Heimberg, R.G. (1991). *A manual for conducting cognitive-behavioral group therapy for social phobia.* Unpublished manuscript, State University of New York at Albany, Center for Stress and Anxiety Disorders.

Heimberg, R.G., Dodge, C.S., & Becker, R.E. (1987). Social phobia. In L. Michelson & M. Ascher (Eds.), *Anxiety and stress disorders: Cognitive behavioral assessment and treatment* (pp. 280–309). New York: The Guilford Press.

Hope, D.A., Holt, C.S., & Heimberg, R.G. (1993). In T.R. Giles (Ed.), *Handbook of effective psychotherapy* (pp. 227–251). New York: Plenum Press.

Lesser, I.M., Rubin, R.T., Pecknold, J.C., Rifkin, A., Swinson, R.P., Lydiard, R.B., Burrows, G.D., Noyes, R., Jr., & DuPont, R.L. Jr. (1988). Secondary depression in panic disorder and agoraphobia. *Archives of General Psychiatry, 45,* 437–443.

Mattick, R.P., & Peters, L. (1988). Treatment of severe social phobia: Effects of guided exposure with and without cognitive restructuring. *Journal of Consulting and Clinical Psychology, 56,* 251–260.

Mattick, R.P., Peters, L., & Clarke, J.C. (1989). Exposure and cognitive restructuring for severe social phobia: A controlled study. *Behavior Therapy, 20,* 3–23.

McGinn, L.K., Young, J.E., & Sanderson, W.C. (1995). When and how to do longer-term therapy . . . without feeling guilty. *Cognitive and Behavioral Practice, 2,* 187–212.

McGinn, L.K., & Sanderson, L.K. (1995). The nature of panic disorder. *In session: Psychotherapy in practice, 1*(3), 7–19.

Noyes, R., Jr., Reich, J., Christiansen, J. Suelzer, M., Pfohl, B., & Coryell, W.A. (1990). Outcome of panic disorder. *Archives of General Psychiatry, 47,* 809–818.

Rachman, S. (1969). Treatment by prolonged exposure to high intensity stimulation. *Behavior Research and Therapy, 7,* 295–302.

Rapee, R.M., Sanderson, W.C., & Barlow, D.H. (1988). Social phobia symptoms across the *DSM-III-Revised* anxiety disorder categories. *Journal of Psychopathology and Behavioral Assessment, 10*(3), 287–299.

Rapee, R.M., Sanderson, W.C., McCauley, P.A., & Di Nardo, P.A. (1992). Differences in reported symptom profile between panic disorder and other *DSM-III-R* anxiety disorders. *Behavior Research and Therapy, 30,* 45–52.

Rathus, J.H., & Sanderson, W.C. (in press). The role of emotion in the psychopathology and treatment of the anxiety disorders. In W. Flack & J. Laird (Eds.), *Emotions in psychopathology.* New York: Oxford University Press.

Rathus, J.H., Sanderson, W.C., Miller, A.L., & Wetzler, S. (1995). Impact of personality functioning on cognitive behavioral treatment of panic disorder. *Journal of Personality Disorders, 9,* 160–168.

Reich, J. (1988). Instruments measuring *DSM-III* and *DSM-III-R* personality disorders. *Journal of Personality Disorders, 1,* 220–240.

Reich, J., & Noyes, R.A. (1987). A comparison of *DSM-III* personality disorders in acutely ill panic and depressed patients. *Journal of Anxiety Disorders, 1,* 123–131.

Riggs, D.S., & Foa, E.B. (1993). Obsessive compulsive disorder. In D.A. Barlow (Ed.), *Clinical handbook of psychological disorders* (pp. 137–188). New York: Guilford Press.

Salkovskis, P.M., & Warwick, H.M.C. (1985). Cognitive therapy of obsessive-compulsive disorder: Treating treatment failures. *Behavioral Psychotherapy, 13,* 243–255.

Sanderson, W.C. (in press). *Symptom focused treatment for a managed care environment.* Northvale, NJ: Jason Aronson.

Sanderson, W.C., & Barlow, D.H. (1990). A description of patients diagnosed with *DSM-III-R* generalized anxiety disorder. *Journal of Nervous and Mental Disease, 178,* 588–591.

Sanderson, W.C., Beck, A.T., & Beck, J. (1990). Syndrome comorbidity in patients with major depression or dysthymia: Prevalence and temporal relationships. *American Journal of Psychiatry, 147,* 1025–1028.

Sanderson, W.C., Beck, A.T., & McGinn, L.K. (1994). Cognitive therapy for generalized anxiety disorder: Significance of comorbid personality disorders. *Journal of Cognitive Psychotherapy, 8,* 13–18.

Sanderson, W.C., Di Nardo, P.A., Rapee, R.M., & Barlow, D.H. (1990). Syndrome comorbidity in patients diagnosed with a *DSM-III-R* anxiety disorder. *Journal of Abnormal Psychology, 99,* 308–312.

Sanderson, W.C., Friedman, T., Asnis, G.M., & Wetzler, S. (1992, November). *Personality disorders in patients with major depression, panic disorder, and generalized anxiety disorder.* Paper presented at the annual meeting of the Association for the Advancement of Behavior Therapy, Boston, MA.

Sanderson, W.C., Raue, P., & Wetzler, S. (1995, August). *Generalizability of cognitive behavior therapy for panic disorder.* Paper presented at the annual meeting of the American Psychological Association, New York City.

Sanderson, W.C., Wetzler, S., Beck, A.T., & Betz, F. (1994). Prevalence of personality disorders among patients with anxiety disorders. *Psychiatry Research, 51,* 167–174.

Sank, L.I., & Shaffer, C.S. (1984). *A therapist's manual for cognitive-behavior therapy in groups.* New York: Plenum Press.

Schwartz, M.S. (1987). *Biofeedback: A practitioner's guide.* New York: Guilford Press.

Turner, S.M. (1987). The effects of personality disorders on the outcome of social anxiety symptom reduction. *Journal of Personality Disorders, 1,* 136–143.

Wolfe, B.E. (1994). Adapting psychotherapy outcome research to clinical reality. *Journal of Psychotherapy Integration, 4,* 160–166.

5

Drug Treatment of Anxiety Disorders with Comorbidity

JUSTINE M. KENT
JACK M. GORMAN

Anxiety disorders affect a significant proportion of the general population, causing distress and impairing functioning. Psychotherapy and drug treatment, alone or in combination, result in significant alleviation of anxiety symptoms. The diagnosis of anxiety disorders, however, is often complicated by other Axis I coexisting disorders such as mood disorders, other anxiety disorders, or substance abuse, or by a co-occurring Axis II personality disorder.

Outcome of anxiety disorder treatment is affected by comorbid conditions, and failure to evaluate a patient for other concomitant psychiatric disorders may result in what appears to be treatment resistance. Comorbid psychiatric conditions affect drug treatment response and must be taken into consideration before a medication trial is deemed ineffective.

MEDICATIONS USED IN THE
PHARMACOLOGIC MANAGEMENT OF ANXIETY

Perhaps the most common causes of treatment resistance in the drug treatment of anxiety disorders are failure to consider comorbid psychiatric disorders, inadequate dose and length of drug trials, and failure to fully assess medical conditions complicating the anxiety presentation. When these factors are taken into consideration, anxiety disorders are highly treatable. There are four major classes of medications used in the management of anxiety: (1) benzodiazepines, (2) cyclic antidepressants, (3) selective serotonin reuptake inhibitors (SSRIs), and (4) noncyclic/atypical agents.

Benzodiazepines

Benzodiazepines remain the most commonly used drugs in the pharmacologic treatment of anxiety. A high therapeutic index and good safety profile, along with established efficacy, have led the benzodiazepines to supplant the barbiturates and other nonbenzodiazepine hypnotics in the treatment of anxiety states. Benzodiazepines are commonly employed in the primary treatment of generalized anxiety disorder (GAD) and panic disorder, and as a second-line treatment for social phobia. The benzodiazepines are generally subdivided according to their duration of action (long acting, intermediate acting, and short acting). All are equally sedating; however, short-acting (short half-life) benzodiazepines are advantageous for brief use as they result in less daytime sedation. Although patients develop tolerance to the sedating effects within one or two weeks, tolerance to the anxiolytic effects is uncommon, and patients, once established at a therapeutic dose, do not usually require increases in dose over the period of treatment.

In general, benzodiazepines are avoided or used as an adjunct in the treatment of patients with histories of organic brain syndromes or histories of substance abuse. If stopped abruptly, they may cause a discontinuation syndrome characterized by increased anxiety, sleep disruption, agitation, headache, nausea, and tremor. Rarely, withdrawal seizures may occur. Because discontinuation symptoms tend to be proportional to the duration of administration of the benzodiazepine, the dose, and the rapidity of discontinuation, it is recommended that benzodiazepines be prescribed at the lowest possible effective dose and for the shortest duration needed for symptom relief. Generally, long-term treatment with a benzodiazepine should continue for two weeks past the time of symptom remission, then be tapered and withdrawn. Discontinuation symptoms can be minimized by a slow taper of a 10 percent reduction in dose every two or three days.

Cyclic Antidepressants

Cyclic antidepressants were first found to have efficacy in treating anxiety beyond their antidepressant effects by Klein and Fink (1962), who reported that imipramine treatment reduced the number of panic attacks in patients with panic disorder. Cyclic antidepressants are now commonly used in the treatment of panic disorder (imipramine), GAD (imipramine, others), and obsessive compulsive disorder (OCD) (clomipramine). They are easy to dose (usually once a day) and do not cause serious withdrawal symptoms when discontinued. Issues affecting compliance include the anticholinergic side effects, the delayed onset of anxiolytic action, sedation, and orthostatic hypotension. In general, these side effects are manageable, and if addressed, do not interfere with treatment.

The anticholinergic side effects such as constipation, urinary retention, dry mouth, weight gain, and sexual dysfunction tend to be more often reported as troubling to patients and are a frequent cause of discontinuation of the cyclic antidepressants. Constipation is easily treated by having patients add a stool softener and increase their fluid intake and the amount of fiber consumed in the diet. Urinary hesitancy may respond to a lowering of the dose or the addition of bethanechol. The antihistamine cyproheptadine can be used to treat sexual dysfunction secondary to the cyclic antidepressants. Desipramine, the cyclic antidepressant with the least anticholinergic effects, may be better tolerated by patients who are particularly sensitive to these side effects. Orthostatic hypotension, affecting primarily the elderly, can be managed by careful instruction of the patient to avoid rapid postural changes, and to wear support hose and increase salt and fluid intake. If necessary, a mineralocorticoid or low-dose amphetamine may be added.

Serotonin Reuptake Inhibitors

The SSRIs have gained in popularity in the treatment of anxiety disorders, as controlled clinical trials have established them to be often as effective as the cyclic antidepressants, but with a superior side effect profile. Selective serotonin reuptake inhibitors are currently being used in the treatment of panic disorder, OCD, and social phobia. The advantages of the SSRIs over the cyclic antidepressants are little to no sedation of patients, less weight gain, no orthostasis, and no significant cardiac or anticholinergic effects. They may, however, be activating, causing an agitation and jitteriness that may initially worsen the patient's anxiety symptoms. This effect is best avoided by starting the SSRIs at small doses and increasing them in small increments. Insomnia may be reduced by morning dosing. Sexual side effects (erectile dysfunction, anorgasmia) are a significant cause of discontinuation of the SSRIs. Sexual functioning may improve with a reduction in dosage. Bethanechol, cyproheptadine, and yohimbine have all been used in the treatment of anorgasmia. In addition, yohimbine may also be effective in treating erectile dysfunction. If sexual side effects persist, a change to an alternative medication is indicated.

Noncyclic/Atypical Antidepressants

Among the noncyclic/atypical agents used as anxiolytics are the monoamine oxidase inhibitors (irreversible and reversible), buspirone, fenfluramine, and the beta-blockers. The monoamine oxidase inhibitors (MAOIs) are useful in the treatment of panic disorder and social phobia. Hesitancy among some clinicians to prescribe MAOIs occurs because patients must adhere to a tyramine-free diet to avoid hypertensive crises. When properly instructed, however, most patients find the diet easy to follow. The MAOI phenelzine appears to be slightly more effective than imipramine and both are shown to be significantly more effective than placebo in the treatment of phobic anxiety (Sheehan, Bach, Ballenger, & Jacobsen, 1980). The most commonly encountered side effects of the MAOIs include orthostatic hypotension, urinary retention, weight gain, sexual dysfunction, insomnia, peripheral edema, and weak anticholinergic effects. Orthostatic hypotension should respond to the measures mentioned above for the tricyclic antidepressants. Other side effects may respond to dose adjustment or require discontinuation of the medication. The reversible MAOIs (brofaromine, moclobemide) have the advantage of fewer side effects and less risk of hypertensive crises despite less stringent dietary restrictions. Their selectivity for the MAO-A isoenzyme and ability to bind reversibly make them more user-friendly for both patient and physician.

Buspirone is an anxiolytic unrelated to the benzodiazepines. Its pharmacologic mechanism of action involves enhancing dopaminergic transmission while antagonizing serotonergic and gamma-amino butyric acid (GABA) neurotransmission. It has a short half-life and requires multiple dosing for effective anxiolytic response, which may take up to four weeks. This delay in response is a disadvantage when compared with the benzodiazepines. However, buspirone has the advantage of fewer side effects and no withdrawal syndrome on discontinuation. Its major uses are in GAD and as an augmentation strategy in OCD and social phobia.

The beta adrenergic receptor antagonists (beta-blockers) are useful in treating the autonomic symptoms that often accompany anxiety, such as rapid heart rate, perspiration, tremor, blushing, and chest tightness. The beta-blocker atenolol was found to be effective in the treatment of social phobia (Gorman, Liebowitz, Fyer, Campeas, & Klein, 1985) in an open trial; however, in the controlled trials that followed, beta-blockers have not been found to be better than placebo (Liebowitz et al., 1992). The current most common clinical use of the beta-blockers is in the treatment of performance anxiety.

ANXIETY DISORDERS COMORBID
WITH OTHER ANXIETY DISORDERS

Generalized Anxiety Disorder (GAD)

Generalized anxiety disorder is characterized by persistent excessive anxiety or worry of at least six months' duration, accompanied by increased autonomic activity/sensitivity and hypervigilance. Often chronic, with a waxing and waning course, it may be associated with significant disability and both social and occupational impairment. Many clinicians believe that GAD is underdiagnosed in the presence of other Axis I disorders, as anxiety is often accepted as naturally occurring with many different disorders yet not distinguished as a discrete entity. The most common comorbid conditions with GAD are depression and other anxiety disorders, particularly panic disorder.

Benzodiazepines have been the mainstay of GAD treatment and are well established in terms of efficacy and safety. They provide immediate relief and can be used long term, although discontinuation should be attempted every six months. Dose escalation has not been found to be a problem in anxiety patients receiving benzodiazepines for many years (Pollack et al., 1993; Rickels, Case, Schweizer, Swenson, & Fridman, 1986).

Although the pharmacologic treatment of GAD with comorbid panic disorder has not been systematically studied, clinical experience suggests that a combination of a tricyclic antidepressant and a benzodiazepine are effective. Although a high-potency benzodiazepine alone may give short-term relief of symptoms of both panic disorder and GAD, relapse may be high following discontinuation. Another option is buspirone in combination with a tricyclic or SSRI. Again, the SSRI should be started at the lowest possible dose and increased gradually to avoid exacerbation of anxiety symptoms. Although there are few studies in the literature including long-term follow-up of patients treated with anxiolytics for GAD, a report by Rickels and Schweizer (1990) of 61 chronically anxious GAD patients who received six months of anxiolytic therapy with either clorazepate or buspirone indicated that at 40-month follow-up, relapse rates were as high as 57 percent (clorazepate) and 25 percent (buspirone). As the relapse rate in panic disorder within the first year after initial treatment has been reported as high as 68 percent (Schweizer, Rickels, & Zavodnick, 1988), serious consideration should be given to long-term maintenance therapy in patients with comorbid GAD and panic disorder. Encouraging is a recent study demonstrating that panic patients, after receiving six months of successful tricyclic treatment, were maintained without relapse on half the dose required initially (Mavissakalian & Perel, 1992). This finding suggests that during the initial phase of treatment in patients with comorbid GAD and panic disorder, a combination of a benzodiazepine and tricyclic could be used, with an attempt to taper off the benzodiazepine within the first six months of treatment while continuing the tricyclic at a reduced dose.

Panic Disorder

Comorbidity with other anxiety disorders, depression, and alcoholism is common in panic disorder. Even patients with uncomplicated panic disorder have significantly impaired social and occupational functioning (Markowitz, Weissman, Ouellette, Lish, & Klerman, 1989); however, comorbidity compounds these difficulties and presents further treatment dilemmas. Several classes of pharmacologic agents are used in the treatment of panic, including the heterocyclic antidepressants, the serotonin reuptake inhibitors, the MAOIs, the benzodiazepines, and other less typical agents. More recently, the SSRIs, due to their lower side-effect profile, have become first-line choices in the treatment of panic disorder, along with the more traditional heterocyclic antidepressants, the benzodiazepines, and the MAOIs. A comparative trial between the SSRI fluvoxamine and the heterocyclic maprotiline showed fluvoxamine to be superior in treating the symptoms of panic disorder (den Boer & Westerberg, 1988). One group (Roy-Byrne, Wingerson, Cowley, & Dager, 1993) has concluded that an advantage of the SSRIs over the tricyclics may be their broader efficacy in other Axis I disorders, suggesting that an SSRI may be a good choice for a patient with another comorbid anxiety disorder.

Obsessive Compulsive Disorder (OCD)

The literature supports a significant association between OCD and other anxiety disorders. In a study examining the lifetime prevalence of other anxiety disorders comorbid with OCD, Rasmussen and Eisen (1988) found rates of 28 percent for simple phobia, 26 percent for social phobia, 17 percent for separation anxiety, and 15 percent for panic disorder. Similarly, in a smaller clinical sample of OCD patients, Austin and colleagues (1990) reported rates at time of interview of 19 percent for simple phobias, 14 percent for panic disorder, and 14 percent for social phobia.

The most commonly employed medications in the treatment of uncomplicated OCD, with proven effectiveness in placebo-controlled studies, are clomipramine (Clomipramine Collaborative Study Group, 1991; Thoren, Asberg, Cronholm, Jornestedt, & Traskman, 1980) and the SSRIs fluvoxamine and fluoxetine (Liebowitz et al., 1989; Price, Goodman, Charney, Rasmussen, & Heninger, 1987). Few studies have attempted to examine the pharmacologic effectiveness of these agents in OCD with comorbid anxiety disorders. A portion of the sample in Austin's group (Austin et al., 1990) was treated with clomipramine in doses of a minimum of 100 mg per day for three months. The group reported that those OCD patients with a history of a comorbid anxiety disorder (particularly panic attacks or panic disorder) benefited most from treatment with clomipramine, suggesting that in those OCD patients who are able to tolerate it, clomipramine may be a good choice when panic disorder is comorbid.

In a retrospective study of 12 OCD patients with comorbid social phobia, Carrasco, Hollander, Schneier, and Liebowitz (1992) found that response of social phobic symptoms occurred in parallel with that of OCD symptoms, and that although the number of subjects was small, patients receiving an MAOI responded at a higher rate (80 percent) than those receiving SSRIs (27 percent). The researchers suggest that OCD patients with comorbid social phobia, particularly the generalized subtype, may be less responsive to treatment with SSRIs than uncomplicated OCD patients. In this group of patients, an MAOI might be considered for first-line therapy.

Social Phobia

Rates of comorbidity of social phobia with other anxiety disorders may be higher than for any other anxiety disorder. One study (Van Amerigan, Mancini, Styan, & Donison, 1991) reported that 70 percent of social phobic patients suffered from at least one other anxiety disorder, with 49 percent having comorbid panic disorder, 32 percent comorbid GAD, 19 percent comorbid simple phobia, and 11 percent obsessive compulsive disorder. Among the best investigated of these comorbid conditions is the relationship between social phobia and panic disorder; however, little is available on the pharmacologic treatment of this comorbidity. Rosenbaum and Pollock (1994) recommend that high-potency benzodiazepines be used as first-line treatment in those patients with comorbid social phobia and panic, followed by MAOIs, SSRIs, and the serotonergic tricyclic, clomipramine.

ANXIETY DISORDERS COMORBID
WITH MOOD DISORDERS

Anxiety symptoms commonly complicate mood syndromes, most notably depression. Any anxiety disorder and any affective disorder may be comorbid, or either the anxiety or the mood symptoms may complicate the primary disorder. Some patients may have histories of both anxiety and mood disorders, but these may not occur simultaneously. Most often, however, patients will manifest both mood and anxiety symptoms together. It is important to attempt to establish whether the primary disorder is affective or anxious whenever possible, as this will influence treatment choices. This distinction can best be made by careful review of the nature and temporal occurrence of the symptoms, which may clarify the clinically dominant disorder.

Anxiety Disorders Comorbid with Depression

Depression and anxiety may be among the most commonly comorbid conditions in all of psychiatry. Patients with a primary diagnosis of an anxiety disorder may become secondarily depressed in response to psychosocial limitations resulting from their anxiety. This condition is often seen in patients with panic disorder, social phobia, and GAD. Anxiety symptoms, on the other hand, may be secondary symptoms to the depressive illness but appear more clinically prominent than the mood symptoms. There is significant overlap in symptoms, for instance, in major depression and GAD: psychomotor agitation/restlessness, fatigue, difficulty concentrating, and sleep disturbance.

Whether the depressive disorder is primary or comorbid with an anxiety disorder, the presence of both depressive and anxious symptoms has significance for prognosis, treatment responsiveness, and functioning. Stavrakaky and Vargo (1986) found that anxiety and depression together may represent a distinct syndrome from either depression or anxiety alone. In their extensive review of the literature, they found these mixed depressed/anxious patients to be more chronically ill, with more severe symptoms, and with poorer treatment outcomes than nonanxious depressed patients. Similarly, Murphy (1986) reported data from the Stirling County study assessing 80 percent of depressed and anxious subjects to have poorer treatment outcomes than those with depression alone. Tollefson, Souetre, Thomander, and Potvin (1993) studied 454 French outpatients in a cross-sectional, naturalistic design to assess the effect of three interventions (no treatment, fluoxetine, tricyclic antidepressant) on functional capacity as measured by work attendance. Comorbid anxiety symptoms were found to contribute to higher Hamilton Depression severity scores, which in turn predicted greater work impairment. Comorbid anxiety was not, however, an independent predictor of work recovery.

Generalized Anxiety Disorder (GAD) and Depression

As mentioned above, the symptoms of GAD overlap those of major depression, and therefore distinguishing two distinct diagnoses in patients suspected of comorbidity is a challenge to the clinician. What is apparent is that GAD and major depression frequently co-occur (Sanderson, Beck, & Beck, 1990). The National Institute of Mental Health (NIMH) Epidemiologic Catchment Area study established a 54 percent rate of comorbid depression or panic in patients with GAD. Clayton et al. (1991) reported that patients with a primary diagnosis of major depression with comorbid GAD have longer treatment courses.

Benzodiazepines have long been established in terms of efficacy and safety as first-line medications for GAD. However, they have been found to have limited use in the treatment of depressive syndromes, with the exception of adjunctive treatment of accompanying anxiety and insomnia. What, then, is the role of benzodiazepines in the treatment of GAD with co-occurring depressive symptoms? The literature suggests that the triazolobenzodiazepines—in particular alprazolam—have specific antidepressant effects that can be distinguished from their antianxiety effects (Feighner, Aden, Fabre, Rickels, & Smith, 1983; Rickels, Feighner, & Smith, 1985; Warner, Peabody, Whiteford, & Hollister, 1988). In a study of the effectiveness of alprazolam versus oxazepam in the treatment of GAD, panic, and social phobia patients with associated symptoms of depression, both medications were found to relieve anxiety and depressive symptoms in all three groups; however, alprazolam proved slightly superior in terms of rapidity of onset of anxiolytic action and in reduction in scores on depressive and anxiety scales (Rimon et al., 1991).

Although the supporting data are limited, it makes clinical sense, when choosing among the benzodiazepines for treatment of GAD, to consider a triazolobenzodiazepine first for patients with accompanying depressive symptoms. Other longer-acting benzodiazepines commonly used in uncomplicated GAD, such as diazepam and clonazepam, could possibly exacerbate the depressive symptomatology, resulting in a partial treatment response with a reduction of anxiety but emergence of a fuller depressive syndrome.

A number of studies comparing the efficacy of benzodiazepines versus tricyclic antidepressants in the treatment of GAD have found that the tricyclics have an anxiolytic efficacy equivalent to the benzodiazepines; however, onset of anxiolytic effect is more delayed (Hoehn-Saric, McLeod, & Zimmerli, 1988; Johnstone et al., 1980; Kahn et al., 1986; Rickels, Downing, Schweizer, & Hassman, 1993). Although Rickels and colleagues (1993) excluded patients with co-occurring major depression in their placebo-controlled study of imipramine, trazadone, and diazepam for the treatment of GAD, they found that of the remaining patients, those with high versus low levels of accompanying depressive symptoms did better with the two antidepressants than with diazepam.

These results suggest that a tricyclic antidepressant is an appropriate first-line medication for GAD complicated by depressive symptoms. The main drawback of using a tricyclic alone is the delayed onset of both anxiolytic and antidepressant effects (two to four weeks). Therefore, a combination of a tricyclic antidepressant and a benzodiazepine may be the most clinically effective. The benzodiazepine should be begun at as low a dose as possible and tapered off once the antidepressant and antianxiety effects of the tricyclic are established. The limited data available appear to support the use of one of the triazolobenzodiazepines, although the choice of antidepressant (imipramine, amitriptyline, desipramine, norpramine) may be less critical.

The azapirones (buspirone, gepirone, ipsapirone), but particularly buspirone, have been established as effective treatments for GAD. In a meta-analysis of eight randomized controlled studies of buspirone in 520 GAD patients, 44 percent to 64 percent were found to have significant depressive symptoms (comorbid major depression patients were excluded), and buspirone was found to be superior to placebo in patients with both low and high levels of accompanying depression (Gammans et al., 1992). An interesting finding is that patients with higher levels of depression showed equal or greater improvement compared to those with less intense depressive symptoms. This result is not surprising in light of the body of data supporting the antidepressant effectiveness of the azapirones in major depression (Jenkins et al., 1990; Rausch, Ruegg, & Moeller, 1990; Rickels, Amsterdam, Clary, Puzzuoli, & Schweizer, 1991; Robinson et al., 1990). Buspirone, because of its superior side effect profile and lack of synergistic depressant effect with alcohol, may also be considered an appropriate first-line choice for GAD patients with depressive symptomatology. However, it has the same drawback as the tricyclics in having a delayed onset of action and therefore should probably be reserved for patients unable to tolerate a combination of a tricyclic and a benzodiazepine. Buspirone, however, may be very useful in the case of a patient who is continuing to abuse alcohol during treatment, or is self-escalating the dose of prescribed benzodiazepine. Because buspirone has no direct interactions with the benzodiazepines, it can be safely combined with a benzodiazepine during a cross-taper. For anxiety symptoms alone, the dose range is between 15 and 45 mg per day; however, with comorbid depressive symptoms, the target dose should be increased by 10 to 15 mg per day for the best overall efficacy.

Panic Disorder and Depression

It is estimated that major depression co-occurs with panic disorder in approximately 40 percent to 50 percent of panic patients (Lydiard, 1991). Some researchers have found rates as high as 75 percent to 80 percent for the presence of primary or secondary depression when the patient has a diagnosis of panic disorder (Barlow, Di Nardo, Vermilyea, B., Vermilyea, J., & Blanchard, 1986; Cloninger, Martin, Clayton, & Guze, 1981; Raskin, Peeke, Dierman, & Pinsker, 1982). Epidemiologic community studies, designed to avoid the bias of studying only patients in specialized treatment centers, also confirm that depression occurs at a higher frequency among panic disorder patients than would be expected based on general occurrence of depression alone (Angst & Dobler-Mikola, 1985; Boyd & Weissman, 1981; Weissman & Myers, 1976; Wittchen, Semler, & von Zerrssen, 1985). Rates are sufficiently high for depression to be considered in the assessment of any patient presenting with a complaint of panic symptoms.

Patients may experience the two disorders as a simultaneous illness, or either may precede the other; however, one of the two disorders is usually established as clinically dominant. Clayton et al.'s review of the literature (1991) suggests that up to one third of depressed patients will have recurrent panic attacks, a point to be noted when depression is dominant. Several studies suggest that depressed panic disorder patients may have more severe panic symptoms than panic patients without comorbid depression (Breier, Charney, & Heninger, 1984; Chambless, 1985; Grunhaus, 1988; Stein & Uhde, 1988; Van Valkenburg, Akiskal, Puzantian, & Rosenthal, 1984). They tend to be more socially anxious and socially impaired. It makes intuitive sense that patients with panic may become secondarily depressed as a result of anticipatory anxiety and agoraphobic symptoms, which often lead to severe constrictions in social functioning and lifestyle. However, in reviewing the literature, Clum and Pendry (1987) found that only half the panic disorder patients felt their depression was secondary to the panic, with the other half reporting symptoms consistent with primary depression. Studies attempting to define the symptomatology of secondary depression associated with panic disorder have found that patients have fewer melancholic features and less weight loss, but more somatization and negative feelings of discouragement and hopelessness (Breier, Charney, & Heninger, 1985; Lesser et al., 1989).

What effect, then, does the presence of comorbid depressive symptoms have on the outcome of pharmacological treatment of panic disorder? The literature suggests that treatment outcome may be different based on whether the depression is primary in clinical prominence or secondary to the panic symptoms. For major depression that is comorbid with panic disorder, the literature supports the conclusion that prognosis is worse for pharmacologic treatment outcome than in panic disorder alone, or panic disorder with secondary depressive symptoms (Maddock & Blacker, 1991; Noyes et al., 1990; Pyke & Kraus, 1988; Van Valkenburg et al., 1984). Keller and associates (1993) investigated the effect of comorbid major depression in the treatment of panic disorder in a randomized trial comparing alprazolam, imipramine, and placebo. They reported that both active medications were superior to placebo in treating depression and anxiety symptoms, although they noted that alprazolam's equivalent efficacy to imipramine in treating depressive symptoms has not been established in patients with more severe levels of comorbid depression. In a nonblind, uncontrolled study of the use of fluoxetine in major depression and panic disorder (Louie, Lewis, & Lannon, 1993), patients with concomitant major depression and panic disorder were able to tolerate only low doses of fluoxetine, although many benefited from treatment at these lower doses (< 20 mg per day).

A study by Maddock and colleagues (1993) was designed to help determine whether the worse prognosis of comorbid panic disorder and major depression is due to the co-occurrence of two disorders with broad symptomatology or to another underlying distinct disorder. These researchers studied a group of 180 nondepressed panic disorder patients, 29 percent of whom had a past history of major depression, in a placebo-controlled trial of four weeks of treatment with adinazolam-SR. They found no significant treatment outcome differences for the patients with past histories of primary, secondary, or single episode major depression versus those patients with no history of comorbid depression. In a small number of patients with histories of recurrent major depression, however, treatment outcome was worse and symptomatology was greater. The researchers concluded that a history of recurrent major depression may be associated with a more severe underlying condition in patients with panic disorder, but that non-depressed panic patients with a history of single episode major depression or secondary depression do not have a worse outcome in short-term treatment with adinazolam-SR than those with no history. They suggest that previous studies, which have concluded that patients with comorbid depression and panic disorder have more severe symptomatology and worse treatment outcomes, may simply reflect the effect of the two concurrent disorders, culminating in a broad array of symptoms.

The majority of investigators have reported no significant differences in treatment responsiveness to pharmacotherapy between panic patients who are secondarily depressed and those who are not depressed (Lesser et al., 1988; Maddock & Blacker, 1991; Maier & Buller, 1988; Maier et al., 1991; Nagy, Krystal, Woods, & Charney, 1989; Van Valkenburg et al., 1984). However, Pyke and Krauss (1988) found that panic disorder patients with secondary depression were less responsive to treatment with alprazolam, but patient compliance with medication dosing was not stringently reported. In sum, these studies suggest that the presence of secondary depression may not be a major factor in choice of antipanic medication, and that selection of drug based on side effect profile is most logical.

Recommendations regarding the pharmacologic treatment of concurrent major depression and panic disorder are limited due to the paucity of controlled pharmacologic studies of this group of patients. However, the findings of Keller and colleagues (1993) suggest that either imipramine or alprazolam may be equally effective in panic patients with mild to moderate co-occurring major depression. In such patients, the choice of medication is again best made by side effect profile and consideration of the onset of action of each medication. An alternative to imipramine and alprazolam is one of the SSRIs, which are rapidly becoming the first-line choice.

Unlike the literature on comorbid major depression, there is a growing body of literature on the drug treatment of panic disorder patients with secondary depression that suggests the presence of comorbid depressive symptoms does not necessarily reduce the anxiolytic and antipanic effects of appropriate pharmacotherapy. In this group of patients with comorbid panic disorder and depression, the best studied of the medications with established efficacy include imipramine and alprazolam (Klerman, 1990; Lesser et al., 1988; Maier et al., 1991; Rosenberg, 1967; Van Valkenburg et al., 1984). One study (Keller et al., 1993) suggests that alprazolam may have an advantage of alleviating phobic symptoms earlier than imipramine; however, both medications were equivalent in reducing phobic symptoms at the eight-week end point of the study. Thus, either of these medications is an appropriate choice for patients with a primary diagnosis of panic disorder with comorbid secondary depression. Although we were unable to find any studies in the literature examining the effectiveness of the MAOIs in this patient population, they are established as a class to be independently effective in the treatment of both panic disorder and major depression; consequently, they are an alternative in patients who do not respond to either imipramine or alprazolam.

Obsessive Compulsive Disorder (OCD) and Depression

As with GAD and panic disorder, OCD is frequently complicated by comorbid depression, which often exacerbates obsessive compulsive symptoms and therefore must be addressed for overall symptom improvement. Rasmussen and Tsuang (1986) found the lifetime prevalence of depression in 44 OCD patients to be 80 percent, with 30 percent of patients having a concomitant major depressive episode at the time of the study. Vallejo, Olivares, Marcos, Bulbena, and Menchon (1992) similarly reported a major depression rate of 31 percent among 26 OCD patients studied during a pharmacological trial.

Currently, the most commonly employed medications in the treatment of OCD are also antidepressants (clomipramine, fluoxetine, fluvoxamine). A number of controlled studies have established the antidepressants, but particularly clomipramine, to be effective in the treatment of OCD versus placebo (Insel et al., 1983; Mavissakalian, Turner, Michelson, & Jacob, 1985; Montgomery, 1980; Thoren et al., 1980). In terms of antiobsessional action, clomipramine has been found to be superior to a number of the other heterocyclic antidepressants, including imipramine, desipramine, amitriptyline, and nortriptyline (Ananth, Pecknold, van den Steen, & Engelsmann, 1979; Insel et al., 1983; Thoren et al., 1980; Volavska, Neizoglu, & Yaryura-Tobias, 1985).

The effectiveness of clomipramine in treating depressive symptoms occurring with OCD is less well studied. Katz and deVeaugh-Geiss (1990) conducted two multicenter double-blind trials of clomipramine versus placebo in 192 patients with OCD, subgrouped into no mood disturbance and concomitant depressive symptoms judged to be secondary to OCD; patients with major depression were excluded. The researchers found that in both trials, clomipramine was superior to placebo in reducing obsessions in both the depressed and nondepressed subgroups. They noted, however, that there was only a slight decrease in scores on the Hamilton Rating Scale for Depression (1 to 2 points), indicating only a mild antidepressant effect.

Vallejo and colleagues (1992) studied a group of 30 OCD patients in a 12-week double-blind trial of clomipramine versus phenelzine. They found that patients improved significantly in both groups, with no therapeutic differences between groups. Thirty-one percent of the patients studied met criteria for a major depressive episode at the time of entry into the study. The researchers found that in both treatment groups depressive symptoms improved earlier than obsessive symptoms, but there was no correlation between early improvement in depressive symptoms and later improvement in OCD symptoms. They suggest that MAOI's may be a valid alternative to treatment with clomipramine, although specific response predictors are yet to be defined. This study population, however, had a superior antidepressant response to both clomipramine and phenelzine compared with the OCD patients studied by Katz and DeVeaugh-Geiss (1990).

The serotonin reuptake inhibitors, specifically fluoxetine and fluvoxamine, have more recently been established in several controlled trials as effective in the treatment of OCD. Hollander and others (1991), however, found in studying a small group of OCD patients that rapid increases in the dose of fluoxetine led paradoxically to an increase in depressive symptoms. They suggest that the combination of fluoxetine and a tricyclic may be helpful in relieving depression associated with OCD. As part of another group of researchers, Hollander and associates (1988) previously suggested that both the noradrenergic and serotonergic systems may be involved in OCD. Hence, combining fluoxetine (serotonergic modifier) with a tricyclic (noradrenergic modifier) may mimic the effects of clomipramine, which has potent effects on both systems.

Goodman and colleagues (1990) compared the efficacy of the serotonin reuptake inhibitor fluvoxamine directly to the efficacy of the noradrenergic reuptake inhibitor desipramine in a sample of OCD patients with varying levels of depression. They found that fluvoxamine was superior to desipramine in alleviating obsessive compulsive symptoms and was also superior to desipramine in relieving symptoms of secondary depression. This, however, was less true for the patients with the most severe depressive symptoms, who responded less well to fluvoxamine. These findings again suggest that although both OCD and depressive symptoms may respond to an SSRI alone, improvement is less likely if the depressive symptoms are severe; in this case, the addition of a tricyclic antidepressant may be necessary.

Caution must be used, however, when combining fluoxetine and a tricyclic, as plasma tricyclic levels may quickly increase, causing untoward side effects. Therefore, careful monitoring of side effects and of plasma tricyclic levels should be done, and the clinician should be prepared to adjust the dose of tricyclic downward as necessary.

Posttraumatic Stress Disorder (PTSD) and Depression

Compared to treatment of the other anxiety disorders, treatment of PTSD has been the subject of only a limited number of controlled pharmacologic studies. Those studies that do exist generally support the efficacy of tricyclic antidepressants and MAOIs. Among researchers, there has been debate as to whether these antidepressants affect mainly the associated depressive symptoms or the primary characteristic symptoms of the disorder.

Kosten, Frank, Dan, McDougle, and Giller (1991) entered 60 male veterans with PTSD into an eight-week, randomized trial of phenelzine versus imipramine versus placebo. By five weeks, both imipramine and phenelzine significantly reduced PTSD symptoms, but the improvement with phenelzine was superior and treatment retention was also better than for patients on imipramine. Interestingly, the initially rated mild-to-moderate depressive symptoms did not improve significantly in either group, suggesting that an antidepressant response was not accountable for the effects found. As this study population did not include patients with more severe levels of depression, the conclusions that can be drawn are limited.

At this time, no specific recommendations can be made regarding the treatment of PTSD with comorbid depression. As several classes of antidepressants have been shown effective in the treatment of uncomplicated PTSD, including the tricyclics (Davidson et al., 1990), MAOIs (Frank, Kosten, Giller, & Dan, 1988), and the SSRI fluoxetine (Davidson, Roth, & Newman, 1991), the choice of medication can be made based on side effect profiles.

Social Phobia and Depression

One group of investigators (Stein, Tancer, Gelernter, Vittone, & Uhde, 1990) reported a history of major depression to be present in 35 percent of social phobic patients. As the symptoms of social phobia cross over with the symptoms of atypical/rejection sensitive depression, some investigators feel that an MAOI has the best chance of effectiveness; however, an SSRI may be the most appropriate first-line therapy given the two side effect profiles (Rosenbaum & Pollack, 1994).

Anxiety Disorders Comorbid with Bipolar Disorder

Although a high rate of comorbidity between depression and anxiety has been well established, less is known about the relationship between bipolar disorder and anxiety. It appears, however, that anxiety is significantly less frequently associated with bipolar disorder than with unipolar depression (Donnelly, Murphy, & Goodwin, 1978; Mezzich, Ahn, Fabrega, & Pilkonis, 1990; Schatzberg et al., 1990). Mezzich and associates (1990) found anxiety disorders to co-occur with bipolar disorder at a lower rate in a community-based sample, in contrast to the high rates of anxiety associated with depression, cited earlier.

A study of 81 outpatients with bipolar disorder (Young, Cooke, Robb, Levitt, & Joffe, 1993), subdivided into low versus high anxiety symptom scores reported that 22 percent of the bipolar patients fell into the high anxiety category. These patients had higher rates of comorbidity, most notably higher rates of suicidal behavior and alcohol abuse. Of interest in terms of treatment responsiveness, the high anxiety-rated bipolar patients had a trend as a group toward lithium nonresponsiveness. When patients were divided on the basis of a concomitant diagnosis of GAD or panic disorder, differences in terms of morbidity and treatment responsiveness were not found. The authors concluded that anxiety symptoms, rather than an anxiety diagnosis per se, appear to predict morbidity and treatment responsiveness. The findings of Young's group suggest that measures of anxiety in bipolar disorder patients may be important to consider in directing treatment. Bipolar disorder patients with significant anxiety symptoms may require a lower threshold for hospitalization due to suicide risk. Although all bipolar patients should be continually assessed for alcohol abuse, those with high levels of anxiety may require additional monitoring and structured treatment programs to stop drinking. However, it is often difficult to make a diagnosis of GAD or other anxiety disorder in a patient who is drinking, as the symptoms may abate or exacerbate when the patient stops drinking. It is best to avoid benzodiazepines in this population as the patients may abuse them. If an adjunctive medication is necessary to control anxiety symptoms, in addition to the mood stabilizer, a low dose antipsychotic or buspirone may be effective without leading to potential abuse.

ANXIETY DISORDERS COMORBID WITH PERSONALITY DISORDERS

The literature suggests that comorbid personality disorders may have a negative effect on treatment response for a wide range of Axis I psychiatric disorders. Most of these data have resulted from studies comparing the effects of personality disorders on the outcome of treatments for depression. Only a limited number of studies have examined the role of personality in the treatment outcomes of anxiety disorders. Clinicians often associate the anxiety disorders with the Cluster C personality disorders, often referred to as the anxious cluster: dependent, avoidant, and obsessive compulsive. The distinction between an Axis I anxiety disorder and an anxious cluster, Axis II personality disorder may not always be clear-cut. However, the anxiety disorders are distinguished as being discrete or episodic illnesses as opposed to the personality disorders, characterized by persistent patterns of behavior and thinking that are maladaptive and inflexible.

The investigation of the co-occurrence of personality disorders with the anxiety disorders has focused primarily on panic disorder, social phobia, and OCD. Because of the sparse data on GAD, PTSD, and specific phobia comorbid with personality disorders, those disorders are not discussed here.

Panic Disorder

The literature on panic disorder comorbid with personality disorders has yielded a variety of results. The majority of studies support the concept that the Cluster C personality disorders are more prevalent in patients with panic disorder; however, all the other personality disorders have also been found, in smaller numbers to be comorbid with panic.

The majority of studies looking at the prevalence rates of personality disorders comorbid with panic disorder have found the rate of any comorbid personality disorder to be approximately 40 percent to 60 percent (Black, Wesner, Gabel, Bowers, & Monahan, 1994; Friedman, Shear, & Frances, 1987; Green & Curtis, 1988; Mavissakalian & Hamann, 1987; Reich, 1988, 1990; Reich & Noyes, 1987; Zimmerman & Coryell, 1989). The most commonly encountered personality disorders corresponded to the Cluster C anxious group. However, Zimmerman and Coryell (1989) found schizotypal, borderline and antisocial personality disorder to be most prevalent in a group of 24 panic and 74 phobic patients. Reich (1990) found schizotypal, histrionic, borderline, dependent, and avoidant personality disorders to be most common among 28 panic disorder patients. In summary, these studies suggest that among panic disorder patients having a comorbid personality disorder, the anxious cluster personality disorders are most typically encountered, with the odd cluster (paranoid, schizoid, schizotypal) being the least common. Antisocial personality disorder was found to coexist with 4.6 percent of panic disorder patients and 1.7 percent of agoraphobics in the Epidemiologic Catchment Area study. This percentage is consistent with the comorbid rate of antisocial personality disorder with other psychiatric conditions. However, it is worth the clinician's effort to probe for the coexistence of anxiety and antisocial personality disorder, as at least one report has found the comorbidity to increase the patient's risk for suicide (Weiss, Davis, Hedlund, & Cho, 1983).

Few studies have examined the prognostic significance of the co-occurrence of panic disorder and personality disorder and its effect on treatment outcome. In those that have, the coexistence of a personality disorder has uniformly been a negative predictor of outcome in both short-term studies (Black, Wesner, Gabel, Bowers, & Monahan, 1994; Green & Curtis, 1988; Reich, 1988) and long-term studies (Mavissakalian & Hamann, 1987; Noyes et al., 1990).

In a study of 66 patients with panic disorder receiving either fluvoxamine, cognitive therapy, or placebo (Black et al., 1994), the presence of any Axis II personality disorder was a significant predictor of negative outcome. This was particularly true of the cognitive treatment group, but was not an important predictor of outcome in the fluvoxamine-treated group. This finding suggests that panic disorder patients with comorbid personality disorders may do better if pharmacotherapy is the primary mode of treatment employed.

Reich (1988) studied 52 patients in a placebo-controlled tricyclic trial, and found that only the presence of a personality disorder in the dramatic cluster (histrionic, narcissistic, antisocial, or borderline) predicted a negative outcome. Green and Curtis (1988) used pharmacotherapy to treat 25 panic disorder patients with and without comorbid personality disorders. They found that both groups responded similarly to treatment, but that those patients with comorbid personality disorders relapsed at a higher rate following treatment.

Mavissakalian and Hamann (1987) enrolled 33 agoraphobic patients in a 16-week trial of combined medication and behavioral therapy. They found that patients with greater numbers of pathologic personality traits were significantly less treatment responsive.

In summary, these few studies overall have found that the co-occurrence of a personality disorder is a negative predictor of outcome. Therefore the question should be raised, does treatment of panic disorder in patients with comorbid personality disorders result in any effective change in personality traits?

Green and Curtis (1988) found that pharmacologic treatment of the panic disorder did not effect any change in personality. Contrarily, Mavissakalian and Hamann (1987) found that successful treatment of agoraphobic patients with combined pharmacologic and behavioral therapy resulted in a reduction of the frequency of personality disorders. Several groups (Green & Curtis, 1988; Mavissakalian & Hamann, 1987) have found the degree of social avoidance present to be associated with poor treatment outcome.

In summary, considering and defining the presence of comorbid personality disorders in patients with panic disorder may aid clinicians in targeting treatment to improve overall patient outcome, although it is unlikely that significant changes in character traits will be achieved. Special treatment considerations should include targeting interventions for social avoidance and impairment as well as suicide prevention in patients with antisocial personality disorder. The data of Black's group (1994) suggest that patients with significant character pathology have higher dropout rates and may be particularly ill-suited to primary trials of cognitive therapy.

Social Phobia

Clinicians continue to have difficulty drawing lines between social phobia and avoidant personality disorder. The *DSM-IV* defines social phobia as "a marked and persistent fear of one or more social or performance situations in which a person is exposed to unfamiliar people or to possible scrutiny by others" (p. 411). The feared situation almost invariably provokes anxiety, the anxiety is felt to be excessive, and the individual fears that he or she will act in a humiliating or embarrassing way. To be differentiated, avoidant personality disorder is defined as "a pervasive pattern of social inhibition, feelings of inadequacy and hypersensitivity to negative evaluation" (p. 662). The *DSM-IV* stresses that this pattern is present in a variety of situations and contexts and that a key component is the fear of criticism, disapproval, or rejection. This is in contrast to social phobia, which tends to be more situationally bound and to have the fear of humiliation, rather than rejection, as primary.

Several small studies looking at the prevalence rates of personality disorders in social phobic patients have found significant rates of comorbidity. Reich, Noyes, and Yates (1989) found that 7 out of 14 social phobics studied had coexistent dependent personality disorder. Of 14 social phobics studied by Turner (1987) with the Minnesota Multiphasic Personality Inventory (MMPI), 7 met criteria for a personality disorder, with schizotypal and avoidant being the most common. When Alnaes and Torgersen (1988) studied 10 social phobics with the SIDP, all met criteria for dependent personality disorder, with nine of 10 meeting criteria for avoidant personality disorder.

What, then, is the role of pharmacologic treatment in effecting change in personality traits in social phobics? The MAOIs, established to be effective in the treatment of social phobia, may effect positive change in avoidant and dependent traits by improving interpersonal sensitivity, as suggested by Liebowitz and colleagues (1988). Whether this change will persist after discontinuation of medication or whether other psychotherapeutic interventions must be made concurrently to maintain improvement needs to be investigated. Reich, Noyes, and Yates (1989) found that although 14 social phobics with avoidant personality traits improved with open treatment with alprazolam, the majority of traits had recurred at follow-up. As with Black's panic disorder patients (Black et al., 1994), Turner (1987) found that social phobics with comorbid personality disorders responded less well to cognitive therapy than those without comorbid personality disorders, and that this result held at one year follow-up. The poor response rate may be an indicator of higher levels of pathology and symptomatology in patients with comorbid personality disorders.

Overall, there are fewer data to confirm the negative predictive value of a comorbid personality disorder in social phobia than in panic disorder. However, these early studies suggest that Cluster C personality disorders are again the most commonly encountered personality disorders in patients with social phobia.

Obsessive Compulsive Disorder (OCD)

Similar to what would appear to be a logical association between social phobia and avoidant personality disorder, many early studies of OCD suggested an association with obsessive compulsive personality disorder (Alnaes & Torgersen, 1988; Rasmussen & Tsuang, 1986; Rosenberg, 1967). However, more recent studies have not found obsessive compulsive personality disorder to be as prominently correlated with OCD as previously thought. Interestingly, OCD patients tend to have personality profiles more similar to panic patients, with greater frequencies of Cluster C traits (Black, Yates, Noyes, Pfohl, & Kelley, 1989; Joffe, Swinson, & Regan, 1988; Mavissakalian, Hamann, & Jones, 1990), and Cluster A traits being least typical, but reported. Mavissakalian and others (1990) compared OCD and panic disorder patients in terms of prevalence and degree of severity of co-morbid personality disorders and found that OCD patients had greater numbers of personality disorder traits than panic/agoraphobic patients, although the distribution among clusters was similar.

These studies in sum suggest that the prevalence of pathologic personality traits among OCD patients is quite high, reported in 50 to 80 percent (Baer et al., 1990; Joffe, Swinson, & Regan, 1988), and that multiple co-occurrent personality disorders are common. However, the data refute the common perception that obsessive compulsive disorder symptoms predict obsessive compulsive personality disorder. In fact, Mavissakalian and colleagues (1990) found that the best predictor of personality disorder in OCD patients was dysphoric mood.

As the co-occurrence of one or more personality disorders in OCD patients is quite common, it is important to examine what is known about the predictive outcome of treatment in these cases. Unfortunately, only three studies have examined the role of personality disorder in outcome of OCD treatment, one being a retrospective chart review.

Mavissakalian and others (1990) studied 27 OCD patients who were entered into a 12-week pharmacologic trial with clomipramine. Fifty-six percent of the patients were found to have at least one personality disorder prior to treatment, with the most common diagnoses being avoidant, histrionic, and dependent. Personality functioning improved posttreatment, with a reduction to 37 percent of patients meeting criteria for one or more personality disorder. The largest changes in personality traits with treatment were among the Cluster C group, especially the avoidant group, in whom there was a decrease from 30 percent to 11 percent. Unexpectedly, this study did not find personality measures significantly correlated with treatment outcome.

This is in contrast to a larger, multicenter prospective trial by Baer and others (1992) in which the presence of multiple personality disorders was a strong predictor of negative outcome after 12 weeks of treatment with clomipramine. Baer found that the severity of OCD symptoms correlated with the number of personality diagnoses assigned. The presence of schizotypal, borderline, or avoidant personality disorder was a poor predictor of outcome, and having any Cluster A personality disorder also correlated with poor outcome.

In a retrospective chart review of 43 OCD outpatients, Jenike, Baer, Minichiello, Schwartz, and Carey (1986) reported a 33 percent prevalence rate of schizotypal personality disorder, which was a negative predictor of treatment outcome. This study is difficult to interpret as standardized personality measures were either not employed or not reported, and the prevalence of other Axis II personality disorders in the sample was not noted.

Because of the scarcity of data currently available, no specific treatment recommendations can be made regarding the treatment of patients with OCD and comorbid personality disorders; however, the clinician should be aware of the high prevalence rate of co-occurring personality disorder in this population. Whether this high prevalence represents a confounding of Axis I and Axis II is yet to be established, but the possibility that the severity of OCD symptoms may contribute to the greater number of personality disorder diagnoses must be considered.

In summary, these findings indicate that a significant number of patients seeking treatment for anxiety disorders will have a comorbid personality disorder that will most likely negatively influence their treatment outcome. Target-specific treatment plans, taking into consideration co-occurring personality disorders, have the best chance of success, with some data supporting the idea that personality traits can be positively modified by appropriate pharmacologic treatment of the Axis I anxiety disorder.

REFERENCES

Alnaes, R., & Torgersen, S. (1988). The relationship between *DSM-III* symptom disorders (Axis I) and personality disorders (Axis II) in an outpatient population. *Acta Psychiatrica Scandinavica, 8,* 485–492.

Ananth, J., Pecknold, J., van den Steen, N., & Engelsmann, F. (1979). Double-blind comparative study of chlorimipramine in obsessive neurosis. *Current Therapeutic Research, 25,* 703–709.

Angst, J., & Dobler-Mikola, A. (1985). The Zurich study V: Anxiety and phobia in young adults. *European Archives of Psychiatry and Neurological Sciences, 235,* 171–178.

Austin, L.S., Lydiard, R.B., Fossey, M.D., Zealberg, J.J., Laraia, M.T., & Ballenger, J.C. (1990). Panic and phobic disorders in patients with obsessive compulsive disorder. *Journal of Clinical Psychiatry, 51,* 456–458.

Baer, L.D., Jenike, M.A., Black, D.W., Treece, C., Rosenfeld, R., & Greist, J. (1992). Effect of Axis II diagnoses on treatment outcome with clomipramine in 55 patients with obsessive compulsive disorder. *Archives of General Psychiatry, 49,* 862–866.

Baer, L., Jenike, M.A., Ricciardi, J.N., Holland, A.D., Seymour, R.J., Minichiello, W.E., & Buttolph, M.L. (1990). Standardized assessment of personality disorders in obsessive-compulsive disorder. *Archives of General Psychiatry, 47,* 826–830.

Barlow, D.H., Di Nardo, P.A., Vermilyea, B.B., Vermilyea, J., & Blanchard, E.B. (1986). Comorbidity and depression among the anxiety disorders: Issues in diagnosis and classification. *Journal of Nervous and Mental Disease, 174,* 63–72.

Black, D.W., Wesner, R.B., Gabel, J., Bowers, W., & Monahan, P. (1994). Predictors of short-term treatment response in 66 patients with panic disorder. *Journal of Affective Disorders, 30,* 233–241.

Black, D.W., Yates, W.R., Noyes, R., Pfohl, B., & Kelley, M. (1989). *DSM-III* personality disorder in obsessive compulsive study volunteers: a controlled study. *Journal of Personality Disorders, 3,* 58–62.

Boyd, J.H., & Weissman, M.M. (1981). Epidemiology of affective disorders. *Archives of General Psychiatry, 38,* 1039–1046.

Breier, A., Charney, D.S., & Heninger, G.R. (1984). Major depression in patients with agoraphobia and panic disorder. *Archives of General Psychiatry, 41,* 1129–1135.

Breier, A., Charney, D.S., & Heninger, G.R. (1985). The diagnostic validity of anxiety disorders and their relationship to depressive illness. *American Journal of Psychiatry, 142,* 787–797.

Carrasco, J.L., Hollander, E., Schneier, F.R., & Liebowitz, M.R. (1992). Treatment outcome of obsessive compulsive disorder with comorbid social phobia. *Journal of Clinical Psychiatry, 53,* 387–391.

Chambless, D.L. (1985). The relationship of severity of agoraphobia to associated psychopathology. *Behavior Research and Therapy, 23,* 305–310.

Clayton, P.J., Grove, W.M., Coryell, W., Keller, M., Hirschfeld, R., & Fawcett, J. (1991). Follow-up and family study of anxious depression. *American Journal of Psychiatry, 148,* 1512–1517.

Clomipramine Collaborative Study Group. (1991). Clomipramine in the treatment of patients with obsessive-compulsive disorder. *Archives of General Psychiatry, 37,* 1281–1285.

Cloninger, C.R., Martin, R.L., Clayton, P., & Guze, S.B. (1981). *A blind follow-up and family study of anxiety neurosis: Preliminary analysis concepts.* New York: Raven Press.

Clum, G.A., & Pendry, D. (1987). Depression symptomatology as a nonrequisite for successful treatment of panic with antidepressant medications. *Journal of Anxiety Disorders, 1*(4), 337–344.

Davidson, J.R.T., Kudler, H., Smith, R., Mahorney, S.L., Lipper, S., Hammett, E., Saunder, W.B., & Cavenar, J.O., Jr. (1990). Treatment of posttraumatic stress disorder with amitriptyline and placebo. *Archives of General Psychiatry, 47,* 259–266.

Davidson, J.R.T., Roth, S., & Newman, E. (1991). Fluoxetine in posttraumatic stress disorder. *Journal of Traumatic Stress, 4,* 419–423.

den Boer, J.A., & Westerberg, G.M. (1988). Effect of serotonin and noradrenaline uptake inhibitor in panic disorder: A double-blind comparative study with fluvoxamine and maprotiline. *Informational Clinical Psychopharmacology, 3,* 59–74.

Donnelly, E.F., Murphy, D.L., & Goodwin, F.K. (1978). Primary affective disorder: anxiety in unipolar and bipolar depressed groups. *Journal of Clinical Psychology, 34,* 621–623.

Feighner, J.P., Aden, G.C., Fabre, L.F., Rickels, K., & Smith, W.T. (1983). Comparison of alprazolam, imipramine, and placebo in the treatment of depression. *Journal of the American Medical Association, 249,* 3057–3064.

Frank, J.B., Kosten, T.R., Giller, E.L., Jr., & Dan, E. (1988). A randomized clinical trial of phenelzine and imipramine for posttraumatic stress disorder. *American Journal of Psychiatry, 145,* 1289–1291.

Friedman, C.J., Shear, M.K., & Frances, A. (1987). *DSM-III* personality disorders in panic patients. *Journal of Personality Disorders, 1,* 132–135.

Gammans, R.E., Stringfellow, J.C., Hvizdos, A.J., Seidehamel, R.J., Cohn, J.B., Wilcox, C.S., Fabre, L.F., Pecknold, J.C., Smith, W.T., & Rickels, K. (1992). Use of buspirone in patients with generalized anxiety disorder and coexisting depressive symptoms. *Neuropsychobiology, 25,* 193–201.

Goodman, W.K., Price, L.H., Delgado, P.L., Palumbo, J., Krystal, J.H., Nagy, L.M., Rasmussen, S.A., Heninger, G.R., & Charney, D.S. (1990). Specificity of serotonin reuptake inhibitors in the treatment of obsessive-compulsive disorder. *Archives of General Psychiatry, 47,* 577–585.

Gorman, J.M., Liebowitz, M.R., Fyer, A.J., Campeas, R., & Klein, D.F. (1985). Treatment of social phobia with atenolol. *Journal of Clinical Psychopharmacology, 5,* 298–301.

Green, M.A., & Curtis, C.G. (1988). Personality disorders in panic patients: Response to termination of antipanic medication. *Journal of Personality Disorders, 2,* 303–314.

Grunhaus, L. (1988). Clinical and psychobiological characteristics of simultaneous panic disorder and major depression. *American Journal of Psychiatry, 145,* 1214–1221.

Hoehn-Saric, R., McLeod, D.R., & Zimmerli, W.D. (1988). Differential effects of alprazolam and imipramine in generalized anxiety disorder: Somatic versus psychic symptoms. *Journal of Clinical Psychiatry, 49,* 293–301.

Hollander, E., Fay, M., Cohen, B., Campeas, R., Gorman, J.M., & Liebowitz, M.R. (1988). Serotonergic and noradrenergic sensitivity in obsessive-compulsive disorder: Behavioral findings. *American Journal of Psychiatry, 145,* 1015–1017.

Hollander, E., Mullen, L., DeCaria, C.M., Skodol, A., Schneier, F.R., Liebowitz, M.R., & Klein, D.F. (1991). Obsessive compulsive disorder, depression, and fluoxetine. *Journal of Clinical Psychiatry, 52,* 418–422.

Insel, T.R., Murphy, D.L., Cohen, R.M., Alterman, I., Kilts, C., & Linnoila, M. (1983). Obsessive-compulsive disorder. A double-blind trial of clomipramine and clorgyline. *Archives of General Psychiatry, 40,* 605–612.

Jenike, M.A., Baer, L., Minichiello, W.E., Schwartz, C.E., & Carey, R.J. (1986). Concomitant obsessive-compulsive disorder and schizotypal personality disorder. *American Journal of Psychiatry, 143,* 530–532.

Jenkins, S.W., Robinson, D.S., Fabre, L.F., Jr., Andary, J.J., Messina, M.E., & Reich, L.A. (1990). Gepirone in the treatment of major depression. *Journal of Clinical Psychopharmacology, 10*(3, suppl.), 77–85.

Joffe, R.T., Swinson, R.P., & Regan, J.J. (1988). Personality feature of obsessive-compulsive disorder. *American Journal of Psychiatry, 145,* 1127–1129.

Johnstone, E.C., Owens, D.G., Frith, C.D., McPherson, K., Dowie, C., Riley, G., & Gold, A. (1980). Neurotic illness and its response to anxiolytic and antidepressant treatment. *Psychological Medicine, 10,* 321–328.

Kahn, R.J., McNair, D.M., Lipman, R.S., Covi, L., Rickels, K., Downing, R., Fischer, S., & Frankenthaler, L.M. (1986). Imipramine and chlordiazepoxide in depressive and anxiety disorders, II: Efficacy in anxious outpatients. *Archives of General Psychiatry, 43,* 79–85.

Katz, R.J., & deVeaugh-Geiss, J. (1990). The antiobsessional effects of clomipramine do not require concomitant affective disorder. *Psychiatry Research, 31,* 121–129.

Keller, M.B., Lavori, P.W., Goldenberg, I.M., Baker, L.A., Pollack, M.H., Sachs, G.S., Rosenbaum, J.F., Deltito, J.A., Leon, A., Shear, K., & Klerman, G.L. (1993). Influence of depression on the treatment of panic disorder with imipramine, alprazolam and placebo. *Journal of Affective Disorders, 28,* 27–38.

Klein, D.F., & Fink, M. (1962). Psychiatric reaction patterns to imipramine. *American Journal of Psychiatry, 119,* 432–438.

Klerman, G.L. (1990). Approaches to the phenomena of comorbidity. In J.D. Maser & C.R. Cloninger (Eds.), *Comorbidity of mood and anxiety disorders* (pp. 13–37). Washington, DC: American Psychiatric Press.

Kosten, T.R., Frank, J.B., Dan, E., McDougle, C.G., & Giller, E.L., Jr. (1991). Pharmacotherapy for posttraumatic stress disorder using phenelzine or imipramine. *Journal of Nervous and Mental Disease, 179*(66), 366–370.

Lesser, I.M., Rubin, R.T., Pecknold, J.C., Rifkin, A., Swinson, R.P., Lydiard, R.B., Burrows, G.D., Noyes, R., & DuPont, R.L. (1988). Secondary depression in panic disorder and agoraphobia. I. Frequency, severity, and response to treatment. *Archives of General Psychiatry, 45,* 437–443.

Lesser, I.M., Rubin, R.T., Rifkin, A., Swinson, R.P., Lydiard, R.B., & Burrows, G.D. (1989). Secondary depression in panic disorder and agoraphobia. II. Dimensions of depressive symptomatology and their response to treatment. *Journal of Affective Disorders, 16,* 49–58.

Liebowitz, M.R., Gorman, J.M., Fyer, A., Campeas, R., Papp, L.A., & Goetz, D. (1988). Pharmacotherapy of social phobia: a placebo controlled comparison of phenelzine and atenolol. *Journal of Clinical Psychiatry, 49,* 252–258.

Liebowitz, M.R., Hollander, E., Schneier, F., Campeas, R., Hatterer, J., Papp, L., Fairbanks, J., Sandberg, D., Davies, S., & Stein, M. (1989). Fluoxetine treatment of obsessive-compulsive disorder: An open clinical trial. *Journal of Clinical Psychopharmacology, 9,* 423–427.

Liebowitz, M.R., Schneier, F., Campeas, R., Hollander, E., Hatterer, J., Fyer, A., Gorman, J., Papp, L., Davies, S., Gully, R., & Klein, D.F. (1992). Phenelzine vs atenolol in social phobia: A placebo-controlled comparison. *Archives of General Psychiatry, 49,* 290–300.

Louie, A.K., Lewis, T.B., & Lannon, R.A. (1993). Use of low-dose fluoxetine in major depression and panic disorder. *Journal of Clinical Psychiatry, 54*(11), 435–438.

Lydiard, R.B. (1991). Coexisting depression and anxiety: Special diagnostic and treatment issues. *Journal of Clinical Psychiatry, 52*(6), 48–54.

Maddock, R.J., & Blacker, K.H. (1991). Response to treatment in panic disorder with associated depression. *Psychopathology, 24,* 1–6.

Maddock, R.J., Carter, C.S., Blacker, K.H., Beitman, B.D., Krishnan, K.R.R., Jefferson, J.W., Lewis, C.P., & Liebowitz, M.R. (1993). Relationship of past depressive episodes to symptom severity and treatment response in panic disorder with agoraphobia. *Journal of Clinical Psychiatry, 54,* 88–95.

Maier, W., & Buller, R. (1988). One-year follow-up of panic disorder: Outcome and prognostic factors. *European Archives of Psychiatry and Neurological Sciences, 238,* 105–109.

Maier, W., Rosenberg, R., Argyle, N., Buller, R., Roth, M., Brandon, S., & Benkert, O. (1991). Subtyping panic disorder by major depression and avoidance behaviour and the response to active treatment. *European Archives of Psychiatry and Clinical Neuroscience, 241,* 22–30.

Markowitz, J., Weissman, M.M., Ouellette, R., Lish, J.D., & Klerman, G.L. (1989). Quality of life in panic disorder. *Archives of General Psychiatry, 46,* 984–992.

Mavissakalian, M., & Hamann, M.S. (1987). *DSM-III* personality disorders in agoraphobia II: Changes with treatment. *Comprehensive Psychiatry, 28,* 356–361.

Mavissakalian, M., Hamann, M.S., & Jones, B. (1990). A comparison of *DSM-III* personality disorders in panic/agoraphobia and obsessive-compulsive disorder. *Comprehensive Psychiatry, 31,* 238–244.

Mavissakalian, M., & Perel, J.M. (1992). Clinical experiments in maintenance and discontinuation of imipramine therapy in panic disorder with agoraphobia. *Archives of General Psychiatry, 49,* 318–323.

Mavissakalian, M., Turner, S., Michelson, L., & Jacob, R. (1985). Tricyclic antidepressants in obsessive-compulsive disorder: antiobsessional or antidepressant agents? II. *American Journal of Psychiatry, 142,* 572–576.

Mezzich, J.C., Ahn, C.W., Fabrega, H., & Pilkonis, P.A. (1990). Patterns of psychiatric comorbidity in a large population presenting for care. In J.D. Maser & C.R. Cloninger (Eds.), *Comorbidity of mood and anxiety disorders* (pp. 189–204). Washington, DC: American Psychiatric Press.

Montgomery, S.A. (1980). Clomipramine in obsessional neurosis: A placebo controlled trial. *Pharmaceutical Medicine, 1,* 189–192.

Murphy, J.E. (1986). Diagnosis screening and demoralization: Epidemiologic implications. *Psychiatric Developments, 2,* 101–133.

Nagy, L.M., Krystal, J.H., Woods, S.W., & Charney, D.S. (1989). Clinical and medication outcome after short-term alprazolam and behavioral group treatment in panic disorder: 2.5-year naturalistic follow-up study. *Archives of General Psychiatry, 46,* 993–999.

Noyes, R., Jr., Reich, J., Christiansen, J., Suelzer, M., Pfohl, B., & Coryell, W. (1990). Outcome of panic disorder: Relationship to diagnostic subtypes and comorbidity. *Archives of General Psychiatry, 47,* 809–818.

Pollack, M.H., Otto, M.W., Tesar, G.E., Cohen, L.S., Meltzer-Brody, S., & Rosenbaum, J.F. (1993). Long-term outcome after acute treatment with alprazolam or clonazepam for panic disorder. *Journal of Clinical Psychopharmacology, 13*(4), 257–263.

Price, L.H., Goodman, W.K., Charney, D.S., Rasmussen, S.A., & Heninger, G.R. (1987). Treatment of severe obsessive-compulsive disorder with fluvoxamine. *American Journal of Psychiatry, 144,* 1059–1061.

Pyke, R.E., & Kraus, M. (1988). Alprazolam in the treatment of panic attack patients with and without major depression. *Journal of Clinical Psychiatry, 49,* 66–68.

Raskin, M., Peeke, V.S., Dierman, W., & Pinsker, H. (1982). Panic and generalized anxiety disorders. *Archives of General Psychiatry, 39,* 687–689.

Rasmussen, S.A., & Eisen, J.L. (1988). Clinical and epidemiologic findings of significance to neuropharmacological trials in OCD. *Psychopharmacology Bulletin, 24,* 466–467.

Rasmussen, S.A., & Tsuang, M.T. (1986). *DSM-III* obsessive-compulsive disorder: Clinical characteristics and family history. *American Journal of Psychiatry, 143,* 317–322.

Rausch, J.L., Ruegg, R., & Moeller, F.G. (1990). Gepirone as a 5-HT agonist in the treatment of major depression. *Psychopharmacology Bulletin, 26,* 169–171.

Reich, J.H. (1988). *DSM-III* personality disorders and the outcome of treated panic disorder. *American Journal of Psychiatry, 145,* 1149–1152.

Reich, J.H. (1990). The effect of personality on placebo response in panic patients. *Journal of Nervous and Mental Disease, 178,* 699–702.

Reich, J.H., & Noyes, R. (1987). A comparison of *DSM-III* personality disorders in acutely ill panic and depressed patients. *Journal of Anxiety Disorders, 1,* 123–131.

Reich, J.H., Noyes, R., & Yates, W. (1989). Alprazolam treatment of avoidant personality traits in social phobic patients. *Journal of Clinical Psychiatry, 50,* 91–95.

Rickels, K., Amsterdam, J.D., Clary, C., Puzzuoli, G., & Schweizer, E. (1991). Buspirone in major depression: a controlled study. *Journal of Clinical Psychiatry, 52,* 34–38.

Rickels, K., Case, G.W., Schweizer, E.E., Swenson, C., & Fridman, R.B. (1986). Low-dose dependence in chronic benzodiazepine users: A preliminary report on 119 patients. *Psychopharmacology Bulletin, 22,* 407–415.

Rickels, K., Downing, R., Schweizer, E., & Hassman, H. (1993). Antidepressants for the treatment of generalized anxiety disorder: A placebo-controlled comparison of imipramine, trazodone, and diazepam. *Archives of General Psychiatry, 50,* 884–895.

Rickels, K., Feighner, J.P., & Smith, W.T. (1985). Alprazolam, amitriptyline, doxepin, and placebo in the treatment of depression. *Archives of General Psychiatry, 42,* 134–141.

Rickels, K., & Schweizer, E. (1990). The clinical course and long-term management of generalized anxiety disorder. *Journal of Clinical Psychopharmacology, 10*(3, suppl.), 101–110.

Rimon, R., Kultalahti, E.R., Kalli, A., Koskinen, T., Lepola, U., Naarala, M., & Tick, E. (1991). Alprazolam and oxazepam in the treatment of anxious outpatients with depressive symptoms: A double-blind multicenter study. *Pharmacopsychiatry, 24,* 81–84.

Robinson, D.S., Rickels, K., Feighner, J., Fabre, L.F., Jr., Gammans, R.C., Shrotriya, R.C., Alms, D.R., Andary, J.J., & Messina, M.E. (1990). Clinical effects of the 5-HT partial agonists in depression: A composite analysis of buspirone in the treatment of depression. *Journal of Clinical Psychopharmacology, 10*(3, suppl.), 67–76.

Rosenbaum, J.F., & Pollock, R.A. (1994). The psychopharmacology of social phobia and comorbid disorders. *Bulletin of the Menninger Clinic, 58*(2, suppl.), 67–83.

Rosenberg, C.M. (1967). Familial aspects of obsessional neurosis. *British Journal of Psychiatry, 19,* 240–253.

Rosenberg, R., Bech, P., Mellergard, M., & Ottosson, J.-O. (1991). Secondary depression in panic disorder: An indicator of severity with a weak effect on outcome in alprazolam and imipramine treatment. *Acta Psychiatrica Scandinavica, 365* (suppl.), 39–45.

Roy-Byrne, P., Wingerson, D., Cowley, D., & Dager, S. (1993). Psychopharmacologic treatment of panic, generalized anxiety disorder, and social phobia. *Psychiatric Clinics of North America, 16*(4), 719–735.

Sanderson, W.C., Beck, A.T., & Beck, J. (1990). Syndrome comorbidity in patients with major depression or dysthymia: Prevalence in temporal relationships. *American Journal of Psychiatry, 147,* 1025–1028.

Schatzberg, A.F., Samson, J.A., Rothschild, A.J., Luciana, M.M., Bruno, R.F., & Bond, T.C. (1990). Depression secondary to anxiety: Findings from the McLean Hospital Research Facility. *Psychological Clinics of North America, 13,* 633–649.

Schweizer, E., Rickels, K., & Zavodnick, S. (1988, August). *Clinical and medication status at one-year follow-up after maintenance treatment of panic disorder.* Paper presented at Collegium Internationale Neuro-Psychopharmacologicum Congress.

Sheehan, D., Bach, M.B., Ballenger, J., & Jacobsen, G. (1980). Treatment of endogenous anxiety with phobic, hysterical, and hypochondriacal symptoms. *Archives of General Psychiatry, 37,* 51–59.

Stavrakaky, C., & Vargo, B. (1986). The relationship of anxiety and depression: A review of the literature. *British Journal of Psychiatry, 149,* 7–16.

Stein, M.B., Tancer, M.E., Gelernter, C.S., Vittone, B.J., & Uhde, T.W. (1990). Major depression in patients with social phobia. *American Journal of Psychiatry, 147,* 637–639.

Stein, M.B., & Uhde, T.W. (1988). Panic disorder and major depression: A tale of two syndromes. *Psychiatric Clinics of North America, 11,* 441–461.

Thoren, P., Asberg, M., Bertilsson, L., Mellstrom, B., Sjoqvist, F., & Traskman, L. (1980). Clomipramine treatment of obsessive-compulsive disorder. II. Biochemical aspects. *Archives of General Psychiatry, 37,* 1289–1294.

Thoren, P., Asberg, M., Cronholm, B., Jornestedt, L., & Traskman, L. (1980). Clomipramine treatment of obsessive-compulsive disorder. I. A controlled clinical trial. *Archives of General Psychiatry, 37,* 1281–1285.

Tollefson, G.D., Souetre, E., Thomander, L., & Potvin, J.H. (1993). Comorbid anxious signs and symptoms in major depression: Impact on functional work capacity and comparative treatment outcomes. *International Clinical Psychopharmacology, 8,* 281–293.

Turner, R.M. (1987). The effects of personality disorder diagnosis on the outcome of social anxiety symptom reduction. *Journal of Personality Disorders, 1,* 136–143.

Vallejo, J., Olivares, J., Marcos, T., Bulbena, A., & Menchon, J.M. (1992). Clomipramine versus phenelzine in obsessive-compulsive disorder. *British Journal of Psychiatry, 161,* 665–670.

Van Amerigan, M., Mancini, C., Styan, G., & Donison, D. (1991). Relationship of social phobia with other psychiatric illness. *Journal of Affective Disorder, 21,* 93–99.

Van Valkenburg, C., Akiskal, H.S., Puzantian, V., & Rosenthal, T. (1984). Anxious depression: Comparisons with panic and major depressive disorders. *Journal of Affective Disorders, 6,* 67–82.

Volavska, J., Neizoglu, F., & Yaryura-Tobias, J. (1985). Clomipramine and imipramine in obsessive-compulsive disorder. *Psychiatry Research, 14,* 83–91.

Warner, M.D., Peabody, C.A., Whiteford, H.A., & Hollister, L.E. (1988). Alprazolam as an antidepressant. *Journal of Clinical Psychiatry, 49,* 148–150.

Weiss, J.M., David, D., Hedlund, J.L., & Cho, D.W. (1983). The dysphoric psychopath: A comparison of 524 cases of antisocial personality disorder with matched controls. *Comprehensive Psychiatry, 24,* 355–369.

Weissman, M.M., & Myers, J. (1976). *The New Haven community survey 1967–1975: depressive symptoms and diagnosis.* Paper presented to the Society for Life History Research in Psychopathology, Fort Worth, TX.

Wittchen, H.-U., Semler, G., & Van Zerrssen, D. (1985). A comparison of two diagnostic methods: Clinical *ICD* diagnosis vs. *DSM-III* and Research Diagnostic Criteria using the Diagnostic Interview Schedule (DIS). *Archives of General Psychiatry, 42,* 677–684.

Young, L.T., Cooke, R.G., Robb, J.C., Levitt, A.J., & Joffe, R.T. (1993). Anxious and non-anxious bipolar disorder. *Journal of Affective Disorders, 29,* 49–52.

Zimmerman, M., & Coryell, W. (1989). *DSM-III* personality disorder diagnoses in a nonpatient sample. *Archives of General Psychiatry, 46,* 682–689.

6

Cognitive Therapy of Mood Disorders with Comorbidity

ROBIN B. JARRETT
DOLORES KRAFT
PAUL SILVER

Diagnostic comorbidity typically creates complexity during treatment. Cognitive therapy for patients who are diagnosed with depression and also have comorbid conditions is no exception to this truism.

In this chapter, the main purpose is to outline how standard cognitive therapy for depression, as defined by Beck, Rush, Shaw, and Emery (1979), is supplemented when the patient with depression suffers from additional syndromes or disorders. The authors articulate hypotheses that have influenced the cognitive therapy they have provided to outpatients who have been diagnosed with major depressive disorder and who also carry one or

The authors gratefully acknowledge the research assistance provided by Greg Graves, M.D., and the care with which Edna Christian, RMT, prepared this manuscript. Thanks are expressed to Kenneth Z. Altshuler, M.D., Stanton Sharp Professor and Chairman, Department of Psychiatry, for his administrative support.

This manuscript was supported, in part, by a research grant from the National Institute of Mental Health (MH-38238-11).

Correspondence concerning this manuscript should be addressed to Robin B. Jarrett, Ph.D., at the Department of Psychiatry, University of Texas Southwestern Medical Center, 5323 Harry Hines Boulevard, Dallas, TX, 75235-9149. Electronic mail may be sent via Internet to rjarrl@mednet.swmed.edu.

more additional psychiatric diagnoses. Specifically, they focus their comments on how they adapt cognitive therapy for outpatients with major depressive disorder who also have anxiety disorders or personality disorders (as defined by the *Diagnostic and Statistical Manual of Mental Disorders* [*DSM-IV*]; American Psychiatric Association [APA], 1994). The word *comorbid* is used to refer to psychiatric diagnoses that may precede, follow, or covary with major depressive disorder. In the discussion of comorbid anxiety disorders, the focus is on concurrent diagnoses. In considering comorbid personality disorders, the focus is on past or future diagnoses, made while the patient was or is euthymic. In the opinion of the authors, this lifetime diagnostic perspective is essential, as most depressions appear to be recurrent, chronic, or both. The authors do not comment on cognitive therapy for patients with depression who present with concurrent substance abuse or dependence because their typical approach has been to refer these patients for additional specialty care in chemical abuse/dependence prior to treating their depression with cognitive therapy. Neither do they focus on cognitive therapy for patients diagnosed with depression who also have additional major medical illnesses.

Investigators who have studied cognitive therapy for depression provide few comments on psychiatric comorbidity. However, practice guidelines have emerged in the field of psychiatric disorders (e.g., APA, 1996, 1995a, 1995b, 1995c, 1993a, 1993b; Depression Guideline Panel, 1993a, 1993b), and this practical development offers opportunities to improve both practice and research for patients with depression and comorbid anxiety or personality disorders. Although practice guidelines frequently do not speak to comorbidity, per se, they offer the clinician a useful overview of treatment methods, which have some consensual validation with varying degrees of empirical validation, when the targeted psychiatric disorder occurs alone. These guidelines can aid the practitioner in surveying possible adjunctive treatment options for the comorbid condition. As always, more research is needed. In the absence of solid data, the authors provide a set of practical hypotheses to drive cognitive therapy for depression for patients with the comorbid conditions.

The authors' working clinical model for diagnosing, treating, and evaluating the course of depression in outpatients has been described previously by Jarrett (1995). The major components of this model are using semistructured clinical interviews, supplemented with medical laboratory screening and consultation to establish *DSM-IV* diagnoses; providing sufficient information regarding the effective treatment alternatives for patients and their families to give informed consent; including expert use of behavioral assessment to provide baseline and longitudinal assessment of symptom severity and target problems; scheduling continued evaluation of the effectiveness and quality of treatment; changing or adding treatments when symptoms do not improve or the patient is noncompliant with the demands of the treatment approach; treating throughout the period of risk of relapse/ recurrence; and conducting longitudinal follow-up to reduce the likelihood of the patient's experiencing a recurrence or developing a chronic syndrome. Also provided here is a description of how cognitive therapy is divided into acute, continuation, and maintenance phases in an attempt to affect the course of the illness (Jarrett & Kraft, in press).

WEIGHING PSYCHIATRIC DIAGNOSES: WHICH TO TREAT FIRST?

In treating patients with depression and comorbid disorders, after a thorough diagnostic evaluation, the clinician must first decide which disorder is primary. In making practical decisions regarding where to initiate treatment, the first step is to decide which disorder or set of problems is the most significant clinically. In doing so, the clinician must determine which disorder is associated with the most impairment in the patient's daily functioning. This evaluation is typically made during the diagnostic phase but evaluation continues so the clinician can decide which disorder results in the most functional impairment after acute phase cognitive therapy begins. In addition, heavy consideration should be given to the patient's perception of the syndrome or problem that is associated with the most distress. This chapter concentrates on cognitive therapy with patients who may have been diagnosed with anxiety disorders or personality disorders but whose depression is the most clinically significant problem. However, when these patients with depression also suffer from comorbid disorders and do not respond to typical antidepressant treatments (including cognitive therapy or pharmacotherapy), they are well served by the clinician who reevaluates to determine which disorder or problem is primary and shifts the focus of treatment.

Practical application of the principles above involves selecting useful dependent measures that are sensitive to change. Among those that are helpful in monitoring the course of depression and its symptoms are the *DSM-IV* criteria for major depressive disorder (MDD) and other comorbid disorders, the Beck Depression Inventory (Beck, Ward, Mendelson, Mock, & Erbaugh,

1961), the Hamilton Rating Scale for Depression (Hamilton, 1960), and the self-report and clinician versions of the Inventory of Depressive Symptoms (Rush et al., 1986). To monitor the occurrence of psychiatric syndromes longitudinally, the Longitudinal Interval Follow-Up Evaluation (LIFE; Keller et al., 1987) is helpful. To monitor the effect of cognitive therapy on other target problems or syndromes, it is useful to assess the deficits or excesses in functioning that are influenced by the symptom, syndrome, or problem. For example, take the unemployed patient diagnosed with depression who wishes to return to work. If the patient with depression cannot drive to job interviews and attributes this deficit to panic attacks on the freeways, during treatment clinicians could track the frequency of panic attacks, drives on the freeway, and job interviews. A self-monitoring tool like a diary might be used to facilitate the frequency count of each. They might examine the extent to which teaching the patient breathing techniques and cognitive restructuring, aimed at decatastrophizing the panic attacks, influences the frequency of the patient's driving on the freeway and attending job interviews.

The Dictionary of Behavioral Assessment Techniques (Hersen & Bellack, 1988) provides a useful reference of possible assessment tools. Only systematic data collection of relevant responses, however, will allow the clinician to discover the extent to which and the circumstances under which, the patient's behavioral deficits and excesses are related. Throughout this chapter, there is emphasis on the importance of functional analysis (Ferster, 1973) and behavioral assessment to conceptualize how best to treat patients with depression and comorbid conditions and how to maintain behavioral gains over time.

UNWINDING FUNCTIONAL RELATIONSHIPS AMONG SYMPTOMS: CONCURRENCE OR COMPLICATION?

In the treatment of patients with major depressive disorder who have comorbid anxiety disorders, personality disorders, and/or nonadaptive interpersonal functioning, the primary skills the cognitive therapist must use are the skills of behavioral assessment and cognitive conceptualization. The cognitive therapist proposes and tests hypotheses regarding functional relationships, or the lack thereof, among the behaviors inherent in the patient's concurrent or lifetime symptoms. By using these skills, the therapist must understand when the techniques initially presented by Beck and colleagues (1979) require supplementation to affect the presenting psychiatric symptoms or interpersonal responses, to improve patient functioning, or to attempt to inoculate patients from relapses or recurrences of the symptoms they have suffered at the time of presentation or over the life span.

In treating patients with depression and comorbid conditions, the cognitive therapist grapples with a basic tension between two competing hypotheses. The first hypothesis is this: The concurrent disorder is related functionally to the patient's depression in such a manner that reductions in the depressive symptoms will also improve the comorbid symptoms. Although the concurrent symptom is not part of the diagnostic criteria for major depressive disorder, the comorbid symptoms improve as the depression improves. Untreated panic attacks, which remit quickly as the patient learns basic cognitive restructuring techniques illustrate this phenomenon. Somehow the panic attacks diminish as other symptoms diminish. Perhaps as the patient learns effective skills for coping with depression, he or she generalizes these to the panic attacks, which are also effectively treated by cognitive therapy. One might think of this hypothesis as the *concomitant symptom hypothesis.*

The second hypothesis is: Although the concurrent problem may worsen the depression, it functions with some autonomy or is severe enough that these concurrent symptoms must be treated using methods that were designed specifically for that disorder, thus supplementing Beckian antidepressant strategies. The authors call this the *complicating symptom hypothesis.* When the concomitant symptom hypothesis is not supported, testing the complicating symptom hypothesis involves adding interventions that treat that specific comorbid disorder effectively. Even when the therapist adds interventions, these are incorporated into the usual conceptual scheme of the cognitive model, logical analysis, and hypothesis testing.

Treatment manuals such as *Cognitive Therapy of Depression* (Beck et al., 1979) can most productively be viewed as conceptual guidelines for treatment, rather than "how-to" outlines or recipes limited to simplistic techniques. The authors avoid viewing a treatment manual as a set of techniques but rather see it as a conceptual, empirically based approach to treating individuals. They approach cognitive therapy as if there is no "modal" patient. In this way, there is no conceptual difficulty in inserting supplemental, empirically based treatment strategies into the cognitive-behavioral model for depression originally outlined by Beck and associates (1979).

In clinical psychology, there is a movement to codify and empirically validate or support specific cognitive-behavioral interventions, which have not only a conceptual foundation but also a technical basis for specific psychiatric disorders (e.g., Sanderson & Woody, 1995). This development will likely improve both research and practice involving patients with depression and other comorbid conditions, as clinicians can be guided by the evidence in selecting the specific interventions that are most likely to reduce comorbid symptoms.

The first necessary skill the therapist must have in testing the concomitant versus the complicating symptom hypothesis is a method for identifying and monitoring the concurrent problem. For example, when the patient presents with depression and panic disorder, the therapist must assess both symptoms over the course of treatment and note the extent to which improvement or worsening in one area influences change or stability in the other.

The second necessary skill the therapist must have in treating patients with depression and comorbid conditions is technical expertise in interventions that will likely result in improvement in the comorbid symptoms. Although this statement appears obvious, therapists can find themselves treating patients whose comorbid symptoms call for therapists to add additional techniques that may not be part of their standard approach. The therapist must be flexible, but more important, broadly trained in a variety of methods that have been empirically supported. Administrators of both doctoral level and continuing educational programs will ultimately serve patients better if they consult the literature when deciding which interventions should be taught. The therapist must be open to considering and active in pursuing pharmacotherapy as a solitary or supplemental treatment (see the aforementioned practice guidelines) when cognitive therapy alone does not produce remission or when cognitive therapy does not reduce patient distress to a manageable level.

CONSIDERATIONS IN COGNITIVE THERAPY FOR PATIENTS WITH MAJOR DEPRESSIVE DISORDER AND COMORBID ANXIETY DISORDERS

Relationships between Mood Disorder and Anxiety Disorders

Mood disorders and anxiety disorders have a high rate of comorbidity. Studies vary in the degree of correlation reported between these two diagnoses depending on whether disorders are diagnosed longitudinally (over the lifetime) or cross-sectionally (at presentation only). For example, of 292 patients presenting for treatment at an anxiety clinic, approximately 30 percent with an anxiety disorder reported at least one past episode of depression during their lifetimes, but only 5 percent of the patients diagnosed with anxiety disorders received a concurrent diagnosis of major depressive disorder (Di Nardo & Barlow, 1990). A second study showed that 44 percent of patients diagnosed with anxiety disorders reported past episodes of depression during the course of their anxiety disorder (Clancy, Noyes, Hoenk, & Slymen, 1978).

Rates of lifetime comorbidity also vary with the specific anxiety and mood disorder examined. Di Nardo and Barlow (1990) found that patients with social phobia and generalized anxiety disorder were the most likely to report at least one past episode of depression during their lifetimes (38 percent to 39 percent) whereas patients with obsessive compulsive disorder and agoraphobia reported a lower rate of past episodes of depression (20 percent and 29 percent, respectively). Only 9 percent of patients with simple phobia reported past depressive episodes. Estimates of comorbidity do range widely in various samples. For example, a second study found that 70 percent of individuals with agoraphobia endorsed a lifetime incidence of major depression (Breier, Charney, & Heninger, 1986). It is estimated that the comorbidity rate for panic disorder and major depressive illness ranges from 64 percent to 75 percent (Barlow, Di Nardo, Vermilyea, Vermilyea, & Blanchard, 1986). The previous estimates all involve clinic samples. Such clinic estimates often inflate the rate of comorbidity because patients with two diagnoses are presumably more distressed and may be more likely to present for treatment than individuals with only one disorder (Regier, Burke, & Burke, 1990).

In the National Institute of Mental Health (NIMH) Epidemiologic Catchment Area Program (NIMH ECA), 20,000 community and institutionalized subjects were diagnosed using structured interviewing. The researchers found that 1.9 percent of the population had a mood disorder with an anxiety disorder in any six-month period, and that 3.6 percent of subjects reported a lifetime history of both diagnoses. These rates indicate that 43 percent of patients with an affective disorder will have a lifetime risk for comorbidity with these two disorders (Regier, Burke, & Burke, 1990).

Using Psychiatric Diagnosis to Aid in Intervention Selection: What Am I Treating?

To understand the effectiveness of standard cognitive therapy for anxiety and depressive symptoms, one must understand the similarities and differences in the cognitive components of and functional relationships between these two disorders. Frequently there is a great deal of overlap in the clinical presentation of anxiety and depression because both are associated with negative cognitions and impaired behavioral functioning. Both result in patients' having depreciated self-concept, negative predictions, and negative bias in the evaluation of current experiences (Beck, 1976; Beck & Emery, 1979, 1985; Beck et al., 1979). At the same time, important differences are revealed in the specific content of these maladaptive cognitions. Beck and Emery (1979) describe several cognitive patterns that distinguish these two disorders. For example, in patients diagnosed with depression, cognitions regarding negative events are frequently attributed to internal, global, and stable factors. In patients diagnosed with anxiety disorders, these negative cognitions may be specific and do not impair as many areas of functioning. Thus, although both anxious and depressed individuals attach unrealistically high probabilities to negative outcomes, anxious individuals often attach these negative expectations to specific events that have not yet occurred. Even with these distinctions, the standard ingredients of cognitive therapy (logical analysis and hypothesis testing) can capably address the cognitive distortions and behavioral avoidance related to both anxiety and depressive symptoms.

Patients with depression who are being treated with cognitive therapy often record mood shifts in their Daily Diary of Dysfunctional Thoughts (Beck et al., 1979); these are frequently labeled anxious-feeling states and are associated with thoughts (or themes) of danger and threat. When cognitive therapists begin treating these depressed patients using the concomitant symptom hypothesis, they must also note the extent to which the anxious mood is a symptom of simple phobia, social phobia, obsessive compulsive disorder, panic disorder with and without agoraphobia, or posttraumatic stress disorder. This assessment is simplified when a thorough psychiatric evaluation precedes treatment.

The therapist should include an assessment of the physiological, cognitive, and behavioral response systems (Street & Barlow, 1994) and how they are interacting with, affected by, or maintaining the anxiety disorder. The physiological system includes monitoring various components of arousal such as heart rate or respiration rate. Cognitive assessment includes the patient's reported severity and understanding of distress as well as the content of panic-related (and usually catastrophic) cognitions. Finally, the therapist must evaluate the patient's level of behavioral avoidance, which is often a key symptom in anxiety disorders. This evaluation will guide the therapist in choosing a method for measuring the target symptom of the comorbid condition causing the most functional impairment. For example, in treating a depressed patient with concurrent obsessive compulsive disorder, it was important to monitor and to reduce her compulsion to make lists of tasks to do rather than actually engaging in the activity.

If the depression appears to be improving but the anxiety disorder is continuing to affect the patient's adaptive functioning, the therapist may move to the complicating symptom hypothesis mentioned previously. That is, he or she may ask which specific interventions for the comorbid anxiety disorder need to be integrated into cognitive therapy for depression. The empirical foundation for the efficacy of cognitive-behavioral therapy is making it easier for therapists to know which techniques for what concurrent anxiety disorders can easily be incorporated into standard Beckian cognitive therapy for depression. Sanderson and Woody (1995) have listed psychological interventions having empirically validated treatment manuals and available training programs, and relevant references are cited in this chapter.

In standard cognitive behavior therapy for depression, the primary interventions involve restructuring the patient's cognitions and other behaviors by a process of logical analysis or by hypothesis testing. If the standard techniques of logical analysis as defined by Beck et al. (1979) do not reduce the symptoms of anxiety, then hypotheses regarding the patient's themes of danger and apprehension can be tested by incorporating independent variables (e.g., from treatment manuals) that target the problematic comorbid symptom. Next is a summary of how this treatment might be implemented with a comorbid anxiety disorder in the treatment of depression.

Panic Disorder

As discussed above, several investigators have published treatment manuals that describe empirically validated treatments for panic disorder. Many of these treatments include a strong cognitive component in restructuring the patient's catastrophic beliefs about the feared situation. In addition to this cognitive restructuring, the primary effective treatment ingredient appears to be graded exposure of the patient to the feared situation. In the case of panic disorder, the patient is exposed to the very symptoms of panic disorder. Effective treatment protocols have been described by Barlow and Cerny (1988), Barlow and Craske (1994), Clark (1989), and Salkovskis and Clark (1991). Because panic disorder can present with or without agoraphobia, the therapist's behavioral assessment will reveal whether or which agoraphobic avoidance complicates treatment and worsens or maintains depressive symptoms.

Several questionnaires are well suited for assessing panic symptoms and can be utilized as the therapist's guide for assessing change in target symptoms. These questionnaires are easily administered to the patient and rely on self-report of panic symptoms (with and without agoraphobia) as the dependent variable. They include the Body Sensations Questionnaire and Agoraphobic Cognitions Questionnaire (Chambless, Caputo, Bright, & Gallagher, 1984) and the Mobility Inventory for Agoraphobia (Chambless, Caputo, Jasin, Gracely, & Williams, 1985). The Fear and Avoidance Hierarchy (FAH) (Street & Barlow, 1994) assesses the degree to which the patient reports fear and avoidance in a variety of situations during daily activities.

Additionally, patients can utilize self-monitoring techniques to evaluate their panic and anxiety symptoms daily. Street and Barlow (1994) describe three self-monitoring techniques that they have utilized in the treatment of anxiety disorders in their clinic. The Panic Attack Record is a small pad the patient carries at all times. Patients record each panic attack by describing its intensity and duration, the number of symptoms experienced, and whether cues were present that triggered the panic attack. Patients completing the Weekly Record of Anxiety and Depression each evening rate the average and maximum levels of anxiety, depression, pleasant feelings, and fear of panic they have experienced throughout each day. In assessing behavioral avoidance, patients using the Daily Activity Monitoring Form record the duration of and level of anxiety they experience during each daily activity.

Other methods of behavioral assessment include observations of patients in their natural environment. This strategy involves recording patients' level of anxiety after asking them to complete activities that induce varying levels of anxiety. Finally, physical symptoms of anxiety can be assessed, although these symptoms have not been as sensitive to capturing therapeutic change (Street & Barlow, 1994).

Once the therapist has completed the initial assessment and chosen a method for evaluating change in the target symptom of the comorbid condition, components of empirically validated treatments for panic can be integrated into the treatment of depression. An important component in treating behavioral avoidance associated with anxiety (e.g., simple phobia, social phobia, and agoraphobia) is in vivo exposure (Barlow & Wolfe, 1981). Here the goal is to develop a systematic plan through which patients can approach and remain in the situations they fear rather than avoid them. Imaginal exposure has proven less effective in reducing patients' agoraphobic avoidance (Emmelkamp & Wessels, 1975). At the same time, for patients with severe anxiety who are also depressed, imagined exposure may be a more comfortable method of breaking the ice. Additionally, it appears that graduated exposure, in which patients begin with situations that are minimally anxiety producing and progress to more difficult situations is superior to flooding or more intensive initial exposure (see Street & Barlow, 1994, for a discussion of why this might be the case).

The focus in the treatment of panic and agoraphobia is no longer limited to exposure-based treatment but has added panic control therapy (Barlow, Craske, Cerny, & Klosko, 1989). Researchers have treated the panic directly in patients with mild agoraphobia with good outcome (Street & Barlow, 1994). Panic control therapy is used both for treating panic alone and panic with mild agoraphobia. It consists of cognitive restructuring, interoceptive exposure—which consists of exposing the patient to somatic symptoms associated with panic attacks—and breathing retraining. Interoceptive exposure involves inducing symptoms of panic in patients through breathing exercises or carbon dioxide inhalation and having patients repeatedly expose themselves to the symptoms of panic. The patients learn to differentiate physical symptoms and panic. Over time, patients learn that these symptoms are not dangerous.

Is Cognitive Therapy Effective in Treating Panic and Depression?

Panic disorder is more severe and results in greater functional impairment when it exists with major depressive disorder (Clum & Pendry, 1987). Patients with coexisting panic disorder and depression are more socially anxious, fearful of criticism, unassertive, chronically anxious, and markedly impaired in many social role areas than are patients with only one of these conditions. They have a higher frequency of panic attacks, experience more intense panic symptoms, and are more afraid of their bodily sensations. This observation has caused some therapists to question whether the treatment for panic and/or depression is significantly reduced in effectiveness in the presence of a comorbid condition.

Evidence for the effectiveness of cognitive-behavioral treatment for patients with primary panic disorder and depression was found by Sokol, Beck, Greenberg, Wright, and Berchick (1989). The intervention involved focused cognitive therapy for panic that recreates the patient's panic symptoms by use of hyperventilation, imagery, or brief exercise. With Socratic methods, the patients were taught to consider noncatastrophic interpretations of their symptoms by questioning their biased, catastrophic thought patterns. Patients learned to control the panic symptoms through breathing exercises, coping self-statements, and refocusing techniques. A manual for the treatment of panic was utilized (Clark & Salkovskis, 1986). Not only were panic symptoms significantly reduced, but depressive symptoms also improved from the moderate (depressive) range to the normal range. Results suggest that use of cognitive-behavioral therapy to treat panic disorder directly can decrease patients' depressive symptoms as well as significantly reduce their symptoms of panic.

LaBerge, Gauthier, Cote, Plamondon, and Cormier (1993) also examined whether cognitive-behavioral treatment is less effective for panic attacks if the patient is also depressed. Their study compared cognitive-behavioral therapy for panic patients with and without secondary depressive disorder. The cognitive-behavioral treatment focused on four components: training in cognitive restructuring, training in breathing control, exposure to physical symptoms of panic, and exposure to anxiety-provoking situations. Cognitive restructuring encouraged the patients to generate more realistic interpretations of their physical symptoms by identifying and then challenging their distorted attributions about their symptoms. Training in breathing control utilized hyperventilation to generate panic symptoms and then allowed the patients to practice gaining control of their breathing. Patients were repeatedly exposed to physical symptoms associated with panic under controlled conditions in the absence of negative consequences. Exposure to anxiety-provoking situations consisted of graduated in vivo exposure to situations the patient had avoided for fear of a panic attack. Treatment resulted in significant improvement in both panic and depressive symptoms. No evidence was found that cognitive therapy was less effective for patients with depression and panic versus those with panic disorder alone.

LaBerge and colleagues offer several hypotheses for why this treatment was successful. A hierarchy with easily attainable subgoals encouraged patients to proceed and reinforced their small strides. Poor homework motivation was overcome by assigning home-based self-exposure exercises the patient could complete in a short time. Thus, depressed patients were able to improve in spite of their tendency to minimize their therapeutic gains because the tasks were constructed in such a way that they could not help noticing their therapeutic gains (LaBerge et al., 1993).

Social Phobia

A number of treatment programs for social phobia have received empirical validation as being effective (e.g., Heimberg & Juster, 1994; Hope & Heimberg, 1993; Turner, Beidel, Cooley, & Woody, 1994). The cognitive therapist might use the Social Phobia and Anxiety Inventory (Beidel,

Turner, Stanley, & Dancu, 1989) or the Index of Social Phobia Improvement (Turner, Beidel, & Wolff, 1994) to evaluate the change in the patient's symptoms of social phobia during the course of treatment. Self-report questionnaires such as the Social Avoidance and Distress Scale (Watson & Friend, 1969) are sensitive to changes in the patient's symptoms. In addition, self-monitoring can be utilized to have the patient record a target behavior related to the phobia (e.g., initiating social contact at a party).

Turner, Beidel, Cooley, and Woody (1994) developed a behavioral treatment program for social phobia that they called social effectiveness therapy. The treatment is designed to reduce social anxiety and fear, reduce avoidance behavior, improve interpersonal skill, increase pleasant social events, and improve self-concept. Treatment components include education regarding social skills training, in vivo and/or imaginal exposure, and programmed practice.

In the treatment of social phobia, the therapist begins by assessing the patient's social skills deficits using in-session role-plays of problematic situations, gathering the patient's self-reports about problematic social interactions, or observing the patient in an actual social situation. Group therapy can be helpful in assessment because it gives the therapist the opportunity to observe the patient's social interactions. The therapist then provides training for social skills deficits that might be contributing to the patient's social phobia. The social skills training could include teaching the patient appropriate conversational skills as well as assertiveness training. Role-plays of problematic scenarios help patients generalize to daily life the skills they learn in the therapy session. The cognitive therapist provides a structure for graded exposure by helping patients develop a hierarchy of feared situations and encourages homework assignments that involve graded exposure to feared social situations. Patients are encouraged to seek out nonevaluative social situations in which to explore distorted automatic thoughts in the comfort of unconditional acceptance. For example, one depressed patient in the authors' clinic who also suffered from social phobia was encouraged to attend weekly Toastmasters meetings in which newcomers are accepted positively and offered repeated practice with constructive feedback.

Simple Phobia

The efficacy of behavioral treatments for simple phobias has been supported. Manuals are available for systematic desensitization (Wolpe, 1990) and exposure therapy (Marks, 1978). Assessment devices include The Fear

Questionnaire (Marks & Mathews, 1979), which measures phobic disturbance, avoidance due to the primary phobia, and a total avoidance score for the 15 most common phobias. The primary treatment for simple phobia is the development of a hierarchy of feared objects/situations and graded exposure to the feared target.

Obsessive Compulsive Disorder

It is common for symptoms of obsessive compulsive disorder to abate with successful treatment for depression. Several investigators have published empirically based manuals that outline the treatment of obsessive compulsive disorder (see Riggs & Foa, 1985; Steketee, 1993). When obsessive compulsive symptoms are severe and long-standing, however, they can interfere with or moderate successful treatment. In this situation, the cognitive therapist continues treating the depressive symptoms and adds treatment components that directly impact the obsessive or compulsive symptoms. First, the therapist identifies a method of monitoring change in these symptoms. Options include a standardized questionnaire or the patient's self-report of how much difficulty the obsessive compulsive symptoms are creating.

Foa, Kozak, Steketee, and McCarthy (1992) have shown that effective behavioral treatment for obsessive compulsive disorder includes exposure and response prevention treatment. Patients are asked to develop a hierarchy of feared situations and/or objects that appear to be related to the obsessive compulsive symptoms. The most common obsessions involve dirt, contamination, aggression, orderliness of inanimate objects, sex, and religion, whereas the most common compulsions are related to cleaning and checking (Akhtar, Wig, Verma, Pershod, & Verma, 1975). Patients are asked to imagine increasingly feared scenes from the previously identified hierarchy, followed by graded in vivo exposure to the feared objects or situations (e.g., shaking hands). The patient is prevented from engaging in ritualistic behavior (e.g., excessive washing or cleaning) during the initial three-week treatment period.

Posttraumatic Stress Disorder

Empirically based programs for the treatment of posttraumatic stress disorder (PTSD) have been published (Meichenbaum, 1994). Treatment planning begins with determining which of the variety of PTSD symptoms (e.g., reexperiencing the traumatic event, avoidance and numbing, and arousal) are causing the most clinical distress for the patient. Assessment can include the PTSD Symptoms Scale (PSS), which is available in both a clinician-rated and self-report version with items measuring severity of PTSD symptoms (Rothbaum, Dancu, Riggs, & Foa, 1990).

Treatments for PTSD include directed therapeutic exposure (Lyons & Keane, 1989), which involves intensive repeated imaginal exposure to a hierarchy of intrusive memories. The goal of this treatment is to reduce the intrusiveness of the traumatic memories. This type of treatment has been found effective for both war veterans and rape victims. The treatment is especially effective when accompanied by stress inoculation training, which focuses on teaching the patient coping skills with which to manage the anxiety. These skills include muscle relaxation, breathing control, thought stopping, cognitive restructuring, guided self-dialogue, covert modeling, and role-playing.

Dancu and Foa (1992) hypothesize that both stress inoculation training and directed therapeutic exposure are important components of the treatment of PTSD and that responsiveness to these techniques may depend on the target symptom. For patients whose primary symptoms include intense arousal, stress inoculation training may be of more benefit than other strategies as it focuses on helping the patient obtain skills to manage the anxiety symptoms. Alternatively, for patients whose primary symptoms are reexperiencing and avoidance, exposure may reduce their symptoms more than other techniques can.

The preceding empirically validated treatment strategies were presented in the context of anxiety disorders. Clinicians trained in cognitive-behavioral therapies for anxiety disorders should be able to add these strategies to standard cognitive therapy for depression when faced with the complicating hypothesis: Symptoms of the comorbid anxiety disorder do not improve with antidepressant cognitive therapy.

CONSIDERATIONS IN COGNITIVE THERAPY FOR PATIENTS WITH MAJOR DEPRESSIVE DISORDER AND COMORBID PERSONALITY DISORDERS AND/OR NONADAPTIVE INTERPERSONAL FUNCTIONING

Standard cognitive therapy for depression as described by Beck and associates (1979) presupposes an adequate premorbid level of interpersonal functioning. Standard cognitive therapy attempts to return the patient to that previously healthy, euthymic level. But what of the patient with personality disorder and/or nonadaptive interpersonal functioning that may precede and overlap with episodes of clinical depression? In other words, what if the patient does not enter therapy with an adequate baseline level of functioning? What if interpersonal difficulties are long-standing?

Personality disorder is best operationalized as specific behaviors that cause distress, discomfort, and other negative consequences for the patient and his or her environment. Considering cognitive therapy's roots in behavioral analysis, the cognitive therapist avoids reifying the construct (i.e., using the diagnosis to *explain* rather than to *describe* the target problem).

To the extent that cognitive therapy is effective for patients diagnosed with depression who also have a confirmed personality disorder, one of the factors influencing efficacy may be the assumptions that the therapist makes about the patient's interpersonal problems, both inside and outside the session. These assumptions are reflected in the way the cognitive therapist structures each session, plans the course of the treatment, and conceptualizes how problematic symptoms interact with each other and influence the patient's environment, and vice versa.

All personality disorders are associated with interpersonal problems. The key to treating patients with major depressive disorder and comorbid personality disorder is operationalizing, assessing, and treating these problematic interpersonal responses. The complication in doing so may be the therapist's affect regarding the patient's problematic interpersonal responses. This affect must be identified and managed. The therapist can use cognitive-behavioral strategies to cope constructively with affect shifts that can occur when interpersonal deficits interfere with standard cognitive therapy.

The authors' hypotheses about treating patients with depression and comorbid personality disorders grow out of their clinical practice within a research program focusing on cognitive therapy for outpatients diagnosed with various subtypes of major depressive disorder. The ideas are speculative and influenced by weekly peer supervision meetings in which the cadre of therapists develop and share strategies they have found useful for a variety of patients with depression, some who also had personality disorders. Additional influences are other cognitive therapists' work on personality disorders. Beck, Freeman, and associates (1990) provide a far more comprehensive discussion of cognitive-behavioral strategies for specific personality disorders than space allows here. Readers are referred to Linehan's (1993) work on borderline personality disorder as an excellent illustration of informed and codified clinical practice currently being subjected to empirical evaluation.

As cognitive therapy is a work in progress rather than a finished product, the following basic approach is meant to inform and guide advanced practice with complex patients while avoiding dogmatic prescriptions. Clinicians reading this will still need to rely on solid theoretical grounding in cognitive therapy as well as their own clinical acumen to further develop approaches consistent with these guidelines. The comments are meant only as an overview of how the authors use the concomitant and complicating symptom hypotheses in cognitive therapy for patients with depression and confirmed personality disorders. Researchers are encouraged to test the hypotheses.

Diagnoses of Personality Disorders during Depression: Wait and See

Prior to and throughout treatment, adequate assessment is imperative. A *DSM-IV* Axis I psychiatric diagnosis is important for delineating target symptoms and establishing baseline data, but a functional analysis is necessary to understand how the patient's symptomatic behaviors are influencing his or her interpersonal relationships, or vice versa. The authors' bias is that any formal assessment of Axis II disorders must be deferred until the Axis I diagnosis has remitted. For example, while the patient is depressed, the clinician defers diagnosing a personality disorder. In other words, until the depression remits, the cognitive therapist avoids relying primarily on in-session interpersonal behavior or self-report to conclude that interpersonal problems are long-standing or likely to continue in the future. The cognitive therapist relies primarily on the concomitant symptom hypotheses until the depression remits.

During the depressive episode, the cognitive therapist's assessment includes collecting data on the patient's long-standing interpersonal problems that are more or less invariant across situations, relationships, and time. The patient's negative depressive cognitive bias prohibits diagnosing a personality disorder until at least remission is achieved. In the meantime, the clinician's assessment produces hypotheses that are tentative and quite subject to revision. At the same time, these hypotheses provide interpersonal targets for change should the complicating symptom hypothesis require activation once remission—or better still, recovery—is achieved. In the presence of a mood disorder, however, the cognitive therapist does note interpersonal styles consistent across situations that may cause distress to the patient and those close to him or her. Although the clinician has not diagnosed personality disorders while the patient is depressed, he or she recognizes the significant comorbidity that can exist between depression and personality disorders.

Mood Disorders and Personality Disorders

The National Institute of Mental Health Treatment of Depression Collaborative Research Program, which examined the relationship between major depressive disorder and four treatment conditions, provided data regarding comorbidity of depression and personality disorders. The *Personality Assessment Form* (Shea, Glass, Pilkonis, Watkins, & Docherty, 1987), which assesses *DSM-III* Axis II personality disorders, was administered to 239 outpatients diagnosed with major depressive disorder. The researchers found that 178 (74 percent) of these patients had at least one personality disorder and 102 (57 percent) had elevated scores on more than one personality disorder. The most common personality disorders were in the anxious-fearful cluster, with 65 percent of the 239 subjects endorsing these items. Next in frequency were the odd-eccentric cluster (20 percent) and the dramatic-erratic cluster (17 percent). Thirty percent of the patients endorsed more than one Axis II cluster (Shea et al., 1990).

Sanderson, Wetzler, Beck, and Betz (1994) found that 50 percent of patients with major depression had an associated personality disorder. Sixty-four percent of these patients diagnosed with depression had a personality disorder from Cluster C (anxious/fearful). Finally, Shea and colleagues (1987) examined the relationship between personality disorders and major depressive disorder and found that 35 percent of the subjects had at least one personality disorder. They also found that an additional 40 percent had a probable personality disorder. Again, the highest frequency of personality disorders was in the anxious-fearful cluster, with the next most frequent being in the paranoid, histrionic, and borderline personality disorders. Clinical characteristics of these subjects revealed that patients with personality disorders had a history of more frequent episodes of depression in addition to a longer duration of their current episode. These patients also reported higher levels of distress.

The preceding rates of personality and mood disorder comorbidity may well be somewhat inflated because personality assessment occurred while the patients were experiencing the symptoms of a major depressive episode. Frequently, patients' self-assessments are more negative or pathological during depressive episodes. For example, in a study on older adults diagnosed with depression, one third of the patients met criteria for a personality disorder when rating their "usual self." In contrast, two thirds received the diagnosis when describing their symptoms during the current episode (Thompson, Gallagher, & Czirr, 1988).

Cognitive Therapy for Interpersonal Deficits: Technique, Relationship, or Both?

In a review of the literature on treatment implications for patients with comorbid depression and personality disorders, Shea, Widiger, and Klein (1992) conclude that, in general, patients with comorbid personality disorders are less responsive to treatments for depression. They state, "The poor treatment response appears to be nonspecific; that is, patients with personality disorders appear to respond less well to most forms of treatment including psychotherapy (*with the possible exception of cognitive therapy*), as well as pharmacotherapy" (p. 864; italics added). Shea and associates (1990) reported that patients with depression and personality disorders, after receiving cognitive therapy, fared as well as or better than patients without a comorbid Axis II diagnosis. The type of personality disorder did not influence the result. Shea's group (1992) speculated that the more favorable treatment response for cognitive therapy could be attributed to a reduced emphasis on interpersonal factors in cognitive therapy and a greater reliance on the patient's independently performing specific techniques.

More investigation is needed to evaluate the extent to which comorbid personality disorder influences response to cognitive therapy for depression. Cognitive therapists rely heavily on relationship factors, yet manage the interpersonal dynamics between the patient and the cognitive therapist in a characteristic manner, relying heavily on the structure of cognitive therapy to cope with affect. The cognitive therapist conceptualizes the patient's depression and interpersonal deficits as a natural concomitant of overlearned habits and distorted thinking rather than as character (i.e., unchangeable) flaws in the patient's core being. Instead of labeling the patient (which could be considered a cognitive error on the therapist's part), the cognitive therapist takes a sympathetic stance, he or she communicates both overtly and covertly the notion that even long-standing interpersonal difficulties present workable problems, subject to rational analysis, cognitive restructuring, hypothesis testing, and behavior modification. The cognitive therapist assumes that the patient *behaves* in a manner that produces interpersonal problems, rather than that the patient *is* the problem. In other words, the interpersonal problem is the problem. This approach encourages optimism and increases motivation for change in both the patient and the therapist. The collaborative stance communicates that the patient is accepted unconditionally and that his or her distorted cognitions need examination and possibly reformulation.

Furthermore, the therapist communicates that the patient generates cognitions, which are associated with distressing affects and behaviors, in an attempt to cope with life; thus his or her underlying motivation is reformulated as understandable and acceptable. (The therapist continually presents data that refute the label of the "bad self.") This therapeutic stance, which is wholly consistent with the cognitive model, provides a nurturing, stable framework for therapy and behavioral change. The therapist avoids reacting emotionally to the patient's problematic in-session behaviors and avoids blaming the patient. Instead, the therapist adapts an objective, analytic stance toward the underlying attributions, affects, and behaviors with the goal of guiding the patient Socratically to consider alternative sources of data and ultimately, to reach a more rational, less disturbed position.

When the patient experiences strong emotional reactions toward the therapist, which is highly likely in patients with an Axis II diagnosis, the cognitive model allows for guided exploration of such *hot cognitions.* In fact, such moments are welcome as opportunities to understand firsthand the patient's phenomenology. Thus, these moments are viewed by the therapist as new learning opportunities to collect data rather than as derailments of therapy. They allow the therapist to handle what psychodynamic therapists call countertransference issues with a consistent structure that can be learned by the patient and generalized to the most important interpersonal relationships—those outside the treatment room.

Equally important is an educated guess at how the patient might attempt to structure his or her relationship with the therapist, typically pulling to recreate the same environmental/interpersonal responses that are associated with negative consequences. These hypotheses guide the therapist in choosing certain alliance-building options over others in order to avoid pitfalls. For example, noting a history of apparent, overly dependent interpersonal relationships in the patient, the therapist may consider delineating clear expectations of boundaries in terms of frequency of session and expected duration of treatment. Although this is typical in cognitive therapy, repeated opportunities to elicit emotions and examine and evaluate automatic thoughts regarding these issues would be important, given the patient's history.

Similarly, whereas feedback in the session is always expected in cognitive therapy, an increased frequency may be even more important with patients who have interpersonal problems. The therapist uses frequent and immediate feedback at the beginning, end, and during the therapy session to teach and to apply cognitive techniques to the emerging hot cognitions generated in the therapy.

Managing Therapist Affect

Although the therapist may be highly trained, such preparation does not render her or him immune from having negative emotions when the patient presents interpersonal obstacles to the therapeutic process or progress. For example, consider the impact on a busy, harried therapist when the patient routinely cancels or misses therapy sessions with little or no advance notice (and then demands immediate rescheduling!). Or consider the patient who spends too much therapy time negatively comparing his or her current therapist to the idealized former therapist.

Therapists can constructively use automatic thought records to help diffuse their negative feelings about the patient's behavior. In addition, the opportunity to participate in routine, weekly peer supervision is invaluable in helping the clinician avoid excessive and interfering emotional reactions toward the patient diagnosed with a personality disorder—a patient who may challenge the therapist's patience during the course of therapy.

Adding To and Emphasizing the
Typical Structure of Cognitive Therapy

In treating patients with depression and confirmed comorbid personality disorders, there are numerous important factors to consider. Among them are the usual nonspecific factors in any psychotherapy such as the nature of the therapeutic relationship, stages of therapy, duration, and frequency of treatment. The same cognitive distortions and maladaptive behaviors that influence the patient's interpersonal life outside therapy will undoubtedly be at play in the interactions with the therapist. The patient's comorbid condition often interferes with the usual course of cognitive therapy for depression. Even so, too few data have been generated regarding many of the unanswered questions, such as these: Are patients with depression and confirmed personality disorders more prone to treatment failure and/or premature dropout? Must cognitive therapy for patients with and without personality disorders vary in length to achieve a similar result? What types of targets are associated with maintaining therapeutic gains? What difficulties arise in trying to set treatment goals with such patients? How should therapy homework be tailored to promote adherence? The authors offer the following hypotheses for clinical scrutiny and empirical evaluation.

Patients drop out of treatment and avoid completing homework when they lose hope. If interpersonal difficulties between patient and therapist are mismanaged, the chance of patient hopelessness and premature termination increases. The cognitive model should be frequently applied in formulating in-session interactions, especially those associated with negative hot cognitions from either the patient, the therapist, or both. The therapist models fearlessness and assertiveness in being willing to examine shared interpersonal interactions in a nondefensive, rational, and forthright manner.

Because there is more to be treated than depression alone, and because time is spent often dealing with interpersonal issues arising out of longstanding habits and cognitive distortion, it is likely that cognitive therapy for patients with depression and comorbid personality disorders will take longer than might be expected to reduce these individuals' functional impairment and to bring them to a stable outcome of reasonable mental health. This reality is often a problem for patients with limited insurance benefits. Time limitations need to be discussed in the very first stages of therapy and brought back into therapeutic focus often enough that the patient does not develop unrealistic expectations. As third party payers press for shorter and shorter durations of treatment, realistic goals include the remission of depressive symptoms and enough training in cognitive therapy techniques for the patient to continue to work on interpersonal difficulties on his or her own after treatment concludes. Self-help manuals (e.g., Burns, 1980; Greenberger & Padesky, 1995) can be useful adjuncts to strengthening such skills, but generally only limited change or learning occurs in patients in the absence of feedback. Also researchers need to generate data on such clinically relevant decisions as duration of treatment, number, and frequency of sessions to educate third party payers regarding the influence of aborted therapy (i.e., too few sessions) on the course of depressive illness.

Setting realistic and measurable treatment goals is the first order of business in standard cognitive therapy, and it is even more important in treating patients with comorbid personality disorders. Because such patients are often prone to painful emotional reactions to their perception of mistreatment, including abandonment by others, the mutual contracting of clear therapy goals is essential from the start. Goal attainments need to be reviewed frequently with the patient and modified as needed. The therapist needs to emphasize that the overarching goal of treatment is to teach the patient enough self-help skills for him or her to continue working independently after therapy ends. The goal is not to solve all the patient's life problems in the course of this treatment. Having clear goals that reflect this aim is essential.

Well-planned homework assignments are absolutely necessary in promoting a positive, therapeutic process and outcome. The patient demonstrates his or her state of readiness for the inevitable end of therapy by being able to carry out self-help homework assignments successfully. Having proficiency in using automatic thought records to control painful, affective reactions to life events is a necessary, fundamental skill for patients. For example, the dependent patient challenges his or her dependency schema by being able to utilize homework. The therapist must be sensitive to signs that the patient is doing the homework to please the therapist rather than to acquire a useful tool, and address that issue directly. The therapist might advise the patient to forgo any homework that appears to be useless rather than completing it to please the therapist. If a patient comes to sessions with homework undone but says it would have been helpful, the therapist might guide him or her through it in the session, making certain that the patient does the work (i.e., hands the pencil to the patient, if needed) and processes any hot cognitions about this interaction as well.

Ideally, treatment ends when the patient's depressive symptoms are fully remitted and the patient has successfully demonstrated mastery of cognitive therapy skills in handling formerly difficult interpersonal interactions. Furthermore, the patient's expectations for the future would be more optimistic and there might even be evidence of new and healthy relationships in the patient's life. In 16 to 20 sessions, however, it may be more likely that the patient's depression may have remitted but that some, perhaps many, interpersonal difficulties remain. Termination may proceed according to the treatment contract agreed to at the outset of therapy unless a new contract is negotiated.

The patient may have considerable affect related to termination. When patients show interpersonal deficits, it is critical that termination issues be discussed from the beginning of treatment and placed on the agenda for at least the last three to four weeks of treatment. Affect and cognitions about termination need to be handled in the same fashion that other hot cognitions were dealt with during the course of therapy. Homework assignments dealing with termination issues are often quite useful. Such assignments might be targeted to help patients recognize their increased coping skills by accepting the termination with a feeling of satisfaction and completion. Stress inoculation exercises are highly useful in ways for the patient to imagine future stressful challenges and select coping strategies prior to the actual occurrence of the stress. Throughout this learning process, the therapist continues to model rational, assertive, and direct communication styles.

SUMMARY

When treating patients diagnosed with depression and comorbid anxiety or hypothetical personality disorders, the clinician first tests the concomitant symptom hypothesis: Treating the depression will improve *both* depressive symptoms and the comorbid condition. If the data do not support this hypothesis, the clinician moves toward the complicating symptom hypothesis: Direct treatment for the comorbid condition must be inserted into standard Beckian cognitive therapy for depression. When depressed patients suffer from comorbid anxiety disorders and the clinician utilizes established treatment protocols, such integration is less complicated than when patients suffer from depression and long-standing interpersonal deficits, for which such protocols remain largely untested.

To work successfully with patients with depression and long-standing interpersonal difficulties, therapists must have a thorough grounding in basic cognitive-behavioral skills, along with an increased emphasis on processing the cognitions and affect occurring in session between therapist and patient. Helping patients to understand the distorted cognitions that are concomitants of maladaptive coping and that impair their relationships with others allows for a nonpejorative, accepting approach by the therapist, which facilitates change. Paradoxically, the cognitive therapist focuses on the therapeutic relationship while increasing the structure of cognitive therapy as a means toward the end of less emotional discomfort and functional impairment in the patient. The primary focus is on treating the patient's depression and helping him or her acquire basic self-help skills while dealing with interpersonal issues as they arise in order to keep the therapy on track. Interpersonal deficits that might predict depressive relapse or recurrence are always candidate targets for behavioral change.

REFERENCES

Akhtar, S., Wig, N.H., Verma, V.K., Pershod, D., & Verma, S. K. (1975). A phenomenological analysis of symptoms in obsessive-compulsive neuroses. *British Journal of Psychiatry, 127,* 342–348.

American Psychiatric Association. (1993a). *Practice guideline for eating disorders.* Washington, DC: Author.

American Psychiatric Association. (1993b). *Practice guideline for major depressive disorders in adults.* Washington, DC: Author.

American Psychiatric Association. (1994). *Diagnostic and statistical manual of mental disorders* (4th ed.). Washington, DC: Author.

American Psychiatric Association. (1995a). *Practice guideline for the treatment of patients with substance use disorders.* Washington, DC: Author.

American Psychiatric Association. (1995b). *Practice guideline for the treatment of patients with bipolar disorder.* Washington, DC: Author.

American Psychiatric Association. (1995c). *Practice guideline for psychiatric evaluation of adults.* Washington, DC: Author.

American Psychiatric Association. (1996). *Practice guidelines.* Washington, DC: Author.

Barlow, D.H., & Cerny, J.A. (1988). *Psychological treatment of panic.* New York: Guilford Press.

Barlow, D.H., & Craske, M.G. (1994). *Mastery of your anxiety and panic-II.* Albany, NY: Graywind.

Barlow, D.H., Craske, M.G., Cerny, J.A., & Klosko, J.S. (1989). Behavioral treatment of panic disorder. *Behavior Therapy, 15,* 431–449.

Barlow, D.H., Di Nardo, P.A., Vermilyea, B.B., Vermilyea, J., & Blanchard, E.B. (1986). Co-morbidity and depression among the anxiety disorders: Issues in diagnosis and classification. *Journal of Nervous and Mental Disease, 174,* 63–72.

Barlow, D.H., & Wolfe, B.E. (1981). Behavioral approaches to anxiety disorder: A report on the NIMH-SUNY Albany research conference. *Journal of Consulting and Clinical Psychology, 49,* 448–454.

Beck, A.T. (1976). *Cognitive therapy and the emotional disorders.* New York: International Universities Press.

Beck, A.T., & Emery, G. (1979). *Cognitive therapy of anxiety and phobic disorders.* Philadelphia: Center for Cognitive Therapy.

Beck, A.T., & Emery, G. (1985). *Anxiety disorders and phobias: A cognitive perspective.* New York: Basic Books.

Beck, A.T., Freeman, A., & Associates. (1990). *Cognitive therapy of personality disorders.* New York: Guilford Press.

Beck, A.T., Rush, J., Shaw, B., & Emery, G. (1979). *Cognitive therapy of depression.* New York: Guilford Press.

Beck, A.T., Ward, C., Mendelson, M., Mock, H., & Erbaugh, J. (1961). An inventory for measuring depression. *Archives of General Psychiatry, 4,* 53–63.

Beidel, D.C., Turner, S.M., Stanley, M.A., & Dancu, C.V. (1989). The Social Phobia and Anxiety Inventory: Concurrent and external validity. *Behavior Therapy, 20,* 417–427.

Breier, A., Charney, D., & Heninger, G.R. (1986). Agoraphobia with panic attacks: Development, diagnostic ability, and course of illness. *Archives of General Psychiatry, 43,* 1029–1036.

Burns, D.D. (1980). *Feeling good: The new mood therapy.* New York: Signet.

Chambless, D.L., Caputo, G.C., Bright, P., & Gallagher, R. (1984). Assessment of fear in agoraphobics: The Body Sensations Questionnaire and the Agoraphobic Cognitions Questionnaire. *Journal of Consulting and Clinical Psychology, 52,* 1090–1097.

Chambless, D.L., Caputo, G.C., Jasin, S.E., Gracely, E.J., & Williams, C. (1985). The Mobility Inventory for Agoraphobia. *Behaviour Research and Therapy, 23,* 35–44.

Clancy, J., Noyes, R., Hoenk, P., & Slymen, D. (1978). Secondary depression in anxiety neurosis. *Journal of Nervous and Mental Disease, 166,* 846–850.

Clark, D.M. (1989). Anxiety states: Panic and generalized anxiety. In D. Hawton, P. Salkovskis, J. Kirk, & D.M. Clark (Eds.), *Cognitive behavior therapy for psychiatric problems* (pp. 52–96). Oxford: Oxford University Press.

Clark, D.M., & Salkovskis, P.M. (1986). *A manual for the cognitive therapy of panic disorder.* Oxford: Oxford University Press.

Clum, G.A., & Pendry, D. (1987). Depression symptomatology as a non-requisite for successful treatment of panic with antidepressant medications. *Journal of Anxiety Disorders, 1,* 337–344.

Dancu, C.V., & Foa, E.B. (1992). Posttraumatic stress disorder. In A. Freeman & F.M. Dattilio (Eds.), *Comprehensive casebook of cognitive therapy* (pp. 79–88). New York: Plenum Press.

Depression Guideline Panel (Ed.). (1993a). *Depression in primary care: Vol. 1. Detection and diagnosis* (Clinical Practice Guideline No. 5, AHCPR Publication No. 93-0550). Rockville, MD: U.S. Department of Health and Human Services.

Depression Guideline Panel (Ed.). (1993b). *Depression in primary care: Vol. 1. Detection and diagnosis* (Clinical Practice Guideline No. 5, AHCPR Publication No. 93-0551). Rockville, MD: U.S. Department of Health and Human Services.

Di Nardo, P.A., & Barlow, D. (1990). Syndrome and symptoms co-occurrence in the anxiety disorders. In J. Maser & C. Cloninger (Eds.), *Comorbidity of mood and anxiety disorder* (pp. 205-238). Washington, DC: American Psychiatric Press.

Emmelkamp, P.G., & Wessels, H. (1975). Flooding in imagination vs. flooding in vivo: A comparison with agoraphobics. *Behaviour Research and Therapy, 13,* 7–15.

Ferster, C.B. (1973). A functional analysis of depression. *Psychologist, 28,* 857–870.

Foa, E.B., Kozak, M.J., Steketee, G.S., & McCarthy, P.R. (1992). Treatment of depression and obsessive-compulsive symptoms in OCD by imipramine and behavior therapy. *British Journal of Clinical Psychology, 31,* 279–292.

Greenberger, D., & Padesky, C.A. (1995). *Mind over mood: A cognitive therapy treatment for clients.* New York: Guilford Press.

Hamilton, M. (1960). A rating scale for depression. *Journal of Neurology, Neurosurgery, and Psychiatry, 23,* 56–62.

Heimberg, R.G., & Juster, H.R. (1994). Treatment of social phobia in cognitive-behavioral groups. *Journal of Clinical Psychiatry, 55,* 38–46.

Hersen, M., & Bellack, A.S. (Eds.). (1988). *The dictionary of behavioral assessment techniques.* New York: Pergamon Press.

Hope, D.A., & Heimberg, R.G. (1993). Social phobia and social anxiety. In D. Barlow (Ed.), *Clinical handbook of psychological disorders: A step-by-step treatment manual* (2nd ed., pp. 99–136). New York: Guilford Press.

Jarrett, R.B. (1995). Comparing and combining short-term psychotherapy and pharmacotherapy for depression. In E.E. Beckham & W.R. Leber (Eds.), *Hand-*

book of depression: Treatment, assessment, and research (pp. 435–464). New York: Guilford Press.

Jarrett, R.B., & Kraft, D. (in press). Prophylactic cognitive therapy for major depressive disorder. *In Session.*

Keller, M.B., Lavori, P.W., Friedman, B., Nielsen, E., Endicott, J., McDonald-Scott, P.M., & Andreasen, N.C. (1987). The longitudinal interval follow-up evaluation: A comprehensive method for assessing outcome in prospective longitudinal studies. *Archives of General Psychiatry, 44,* 540–548.

LaBerge, B., Gauthier, J.G., Cote, G., Plamondon, J., & Cormier, H.J. (1993). Cognitive-behavioral therapy of panic disorder with secondary major depression: A preliminary investigation. *Journal of Consulting and Clinical Psychology, 61,* 1028–1037.

Linehan, M.M. (1993). *Cognitive-behavioral treatment of borderline personality disorder.* New York: Guilford Press.

Lyons, J.A., & Keane, T.M. (1989). Implosive therapy for the treatment of combat-related PTSD. *Journal of Traumatic Stress, 2,* 137–152.

Marks, I.M. (1978). *Living with fear.* New York: McGraw-Hill.

Marks, I.M., & Matthews, A.M. (1979). Brief standard self-rating for phobic patients. *Behaviour Research and Therapy, 17,* 263–267.

Meichenbaum, D. (1994). *A clinical handbook/practical therapist manual for assessing and treating adults with post-traumatic stress disorder (PTSD).* Ontario, Canada: Institute Press.

Regier, D., Burke, J., & Burke, K. (1990). Comorbidity of affective and anxiety disorders in the NIMH epidemiologic catchment area program. In J. Maser & R. Cloninger (Eds.), *Comorbidity of mood and anxiety disorders* (pp. 113–122). Washington, DC: American Psychiatric Press.

Riggs, D.S., & Foa, E.B. (1985). Obsessive compulsive disorder: A step by step treatment manual. In D.H. Barlow (Ed.), *Clinical handbook of psychological disorders* (pp. 189–239). New York: Guilford Press.

Rothbaum, B.O., Dancu, C.V., Riggs, D., & Foa, E.B. (1990, September). *The PTSD symptom scale.* Paper presented at the European Association of Behaviour Therapy Congress on Behaviour Therapy, Paris.

Rush, A.J., Giles, D.E., Schlesser, M.A., Fulton, C.L., Weissenburger, J.E., & Burns, C.T. (1986). The Inventory for Depressive Symptomatology (IDS): Preliminary findings. *Psychiatry Research, 18,* 65–87.

Salkovskis, P.M., & Clark, D.M. (1991). Cognitive treatment of panic disorder. *Journal of Cognitive Psychotherapy, 3,* 215–226.

Sanderson, W.C., Wetzler, S., Beck, A.T., & Betz, F. (1994). Prevalence of personality disorders among patients with anxiety disorders. *Psychiatry Research, 51,* 167–174.

Sanderson, W.C., & Woody, S. (1995). Manuals for empirically validated treatments. *The Clinical Psychologist, 48,* 7–10.

Shea, M.T., Glass, D., Pilkonis, P.A., Watkins, J., & Docherty, J.P. (1987). Frequency and implications of personality disorder in a sample of depressed outpatients. *Journal of Personality Disorder, 1,* 27–42.

Shea, M.T., Pilkonis, P.A., Beckham, E., Collins, J.F., Elkin, I., Sotsky, S.M., &

Docherty, J.P. (1990). Personality disorders and treatment outcome in the NIMH treatment of depression collaborative research program. *American Journal of Psychiatry, 147,* 711–718.

Shea, M.T., Widiger, T.A., & Klein, M.H. (1992). Comorbidity of personality disorders and depression: Implications for treatment. *Journal of Consulting and Clinical Psychology, 60,* 857–868.

Sokol, L., Beck, A.T., Greenberg, R.L., Wright, F.D., & Berchick, R.J. (1989). Cognitive therapy of panic disorder: A nonpharmacological alternative. *Journal of Nervous and Mental Disease, 177,* 711–716.

Steketee, G. (1993). *Treatment of obsessive compulsive disorder.* New York: Guilford Press.

Street, L.L., & Barlow, D.H. (1994). Anxiety Disorders. In L.W. Craighead, W.E. Craighead, A.E. Kazdin, & M.J. Mahoney (Eds.), *Cognitive and behavioral interventions: An empirical approach to mental health problems* (pp. 71–87). Needham Heights, MA: Allyn & Bacon.

Thompson, L.W., Gallagher, D., & Czirr, R. (1988). Personality disorder and outcome in the treatment of late-life depression. *Journal of Geriatric Psychiatry, 21,* 133–146.

Turner, S.M., Beidel, D.C., Cooley, M.R., & Woody, S.R. (1994). A multicomponent behavioral treatment for social phobia: Social effectiveness therapy. *Behaviour Research & Therapy, 32,* 381–390.

Turner, S.M., Beidel, D.C., & Wolff, P.L. (1994). A composite measure to determine improvement following treatment for social phobia: The Index of Social Phobia Improvement. *Behaviour Research & Therapy, 32,* 471–476.

Watson, D., & Friend, R. (1969). Measurement of social-evaluative anxiety. *Journal of Consulting and Clinical Psychology, 33,* 448–457.

Wolpe, J. (1990). *Practice of behavior therapy* (4th ed.). New York: Pergamon Press.

7

Pharmacotherapy of
Major Depressive Disorder
with Comorbidity

GREGORY M. ASNIS
IMRAN FAISAL

In this chapter, the authors review whether certain comorbid conditions of major depression affect its pharmacotherapy. Specifically, they examine these questions: Does a particular comorbid illness influence which antidepressant to use and its specific dose titration and dose range? Does a comorbid illness determine whether additional psychotropic medications are to be coadministered with an antidepressant? The particular comorbid conditions of major depression that are reviewed are anxiety disorders, dysthymia, and personality disorders.

REVIEW OF PHARMACOTHERAPY
OF MAJOR DEPRESSION

The pharmacotherapy of major depression has revolutionized the treatment of this illness, with the choice of antidepressants expanding greatly since their appearance 40 years ago. The late 1950s brought the introduction of tricyclic antidepressants (TCAs) and monoamine oxidase inhibitors

(MAOIs). These were followed by heterocyclics (e.g., trazodone), selective serotonin reuptake inhibitors (SSRIs, e.g., fluoxetine), selective serotonin and norepinephrine reuptake inhibitors (SSNRIs, e.g., venlafaxine), and most recently the serotonin modulators (e.g., nefazodone). Regardless of which specific antidepressant is administered, the response rate among patients is approximately 70 percent to 80 percent. The SSRIs, SSNRIs, and the serotonin modulators have come to be preferred over the TCAs, MAOIs, and heterocyclics because they are better tolerated by patients.

Certain aspects of the major depression can help provide the clinician with a rational choice as to which antidepressants to initially consider. First, if a patient with major depression has a psychotic subtype, the use of any one of the aforementioned antidepressants in conjunction with a neuroleptic (an antipsychotic medication) is required for best results (Spiker et al., 1985). Second, if atypical features are present (mood reactivity with at least two of the following four atypical features: hypersomnia, hyperphagia, leaden paralysis, rejection sensitivity), TCAs should not be used, as prior studies have found them no better than placebo in these cases. The MAOIs may be the drug of choice, being superior to TCAs (Liebowitz et al., 1984). Unfortunately, MAOIs have problematic side effects similar to those of TCAs; also, a patient taking MAOIs must follow dietary restrictions (low tyramine diet). Clinicians have tried SSRIs in atypical depression as they are better tolerated than MAOIs. Some success was reported, although comprehensive trials using SSRIs for this condition have not yet been carried out. Third, other important considerations in selecting an antidepressant are a patient's prior response to a specific antidepressant in a previous depressive episode and whether a family member had a good or poor response to a specific antidepressant.

In determining whether a specific antidepressant is effective for major depression or its specific comorbid condition, a few pharmacological principles are important. First, an antidepressant must be prescribed at a high enough dose to be effective. In the past, most failures in antidepressant treatment have been attributed to ineffective doses. In addition, an antidepressant must be prescribed for a sufficient period of time. In the recent past, 4 to 6 weeks was felt to be an adequate time in which to assess efficacy. With the advent of SSRIs, it now appears that some depressed patients, particularly the elderly, may need treatment periods of 6 to 10 weeks to respond. After obtaining an acute response, the antidepressant should be continued at a full dose for at least 3 to 6 months (the continuation phase) to minimize the risk of relapse. For depressed patients with a history of frequent recurrences of depression, the antidepressant may need to be continued for an additional 6 months to 5 years (maintenance phase) (Kupfer, Frank, & Perel, 1992). When antidepressants are to be discontinued, they should be withdrawn gradually to avoid inducing withdrawal symptoms or a relapse of the depression.

EFFECT OF COMORBID ILLNESSES

As a general pharmacotherapeutic principle, it is simpler and easier to use a single medication that might treat multiple disorders than to utilize a polypharmacy approach. The latter is more likely to be associated with increased side effects and pharmacokinetic interactions, complicating treatment. Because antidepressants have antianxiety, antipanic, and antiobsessional properties, one antidepressant may be successful in treating a number of anxiety and depressive disorders. Nonetheless, the clinician occasionally has to use multiple medications for major depression with comorbid conditions for the most efficacious treatment.

ANXIETY DISORDERS

Panic Disorder (PD)

The recent estimates of panic disorder in the general population are a one-year and lifetime prevalence rate of 2.3 percent and 3.5 percent, respectively (Kessler et al., 1994). Approximately 20 percent of patients with major depressive disorder currently also fulfill criteria for panic disorder (Lydiard, 1991; Sanderson, Beck, & Beck, 1990); the lifetime prevalence of major depression in panic patients is even higher averaging around 50 percent (Barlow, Di Nardo, Vermilyea, Vermilyea, & Blanchard, 1986; Breier, Charney, & Heninger, 1984). The co-occurrence of major depression and panic appears to represent a more severe form of illness than caused by either alone (Grunhaus, Pande, Brown, & Greden, 1994); patients with both disorders tend to have more physical, psychological, and functional impairment and are at increased risk of suicide (Reich et al., 1993). Therefore, an appropriate diagnosis with early and aggressive intervention is particularly important for this group of patients.

Several classes of drugs have shown clinical effectiveness in both major depression and panic disorder, including TCAs, MAOIs, and SSRIs (Raj & Sheehan, 1995). Paroxetine recently became the first SSRI (and the only drug other than alprazolam) to be approved by the Food and Drug Administration (FDA) for the treatment of panic disorder. In treating a depressed patient with panic disorder, we would recommend an initial trial of a TCA (for example, imipramine, desipramine, or nortriptyline) or one of the SSRIs because of their safety, ease of administration, and low side effects in contrast to an MAOI. The TCAs have been studied for a much longer period of time, but there is substantial evidence of the efficacy of the SSRIs in each individual disorder—that is, major depression and panic (Schneier, et al., 1990; Sheehan, Dunbar, & Fuell, 1992). Trazodone, bupropion, maprotiline, venlafaxine, and nefazodone have been ineffective or not thoroughly assessed in the treatment of panic disorder. Therefore, they should be avoided as a first-line treatment in major depression comorbid with panic disorder.

In the treatment of panic disorder alone or comorbid with major depression, dosage of antidepressants is critical. If the dose is increased at increments that are too high and too fast, a subgroup of panic disorder patients (approximately 25 percent) will experience the jitteriness syndrome, an overactivation in which these patients feel overly nervous and develop insomnia, diarrhea, and frequently a worsening of their panic attacks (Pohl, Yergani, & Balon, 1988). This unpleasant condition leads many patients to discontinue their medications and/or become noncompliant, believing the cure is worse than the disease. Some clinicians have suggested that patients will adapt within a short time (days to weeks), but other clinicians' experience suggests that this state is not easily adapted to and that patients do not tolerate it. Dosage is a critical issue as the ultimate dose of antidepressant for most panic patients is similar to that for major depression. The main approach to avoiding the jitteriness syndrome is to increase the antidepressant dose slowly. For example, a dose of 10 mg of nortriptyline or imipramine or 2.5 mg to 5.0 mg of fluoxetine is initiated instead of the usual starting dose for major depression (e.g., 50 mg of nortriptyline or imipramine or 20 mg of fluoxetine). Subsequently, increases can occur every five to seven days. Clearly, this conservative approach does increase the time to reach adequate doses. Alternatively, higher, more routine doses of antidepressants can be initiated as in the treatment of major depression, in conjunction with a minor tranquilizer. This approach may prevent the jitteriness syndrome, or the addition of benzodiazepines after the jitteriness develops can lead to its resolution. Antidepressants typically have a delayed onset of action (four to six weeks) in both major depression and panic disorder. Recently, an SSRI, fluvoxamine, was shown to have an onset of action within two weeks in the treatment of panic disorder. With antidepressant treatment, some antianxiety effects may be seen within days, but the main effect becomes clinically significant only after weeks.

Although benzodiazepines alone, particularly alprazolam, have been used successfully in panic disorder, it is highly recommended that they not be used without antidepressants in the treatment of major depression comorbid with panic disorder. They have been shown to induce or exacerbate depression in over 30 percent of patients with panic disorder (Lydiard, Laraia, Ballenger, & Howell, 1987). The rationale for using benzodiazepines is to provide more immediate relief of the comorbid panic disorder condition. Patients with major depression comorbid with panic disorder are at a higher risk for suicidal behavior than patients with major depression without comorbid panic disorder. The presence of anticipatory anxiety and panic attacks in depressed patients is believed to increase the morbidity and mortality of this group. Therefore, benzodiazepines may be beneficial in the early stages of treatment while the antidepressants have not yet started to have their effect. If benzodiazepines are used in combination with the antidepressants, the clinician should attempt to discontinue benzodiazepine treatment slowly after approximately six to eight weeks of antidepressant treatment when the latter is having a significant clinical effect. Benzodiazepines are usually unnecessary after this time, and more chronic use may lead to dependence and potential withdrawal issues. Of the benzodiazepines, lorazepan, alprazolam, and clonazepam are effective in panic disorder (Raj & Sheehan, 1995). Clonazepam is recommended because it has a longer half-life leading to fewer fluctuations in blood levels and thus less potential for breakthrough panic symptoms or benzodiazepine withdrawal. Although the use of benzodiazepines in major depression comorbid with panic disorder should be temporary, there will be a subgroup of patients who need antidepressants coadministered with long-term use of benzodiazepines.

In summary, the following clinical guidelines are recommended for the treatment of depression comorbid with panic disorder:

1. The use of an SSRI or a TCA is the first treatment of choice, with preference for an SSRI. The initial dose should be low, with slow upward adjustments to avoid the jitteriness syndrome.
2. Benzodiazepines, particularly clonazepam, can be added to the above treatment if panic attacks or anxiety are severe, as these symptoms are rapidly responsive to this treatment. If these symptoms are not healed, they can increase the suicidal risk for the patient.

3. Benzodiazepines should never be used alone because of their potential depressogenic effects and should be withdrawn after six to eight weeks to avoid potential dependence and withdrawal issues.
4. Benzodiazepines also are helpful for the jitteriness syndrome.

Generalized Anxiety Disorder (GAD)

General anxiety disorder (GAD) has a one-year and a lifetime prevalence in the general population of 5.1 percent and 3.1 percent, respectively (Kessler et al., 1994). Although anxiety symptoms are highly prevalent in major depression, occasionally they are prominent and persistent, satisfying a comorbid diagnosis of GAD. The diagnostic criteria of GAD have undergone a number of changes from *DSM-III* through *DSM-IV.* Although somatic anxiety symptoms (e.g., tremor) are part of the symptom clusters, cognitive symptoms (e.g., worrying) have become the central core feature. Approximately 40 percent of patients with major depression currently also have a GAD diagnosis (Sanderson et al., 1990).

A major treatment question for this chapter is whether the presence of GAD alters and/or complicates the treatment of the patient with major depression. The ideal goal of the clinician is to use a medication that treats multiple diagnoses in contrast to the use of individual medications for each diagnosis that might be present. The mainstay treatments of major depression—antidepressants—have been briefly evaluated in the treatment of GAD. Kahn and associates (1986) and Hoehn-Saric, McLeod, and Zimmerli (1988) found that TCAs were as effective as benzodiazepines, with both being superior to placebo in the treatment of GAD; TCAs had a delayed onset of action (three to four weeks) in contrast to a more immediate effect of benzodiazepines. Interestingly, the study by Hoehn-Saric and colleagues (1988) produced a differential response: The TCA, imipramine, was more effective on psychic anxiety whereas the benzodiazepine, alprazolam, was more effective on somatic anxiety. Non-TCA antidepressants—the SSRIs, venlafaxine and nefazodone—have been found to have significant antianxiety properties in major depression, but none of these non-TCA antidepressants have been formally studied in GAD. We recommend, in particular, the use of a TCA or SSRI (although venlafaxine or nefazodone are options) for a period of 4 to 10 weeks in the treatment of a depressed patient with comorbid GAD. As recommended in the prior section on panic disorder, antidepressants should be initiated cautiously at a reduced dose because of the potential initial anxiogenic effect of these medications. Although the full jitteriness syndrome has not been described in GAD, antidepressants, particularly the SSRIs, may initially be anxiogenic. The final dose should be a full antidepressant dose. Although antidepressants are recommended as a first line of treatment for depressed patients with comorbid GAD (as monotherapy is preferred), only benzodiazepines and buspirone are FDA approved for GAD.

If GAD symptoms persist despite a response of the major depression disorder to antidepressants, the addition of buspirone or benzodiazepines is a reasonable choice. Clearly, benzodiazepines are the most well studied and efficacious drugs in the treatment of GAD. Similar to use in those patients with major depression comorbid with panic disorder, benzodiazepines should be coadministered only with antidepressants; they should then be slowly discontinued after six to eight weeks to avoid dependence and withdrawal issues as well as potential depressogenic effects. When benzodiazepines are prescribed, the long-acting ones, such as clonazepam and diazepam, are preferred.

Buspirone is a partial 5-HT1A receptor agonist that has been found in a number of clinical studies to be highly effective in the treatment of GAD and equivalent to various benzodiazepines studied. Buspirone's side effect profile is devoid of sedative and psychomotor effects. Furthermore, the drug does not induce dependence or withdrawal symptoms, a characteristic that makes this antianxiety medication appealing. Although buspirone has not undergone clinical trials in major depression, some reports suggest a few antidepressant properties at higher doses (60 to 90 mg) (Robinson, Alms, Shrotriya, Messina, & Wickramaratne, 1989). It appears that GAD patients who have never been exposed to benzodiazepines respond particularly well to buspirone, in contrast to patients who have had prior benzodiazepine exposure. The other important characteristic of buspirone is that, similar to antidepressants, it has a delayed onset of action of four to six weeks. Because of its short half-life, buspirone should be administered twice or three times a day. A total dose of 45 to 75 mg frequently is indicated (Gammans et al., 1992).

In summary, the following clinical guidelines are recommended for the treatment of the depressed patient comorbid with GAD:

1. Start off with a TCA or SSRI at a low dose, slowly increasing the dose to avoid inducing further anxiety. Begin with the expectation that one drug will help both conditions.
2. If anxiety is very severe or resistant to antidepressant treatment, add buspirone or a long-acting benzodiazepine.

3. Treatments should be longer than for major depression alone, at least 6 to 12 months.

Obsessive Compulsive Disorder

Obsessive compulsive disorder (OCD) has a one-year and lifetime prevalence in the general population of 2.5 percent and 1 percent, respectively (Regier et al., 1993). The disorder is frequently a comorbid illness with major depressive disorder. Approximately a third of depressed patients currently meet criteria for OCD (Sanderson et al., 1990). This disorder consists of obsessive thoughts (obsessions) and/or ritualistic behavior (compulsions) that are accompanied by anxiety, particularly when patients confront their symptoms. The disorder is frequently chronic and disabling (Karno, Golding, & Sorenson, 1988).

To understand how the presence of OCD may alter the psychopharmacological treatment of major depression, one must review some key psychopharmacological findings of OCD. First, OCD is an anxiety disorder with predominantly serotonergic dysfunction. Antidepressants that mainly potentiate serotonin—such as clomipramine, a TCA, and the SSRIs—have been found superior to placebo in the treatment of OCD. In contrast, antidepressants that potentiate norepinephrine—such as desipramine or nortriptyline (a TCA)—are ineffective (DeVeaugh-Geiss, 1993). These results are quite different from results in the treatment of major depression, where there is no preferential response to serotonin or norepinephrine potentiating antidepressants. Second, the dose and duration of antidepressants in the treatment of OCD differ markedly from those seen in the treatment of major depression or other anxiety disorders. In contrast to treatment for panic disorder and other anxiety disorders, treatment for OCD patients can be initiated with a standard antidepressant dose. These patients seem able to tolerate any anxiogenic effects of the medication. It appears that the dose of antidepressant medication needed as a response to OCD is frequently much higher than for other disorders. In particular, a dose of 60 to 80 mg per day of fluoxetine is frequently necessary to treat OCD, in contrast to the usual dose of 20 mg of fluoxetine in the treatment of major depression. Furthermore, the duration of treatment necessary for a response also is longer in OCD in comparison to major depression. Studies have suggested that up to 12 weeks of treatment may be necessary, with most patients needing a minimum of 6 weeks prior to a significant response (Clomipramine Collaborative Study Group, 1991). Third, it is important for the clinician to realize that although OCD is responsive to treatment, it is only partially responsive, with symptom reduction occurring on the average to less than 50 percent of baseline levels. In addition, when treatments are discontinued, OCD patients frequently experience a rapid relapse of their disorder. These observations further highlight the chronicity and dysfunctional aspects of OCD (Pigott, Grady, & Rubenstein, 1993). As an interesting note, there is a low placebo response rate in OCD (Clomipramine Collaborative Study Group, 1991).

Concerning the serotonin potentiating antidepressants, one comparative report suggests increased efficacy for clomipramine over fluoxetine, fluvoxamine, or sertraline (DeVeaugh-Geiss, 1993). A major limiting factor to clomipramine is its high rate of side effects, such as sedation and dry mouth, which are particularly bothersome to patients. In general, the SSRIs are better tolerated.

Although studies evaluating specific treatments for major depression comorbid with OCD are lacking, clinical experience suggests the following guidelines:

1. A serotonin potentiating antidepressant should be used. The SSRIs are usually better tolerated than clomipramine, a TCA.
2. The ultimate antidepressant dose frequently needs to be higher than that used in major depressive disorder.
3. The clinician may have to wait up to 12 weeks at an adequate dose to obtain a satisfactory clinical response.
4. The presence of OCD predicts a more chronic illness, a longer-term treatment, and a poorer response to therapy.

Social Phobia

Social phobia has recently received much attention, being a common disorder with a lifetime and one-year prevalence rate in the general population of 13.3 percent and 7.9 percent, respectively (Kessler et al., 1994). In addition, 5.2 percent of patients with major depression currently also have a comorbid social phobia (Sanderson et al., 1990). Unfortunately, the disorder is frequently unrecognized and therefore untreated. A patient with social phobia experiences intense anxiety in social situations, with frequently a fear of embarrassment or humiliation accompanied by marked avoidance and sometimes panic attacks. This condition is highly problematic, as social phobia is often a chronic illness with significant functional impairment (Liebowitz, Gorman, Fyer, & Klein, 1985).

The pharmacological treatment of social phobia alone has begun to be significantly studied. The MAOIs have been the best-studied medications for social phobia. In a large, double-blind, placebo-controlled study, phenelzine was found to be significantly more effective (66 percent response rate) than a beta-blocker, atenolol, or placebo (each with a 33 percent response rate) (Liebowitz et al., 1992). The dose range necessary for response and duration of treatment is similar to that for the treatment of major depression. Unfortunately, the MAOIs have many side effects and require dietary restrictions. Initial trials with reversible MAOIs (binding only the A isoenzyme of monoamine oxidase) such as moclobemide (Versiani et al., 1992) and brofaromine (van Vliet, den Boer, & Westenberg, 1994), which are not marketed in the United States, have been promising but need further study. These reversible MAOIs have fewer side effects and no dietary restrictions.

The SSRIs have also been effective in social phobia in a few uncontrolled and controlled studies (van Vliet, den Boer, & Westenberg, 1994). In addition, high-potency benzodiazepines, such as clonazepam (Davidson et al., 1993), have also been effective in social phobia. In contrast, beta-blockers such as atenolol have been ineffective in the treatment of social phobia (Liebowitz et al., 1992). It does appear that beta-blockers may be effective in the treatment of social phobia of the nongeneralized type, such as performance anxiety—for example, giving speeches. Administration of 10 to 40 mg propranolol 30 to 60 minutes prior to a performance diminishes anxiety and decreases avoidance (Brantigan, Brantigan, & Joseph, 1982; Lockwood, 1989). The TCAs and buspirone have not been well studied in social phobia, but clinical experience suggests that they have minimal efficacy.

Although the pharmacotherapy of major depression comorbid with social phobia has not been studied, a few clinical guidelines are offered:

1. The treatment of choice tends to be an SSRI because of its efficacy and lack of side effects, compared to an MAOI.
2. The MAOIs, perhaps the most effective of the treatments, are the recommended treatment if SSRIs are not tolerated or are ineffective.
3. The dose and duration of SSRIs and MAOIs are similar to those for major depression.
4. High-potency benzodiazepines are also effective. They can be added to a treatment course with an SSRI or an MAOI if social phobia remains a problem. The clinician must be cautious about any depressogenic effects or dependence and withdrawal consequences of the benzodiazepines.
5. Beta-blockers, although ineffective for social phobia of the generalized type, may be helpful for the nongeneralized type (performance

anxiety). The clinician may add this to an SSRI or MAOI if performance anxiety remains after an adequate antidepressant treatment course. The clinician must be cautious about any depressogenic effects secondary to a beta-blocker.

Posttraumatic Stress Disorder

Posttraumatic stress disorder (PTSD) has a lifetime prevalence in the general population of approximately 1 to 3 percent (Davidson, Hughes, Blazer, & George, 1991; Helzer, Robins, & McEvoy, 1987). It is a complex disorder involving three symptom clusters: intrusive symptoms, such as recurring dreams; avoidance symptoms, such as emotional numbing; and hyperarousal symptoms, such as anxiety. It is not surprising that over 80 percent of patients have at least one comorbid disorder (Breslau, Davis, Andreski, & Peterson, 1991). Studies assessing the prevalence of PTSD in patients with major depression have been lacking. Underlying this inadequacy is the failure of the National Comorbidity Study to evaluate for PTSD. Nonetheless, major depression is known to be a frequent comorbid disorder (approximately 20 percent) within PTSD patients. In addition, PTSD is associated with marked dysfunction as well as alcoholism and drug abuse.

In double-blind placebo-controlled trials, TCAs and MAOIs were highly effective in the treatment of PTSD. In particular, amitriptyline (Davidson et al., 1993) and imipramine (Frank, Kosten, Giller, & Dan, 1988) of the TCAs and phenelzine (Kosten, Frank, Dan, McDougle, & Giller, 1991) of the MAOIs were superior to placebo.

Although no controlled trials have been published on SSRIs, open studies (Nagy, Morgan, Southwick, & Charney, 1993) and clinical experience suggest that SSRIs are highly effective in PTSD. This, if true, is important, as this group of medications is highly tolerated and effective in many of the comorbid conditions of PTSD, such as major depression and panic disorder. These antidepressants should be prescribed in doses similar to those for major depression. Dose titration should be slow, particularly in PTSD patients who also have concurrent panic attacks or comorbid panic disorder.

Mood stabilizers such as carbamazepine appear to be helpful in treating anger and aggressive outbursts sometimes manifested in PTSD patients, particularly in Vietnam veterans (Lipper et al., 1986). More studies need to be conducted, as mood stabilizers also have antidepressant effects and may thus be particularly beneficial to depressed patients with comorbid PTSD. Benzodiazepines are commonly prescribed in PTSD for its anxiety symptoms.

Some clinicians are particularly loath to use benzodiazepines in PTSD as they not only can be depressogenic but can increase anger and disinhibition of emotions (Feldman, 1987). In addition, because alcoholism and drug abuse are frequent comorbid conditions, benzodiazepine administration is a significant risk in PTSD patients. In treating PTSD, clinicians should give patients longer-term treatment, perhaps up to one year in duration (Sutherland & Davidson, 1994). Months of treatment may be required for the symptoms of PTSD to fully respond. Medications are particularly helpful in treating the positive symptoms of PTSD, such as flashbacks or reexperiencing the trauma. The negative symptoms of PTSD, such as avoidance, can be resistant to medication and may best respond to behavior therapy approaches (Silver, Sandberg, & Hales, 1990).

Although the pharmacotherapy of patients with major depression comorbid with PTSD has not been well studied, the following clinical guidelines are offered:

1. One of three antidepressants—SSRIs, TCAs, or MAOIs—should be the treatment of choice. The authors prefer to initiate treatment with an SSRI because these drugs have such a favorable side effect profile.
2. If PTSD is still nonresponsive despite a response of the major depressive episode, a mood stabilizer should be added, particularly if anger or aggressive outbursts are a core problem. Occasionally, benzodiazepines may be coadministered with antidepressants, but with caution because of their depressogenic and anger-inducing properties.
3. Symptoms of PTSD may take months to respond to treatment. Medications should be administered for periods approaching one year; PTSD patients are vulnerable to an early relapse if medications are not given for a sufficient time.

DYSTHYMIA

Dysthymia is another *DSM-IV* Axis I mood disorder separate from major depressive disorder. It is a highly prevalent disorder with a lifetime and one-year prevalence of 6.5 percent and 2.5 percent, respectively (Kessler et al., 1994). It is now clear that this chronic illness (of at least two years' duration that usually has an onset before age 21) can cause marked physical and social impairment. De Lisio, Maremmani, and Perugi (1986) found that impairment caused by dysthymia was even worse than that caused by major depression, and the Medical Outcomes Study found that major depressive disorder comorbid with dysthymia had greater impairment than major depressive disorder without comorbid dysthymia (Wells, Burnam, Rogers, Hays, & Camp, 1992). Dysthymia is also associated with a high rate of suicidal behaviors, comparable to major depression. Asnis et al. (1993) found that 30 percent of outpatients with major depression and 35 percent with dysthymia had a history of suicide attempts. For a diagnosis of dysthymia, a patient must have a depressed mood, compared with major depressive disorder where anhedonia may suffice. Some of the symptoms of dysthymia and major depressive disorder overlap: dysfunctions in sleep, appetite, weight, and energy. It is not surprising that when a dysthymic patient has a worsening of the disorder, with the addition of one or two symptoms such as loss of interest and suicidal ideation, the patient subsequently develops a superimposed major depressive disorder. Horwath, Johnson, Klerman, and Weissman (1992), using the Epidemiologic Catchment Area data, found that patients with dysthymia who had no history of major depression had a 5.5 times increased risk of developing major depressive episode in one year follow-up than subjects without a history of dysthymia or major depression.

There is high comorbidity between major depressive disorder and dysthymia. Keller and Shapiro (1982) originally described this phenomenon of *double depression,* finding that 25 percent of their study subjects with major depressive disorder (n = 101) had double depression. Similarly, Sanderson and colleagues (1990) evaluated 197 patients with major depressive disorder and found that 24 percent had a comorbid diagnosis of dysthymia. In the *DSM-IV* field trial for dysthymia, major depression, and minor depression, Klein (1992) found that 62 percent of the subjects with dysthymia who were interviewed also met a current diagnosis of major depression; 80 percent of them had a lifetime history of major depression.

The effect of comorbidity of dysthymia on major depressive disorder is an important issue. First, patients with double depression had a significantly greater social impairment than patients with only major depressive disorder in a six-month follow-up study (Klein, Taylor, Harding, & Dickstein, 1988). Earlier studies suggested that in double depression, if recovery occurs in the major depressive episode only, patients will experience a high rate of relapse, apparent at one-year and two-year periods of follow-up. It appears that the longer the history of the dysthymic process, the greater is the chance of relapse of the major depressive disorder (Keller, Lavori, Endicott, Coryell, & Klerman, 1983; Keller et al., 1992). Nonetheless, whether double depression affects the outcome and response to treatment is still uncertain from the above studies as they were naturalistic, with the treatment frequently being uncontrolled. Despite this shortcoming, the recommendation is that dysthymia be treated aggressively.

Pharmacotherapy studies have now clearly demonstrated that dysthymia, either in its pure form or as part of a double depression, is responsive to various antidepressant treatments. The TCAs, particularly imipramine and desipramine, were shown by the Cornell group (Kocsis et al., 1988; Marin, Kocsis, Frances, & Parides, 1994) to be highly effective in double depression as well as pure dysthymia. Interestingly, the pure dysthymia group had a higher remission rate than the double depression group—70 percent versus 52 percent—but the difference was not statistically significant (Marin et al., 1994). Unfortunately, the only placebo-controlled study was that of Kocsis and others (1988), which evaluated imipramine in people with chronic depression, with 96 percent of those with dysthymia having a major depression. Although there was a clear drug effect (59 percent on drug versus 13 percent on placebo), a pure dysthymia or major depression alone group was not included (Kocsis et al., 1988). The MAOIs have also been evaluated in double depression and pure dysthymia, and both reversible (such as moclobemide) and irreversible MAOIs (such as phenelzine) are effective. Last, medications that modulate the serotonin system are also effective. In a number of open trials and at least one controlled study using fluoxetine, an SSRI, in pure dysthymia and double depression (Hellerstein et al., 1993; Lapierre, 1994), an overall response rate of 60 percent to 70 percent has been documented. Finally, there are three studies (Bakish et al., 1993; Bersani et al., 1991; Reyntjens, Goelders, Hoppenbrouwers, & Bussche, 1986) that found ritanserin—a 5HT2 antagonist—useful in pure dysthymia/double depression.

Once again, as to whether the presence of dysthymia alters the pharmacotherapy of major depression, it appears not. In fact, the pharmacotherapeutic response in dysthymia with or without concomitant major depression appears equivalent to that in major depression alone. Also, the presence of dysthymia does appear to predict a low placebo response and an increased sensitivity to antidepressant side effects (Lapierre, 1994). In addition, the presence of dysthymia in major depression may suggest a course of treatment of at least one year in duration (Aronson & Shukla, 1989).

It appears that in controlled clinical trials, the presence of comorbid dysthymia does not have a negative impact, at least on the acute pharmacotherapeutic response to major depression. Whether the presence of dysthymia truly has a negative impact on relapse rates, as suggested by Keller and colleagues in naturalistic studies, awaits more careful prospective studies.

Thus, the following clinical guidelines can be offered in treating the patient with major depressive disorder with comorbid dysthymia:

1. For the most part, the clinician should treat double depression pharmacologically no differently than he or she would treat major depression alone. The dose and its titration follow the same principles recommended for major depression without comorbidity.
2. Clinicians should follow the same guidelines in choosing a specific antidepressant as they would in selecting one for major depression alone. The dose and duration of treatment, need for continuation, and maintenance treatment are similar to those for major depression. An SSRI, particularly fluoxetine, is the treatment of choice in double depression, as the SSRIs have been shown to be helpful in both dysthymia and major depression and are well tolerated. The TCAs and MAOIs are convenient alternatives.
3. Duration of treatment may have to be increased slightly to at least one year to decrease the potential for relapse.

PERSONALITY DISORDERS

Personality disorders recognized by *DSM-IV* as Axis II disorders are widely prevalent. Having an onset usually in adolescence or adulthood, they lead to distress and impairment. Patients with major depression have significant comorbidity with various personality disorders, even though the recent Epidemiological Catchment Area study (Regier et al., 1993) and National Comorbidity Survey (Kessler et al., 1994) inadequately evaluated personality disorders per se. The percentage of depressed patients who meet criteria of a personality disorder ranges from 10 percent to 100 percent, with an average of 50 percent (Fabrega, Mezzich, Mezzich, & Coffman, 1986; Joffe & Regan, 1988; Sanderson, Wetzler, Beck, & Betz, 1992). The marked variability of the rates probably relates to methodological issues, such as whether a self-rating scale or structured scale was used—the self-rating scale being associated with higher rates—whether the respondents were inpatients or outpatients—the inpatients being more severely ill, with a higher prevalence rate of personality disorders—and other differences.

Sanderson and associates (1992) conducted a comprehensive study assessing comorbid Axis II diagnoses in 197 patients with major depressive disorder. They utilized a structured clinical interview for *DSM-III-R* to determine comorbid Axis I and Axis II disorders. Fifty percent of the major depressive disorder group had been diagnosed with one personality disorder, and 13 percent had two personality disorders. The most commonly diagnosed personality disorders were from Cluster C (i.e., anxious and fearful)—in particular, avoidant and dependent personalities.

Despite this high comorbidity of personality disorders in patients with major depressive disorder, a word of caution is in order. Some have argued that making a diagnosis of a personality disorder in a patient with major depressive disorder may not be totally valid. There are studies indicating that depression itself may lead to changes in a person's self-perception, cognition, and behavior, making personality disorder diagnosis unreliable. Stuart, Simons, Thase, and Pilkonis (1992) treated 53 depressed patients (14 with and 39 without Axis II diagnoses) and concluded that pretreatment (Axis II) diagnoses were not confirmed after successful treatment with cognitive-behavioral therapy. Joffe and Regan (1988, 1989) treated 42 depressed patients, all of whom had Axis II diagnoses, with TCAs and found significant differences in personality traits and diagnoses between patients in the depressed and remitted state. Thus, a definitive Axis II diagnosis in the presence of a major depressive episode may be possible only after successful treatment of the depressed patient (Akiskal, Hirshfeld, & Yerevenian, 1983).

What effect does a comorbid personality disorder have on the course and treatment of major depressive disorder? Such patients tend to be more severely ill than depressed patients without comorbid personality disorders; they have higher depression and anxiety scores (Sanderson et al., 1992) and have increased suicidal behaviors (Kaplan, Sanderson, Wetzler, Asnis, & McGinn, 1995).

Most specifically, the effect of comorbid personalities in general is negative on the psychopharmacological antidepressant treatment of major depressive disorder. These findings transcend which comorbid Axis II diagnosis coexists, as the presence of the eccentric, dramatic, and anxious clusters all have been shown in most studies to have a negative impact on treatment for major depression (Reich & Green, 1991). Not only does comorbid personality disorder have a negative effect on active psychopharmacological treatments for major depression, but it also appears to have a negative effect on placebo response (Weissman, Prusoff, & Klerman, 1978) as well as on response to electroconvulsive therapy, a nonpharmacological somatic treatment (Zimmerman, Coryell, Pfohl, Corenthal, & Stangl, 1986).

Of the specific antidepressants evaluated in major depressive disorder comorbid with a personality disorder, the most consistent findings have been that TCAs are less effective than in patients with major depressive disorder without a comorbid personality disorder (Reich & Green, 1991; Shea et al., 1990; Shea, Widiger, & Klein, 1992). These patients also appear to be intolerant of TCA side effects or tend to have paradoxical responses leading to noncompliance or discontinuation of treatment (Soloff, George, Nathan, Schulz, & Perel, 1986a). The MAOIs, earlier thought not to be helpful in depressed patients with comorbid personality disorders (Reich & Green, 1991; Tyrer, Casey, & Gall, 1983), now appear helpful in certain clinical combinations of depression and personality disorders/traits. For patients with atypical depression who have borderline and labile personality traits (Liebowitz et al., 1988) or borderline personality (Parsons, Quitkin, & McGrath, 1989), the MAOIs were significantly superior to imipramine or placebo.

Patients with borderline and schizotypal personality disorders, particularly those with marked schizotypal features, and/or psychotic features have responded to small doses of a nonsedating neuroleptic such as trifluoperazine (Cowdry & Gardner, 1988), thiothixene (Goldberg et al., 1986), or haloperidol (Soloff et al., 1986b). It is likely that some depressed patients with comorbid borderline and/or schizotypal personality would benefit from adjunctive treatment with low-dose neuroleptics.

Serotonin dysfunction and particularly patients' response to SSRIs have been a recent focus in understanding and treating personality disorders (Siever & Davis, 1991). A number of investigators have found that personality disorders with the dimensions of impulsivity and aggression—for example, borderline personality—respond well to SSRIs (Norden, 1989; Siever & Davis, 1991). These personality disorders/dimensions have also been reported to respond to mood stabilizers (Cowdry & Gardner, 1988). Thus, a depressed patient with impulsive and aggressive personality dimensions may be best treated with an SSRI and/or a mood stabilizer.

As reviewed in this section of the chapter, only a few investigators have studied the psychopharmacology of personality disorders, and even fewer have studied the effect of personality disorders on the actual treatment of major depression. Nonetheless, the following clinical guidelines are offered for treating depressed patients with comorbid personality disorders:

1. As the presentation of a personality disorder may be affected by a concurrent major depressive episode, it is wise, if possible, to reevaluate the patient after remission of the depressive episode before establishing a clear diagnosis with specific treatments.

2. TCAs should be avoided because of their lack of effectiveness as well as patient intolerance of their side effects and their occasional paradoxical effects.

3. The MAOIs are effective, particularly in atypical depression with borderline personality. A careful evaluation should be undertaken to ensure that patients will be compliant—as they need to follow a special diet—and are not impulsive or suicidal, as these medications can easily lead to death when taken as an overdose.

4. If a patient has significant psychotic features or severe schizotypal features, a low-dose, nonsedating neuroleptic may be helpful as an adjunct to antidepressant treatment.

5. The presence of prominent aggression and impulsivity may respond to an SSRI or a mood stabilizer. Thus, the initial choice of an SSRI as an antidepressant with the potential addition of a mood stabilizer is suggested.

CONCLUSION

Major depression has a significant comorbidity with a number of psychiatric disorders. As reviewed in this chapter, over 50 percent of depressed patients have comorbid anxiety disorders, personality disorders, or other depressive disorders such as dysthymia. The presence of comorbidity usually predicts a more chronic and severe depressive illness that may be less responsive to treatment.

Reviewed in this chapter was the way each comorbid condition affects the treatment of major depression, followed by clinical guidelines and strategies for appropriate treatment. Almost all clinical trials have been conducted in major depression without comorbidity. Because comorbidity is often the rule and not the exception, the authors recommend that clinical trials will now be conducted to assess various treatments in major depression with comorbidity. Clinical recommendations will then be based on scientific findings. Until that time, this chapter may provide the clinician with a rational guide to the treatment of major depression with comorbidity.

REFERENCES

Akiskal, H.S., Hirshfeld, R.M., & Yerevenian, B.I. (1983). The relationship of personality to affective disorder: A critical review. *Archives of General Psychiatry, 40,* 801–810.

Aronson, T.A., & Shukla, S. (1989). Long-term continuation antidepressant treatment: A comparison study. *Journal of Clinical Psychiatry, 50,* 285–289.

Asnis, G.M., Friedman, T.A., Sanderson, W.C., Kaplan, M.L., van Praag, H.M., & Harkavy-Friedman, J.M. (1993). Suicidal behaviors in adult psychiatric outpatients, I: Description and prevalence. *American Journal of Psychiatry, 150,* 150–112.

Bakish, D., Lapierre, Y.D., Weinstein, R., Klein, J., Wiens, A., Jones, B., Horn, E., Browne, M., Bourget, D., Blanchard, A., Thibandeau, C., Wadell, C., & Raine, D. (1993). Ritanserin, imipramine and placebo in the treatment of dysthymic disorder. *Journal of Clinical Psychopharmacology, 6,* 409–415.

Barlow, D.H., Di Nardo, P.A., Vermilyea, D.A., Vermilyea, J., & Blanchard, E.B. (1986). Comorbidity and depression among the anxiety disorders. *Journal of Nervous and Mental Disease, 174,* 63–72.

Bersani, A., Pozzi, F., Marini, S., Grispini, A., Pasini, A., & Ciani, N. (1991). 5HT-2 receptor antagonism in dysthymic disorder: A double-blind, placebo-controlled study with ritanserin. *Acta Psychiatrica Scandinavica, 83,* 244–248.

Brantigan, C.O., Brantigan, T.A., & Joseph, N. (1982). Effect of B-blockade and B-stimulation on stage fright. *American Journal of Medicine, 72,* 88–94.

Breier, A., Charney, D.S., & Heninger, G.R. (1984). Major depression in panic disorder. *Archives of General Psychiatry, 41,* 1125–1139.

Breslau, N., Davis, G.C., Andreski, P., & Peterson, E. (1991). Traumatic events and posttraumatic stress disorder in an urban population of young adults. *Archives of General Psychiatry, 48,* 216–222.

Clomipramine Collaborative Study Group. (1991). Clomipramine in the treatment of patients with obsessive compulsive disorder. *Archives of General Psychiatry, 48,* 730–738.

Cowdry, R.W., & Gardner, D.L. (1988). Pharmacotherapy of borderline personality disorder: Alprazolam, carbamazepine, trifluoperazine and tranylcypromine. *Archives of General Psychiatry, 45,* 111–119.

Davidson, J.R.T., Hughes, D.L., Blazer, D.G., & George, L.K. (1991). Posttraumatic stress disorder in the community: An epidemiological study. *Psychological Medicine, 21,* 713–721.

Davidson, J.R.T., Potts, N., Richichi, E., Krishnan, R., Ford, S.M., Smith, R., & Wilson, W.H. (1993). Treatment of social phobia with clonazepam and placebo. *Journal of Clinical Psychopharmacology, 13,* 423–428.

De Lisio, G., Maremmani, I., & Perugi, G. (1986). Impairment of work and leisure in depressed outpatients. *Journal of Affective Disorders, 10,* 79–84.

deVeaugh-Geiss, J. (1993). Diagnosis and treatment of obsessive compulsive disorder. *Annual Review of Medicine, 44,* 53–61.

Fabrega, H., Mezzich, J., Mezzich, A., & Coffman, G. (1986). Descriptive validity of *DSM-III* depressions. *Journal of Nervous and Mental Diseases, 174,* 573–584.

Feldman, T.B. (1987). Alprazolam in the treatment of post traumatic stress disorder. *Journal of Clinical Psychiatry, 48,* 216–217.

Frank, J.B., Kosten, T.R., Giller, E.L., & Dan, E. (1988). A randomized clinical trial of phenelzine and imipramine for post-traumatic stress disorder. *American Journal of Psychiatry, 145,* 1289–1291.

Gammans, R.E., Stringfellow, J.C., Hvizdos, A.J., Seidehamel, R.J., Cohn, J.B., Wilcox, C.S., & Fabre, L.F. (1992). Use of buspirone in patients with generalized anxiety disorder and coexisting depressive symptoms. A meta-analysis of eight randomized controlled studies. *Neuropsychobiology, 25,* 193–201.

Goldberg, S.C., Shulz, S.C., Shulz, P.M., Resnick, R.J., Hamer, R.M., & Friedel, R.O. (1986). Borderline and schizotypal personality disorders treated with low-dose thiothixene versus placebo. *Archives of General Psychiatry, 43,* 680–686.

Grunhaus, L., Pande, A.C., Brown, M.B., & Greden, J.F. (1994). Clinical characteristics of patients with concurrent major depressive disorder and panic disorder. *American Journal of Psychiatry, 151,* 541–546.

Hellerstein, D.J., Yanowitch, P., Rosenthal, J., Samstag, L.W., Maurer, M., Kasch, K., Burrows, L., Poster, M., Cantillon, M., & Winston, A. (1993). A randomized double-blind study of fluoxetine versus placebo in the treatment of dysthymia. *American Journal of Psychiatry, 150,* 1169–1175.

Helzer, J.E., Robins, L.N., & McEvoy, L. (1987). Post traumatic stress disorder in the general population: Findings of the epidemiological catchment area survey. *New England Journal of Medicine, 317,* 1630–1634.

Hoehn-Saric, R., McLeod, D.R., & Zimmerli, W.D. (1988). Differential effects of alprazolam and imipramine in generalized anxiety disorder: Somatic versus psychic symptoms. *Journal of Clinical Psychiatry, 49,* 293–301.

Horwath, E., Johnson, J., Klerman, G.L., & Weissman, M.M. (1992). Depressive symptoms as relative and attributable risk factors for first-onset major depression. *Archives of General Psychiatry, 49,* 817–823.

Joffe, R.T., & Regan, J.J. (1988). Personality and depression. *Journal of Psychiatry Research, 22,* 279–286.

Joffe, R.T., & Regan, J.J. (1989). Personality and depression: A further evaluation. *Journal of Psychiatry Research, 23,* 299–301.

Kaplan, M.L., Sanderson, W.C., Wetzler, S., Asnis, G.M., & McGinn, L.K. (1995, April). *Personality disorder, generalized anxiety disorders.* Paper presented at the National Conference on Anxiety Disorders, Pittsburgh.

Karno, M., Golding, S.B., & Sorenson, S.B. (1988). The epidemiology of obsessive-compulsive disorder in five U.S. communities. *Archives of General Psychiatry, 45,* 1094–1099.

Keller, M.B., Lavori, P.W., Endicott, J., Coryell, W., & Klerman, G.L. (1983). "Double Depression": Two year follow up. *American Journal of Psychiatry, 140,* 689–694.

Keller, M.B., Lavori, P.W., Mueller, T.I., Endicott, J., Coryell, W., Hirschfeld, R.M., & Shea, T. (1992). Time to recovery, chronicity and levels of psychopathology in major depression: A 5-year follow-up of 431 subjects. *Archives of General Psychiatry, 49,* 809–816.

Keller, M.B., & Shapiro, R.W. (1982). "Double Depression": Superimposition of acute depressive episodes on chronic depressive disorders. *American Journal of Psychiatry, 139,* 438–442.

Kessler, R.C., McGonagle, K.A., Zhao, S., Nelson, C.B., Hughes, M., Eshleman, S., Wittchen, H., & Kendler, K.S. (1994). Lifetime and 12-month prevalence of *DSM-III-R* disorders in the United States: Results from the national comorbidity survey. *Archives of General Psychiatry, 51,* 8–19.

Klein, D.N. (1992, May). DSM-IV *field trial for major depression, dysthymia, depressive personality and minor depression.* Paper presented at the Annual Meeting of the American Psychiatric Association, Washington, DC.

Klein, D.N., Taylor, E.B., Harding, K., & Dickstein, S. (1988). Double depression and episodic major depression: Demographic, clinical, familial, personality and socioenvironmental characteristics and short-term outcome. *American Journal of Psychiatry, 145,* 1226–1231.

Kocsis, J.H., Frances, A.J., Voss, C., Mann, J.J., Mason, B.J., & Sweeney, J. (1988). Imipramine treatment for chronic depression. *Archives of General Psychiatry, 45,* 253–257.

Kosten, T.R., Frank, J.B., Dan, E., McDougle, C.J., & Giller, E.L. (1991). Pharmacotherapy for post-traumatic stress disorder using phenelzine or imipramine. *Journal of Nervous and Mental Disorders, 179,* 366–370.

Kupfer, E.J., Frank, E., & Perel, J.M. (1992). Five-year outcome for maintenance therapies in recurrent depression. *Archives of General Psychiatry, 49,* 769–773.

Lapierre, Y.D. (1994). Pharmacological therapy of dysthymia. *Acta Psychiatrica Scandinavica, 89* (suppl. 383), 42–48.

Liebowitz, M.R., Gorman, J.M., Fyer, A.J., & Klein, D.F. (1985). Social phobia: Review of a neglected anxiety disorder. *Archives of General Psychiatry, 42,* 729–736, 1985.

Liebowitz, M.R., Quitkin, F.M., Stewart, J.W., McGrath, P.J., Harrison, W.M., Markowitz, J.S., Rabkin, J.G., Tricamo, E., Goetz, D.M., & Klein, D.F. (1988). Antidepressant specificity in atypical depression. *Archives of General Psychiatry, 45,* 129–137.

Liebowitz, M.R., Quitkin, F.M., Stewart, J.W., McGrath, P.J., Harrison, W., Rabkin, J., Tricamo, E., Martowitz, J.S., & Klein, D.F. (1984). Phenelzine versus imipramine in atypical depression. *Archives of General Psychiatry, 41,* 669–677.

Liebowitz, M.R., Schneier, F., Campeas, R., Hallander, E., Hatterer, J., Fyer, A., Gorman, J., Papp, L., Davies, S., Gully, R., & Klein, D.F. (1992). Phenelzine versus atenolol in social phobia: A placebo-controlled study. *Archives of General Psychiatry, 49,* 290–300.

Lipper, S., Davidson, J.R.T., Grady, T.A., Edinger, J.D., Hammett, E.B., Mahorney, S.L., & Cavener, J.O. (1986). Preliminary study of carbamazepine in post-traumatic stress disorder. *Psychosomatics, 27,* 849–854.

Lockwood, A.H. (1989). Medical problems of musicians. *New England Journal of Medicine, 320,* 221–227.

Lydiard, B. (1991). Coexisting depression and anxiety: Special diagnostic and treatment issues. *Journal of Clinical Psychiatry, 51* (6, suppl.), 48–54.

Lydiard, R.B., Laraia, M.T., Ballenger, J.C., & Howell, E.F. (1987). Emergence of depressive symptoms in patients receiving alprazolam for panic disorder. *American Journal of Psychiatry, 144,* 664–665.

Marin, D.B., Kocsis, J.H., Frances, A.J., & Parides, M. (1994). Desipramine for treatment of "pure dysthymia" versus "double depression." *American Journal of Psychiatry, 151,* 1079–1080.

Nagy, L.M., Morgan, C.A., Southwick, S.M., & Charney, D.S. (1993). Open prospective trial of fluoxetine for post-traumatic stress disorder. *Journal of Clinical Psychopharmacology, 13,* 107–113.

Norden, M.J. (1989). Fluoxetine in borderline personality disorder. *Progress in Neuropsychopharmacology and Biological Psychiatry, 13,* 885–893.

Parsons, B., Quitkin, F.M., & McGrath, P.J. (1989). Phenelzine, imipramine and placebo in borderline patients meeting criteria for atypical depression. *Psychopharmacology Bulletin, 25,* 524–534.

Pigott, T.A., Grady, T.A., & Rubenstein, C.S. (1993). Obsessive-compulsive disorder and trichotillomania. In D.L. Dunner (Ed.), *Current psychiatric therapy* (pp. 282–287). Philadelphia: W.B. Saunders.

Pohl, R., Yergani, V.K., & Balon, R. (1988). The jitteriness syndrome in panic disorder patients treated with antidepressants. *Journal of Clinical Psychiatry, 49,* 100–104.

Raj, B.A., & Sheehan, D.V. (1995). Somatic treatment strategies in panic disorder. In G.M. Asnis & H.M. van Praag (Eds.), *Panic disorder* (pp. 279–311). New York: Einstein Psychiatry Series.

Regier, D.A., Narrow, W.E., Rae, D.S., Manderscheid, R.W., Locke, B.Z., & Goodwin, F.K. (1993). The de facto U.S. mental and addictive disorder service system: Epidemiologic Catchment Area prospective one-year prevalence rates of disorders and services. *Archives of General Psychiatry, 50,* 85–95.

Reich, J.H., & Green, A.I. (1991). Effect of personality disorders on outcome of treatment. *Journal of Nervous and Mental Diseases, 179,* 74–82.

Reich, J., Warshaw, M., Peterson, L.G., White, K., Keller, M., Lavori, P., & Yonkers, K.A. (1993). Comorbidity of panic and major depressive disorder. *Journal of Psychiatry Research, 27,* 23–33.

Reyntjens, A., Goelders, Y.G., Hoppenbrouwers, M.J.A., & Bussche, G.V. (1986). Thymostenic effects of ritanserin (R 55667), a centrally acting serotonin S2 blocker. *Drug Development and Research, 8,* 205–211.

Robinson, D.L., Alms, D.R., Shrotriya, R.C., Messina, M., & Wickramaratne, P. (1989). Serotonergic anxiolytics and treatment of depression. *Psychopathology, 22,* 27–36.

Sanderson, W.C., Beck, A.T., & Beck, J. (1990). Syndrome comorbidity in patients with major depression and dysthymia: Prevalence and temporal relationships. *American Journal of Psychiatry, 147,* 1025–1028.

Sanderson, W.C., Wetzler, S., Beck, A.T., & Betz, F. (1992). Prevalence of personality disorders in patients with major depression and dysthymia. *Psychiatry Research, 42,* 93–99.

Schneier, F.R., Liebowitz, M.R., Davies, S.O., Fairbanks, J., Hollander, E., Campeas, R., & Klein, D.F. (1990). Fluoxetine and panic disorder. *Journal of Clinical Psychopharmacology, 10,* 119–121.

Shea, M.T., Pilkonis, P.A., Beckam, E., Collins, J.F., Elkin, I., Sotsky, S.M., & Docherty, J.P. (1990). Personality disorder and treatment outcome in the

NIMH treatment of depression collaborative research program. *American Journal of Psychiatry, 147,* 711–718.

Shea, M.T., Widiger, T.A., & Klein, M.H. (1992). Comorbidity of personality disorders and depression: Implications for treatment. *Journal of Consulting and Clinical Psychology, 60,* 857–868.

Sheehan, D., Dunbar, G.C., & Fuell, D.L. (1992). The effect of paroxetine on anxiety and agitation: A pooled analysis including data from 4668 patients. *Psychopharmacology Bulletin, 28,* 139–143.

Siever, L.J., & Davis, K.L. (1991). A psychobiological perspective on the personality disorders. *American Journal of Psychiatry, 148,* 1647–1658.

Silver, J.M., Sandberg, D.P., & Hales, R.E. (1990). New approaches in the pharmacotherapy of post-traumatic stress disorder. *Journal of Clinical Psychiatry, 51* (10, suppl.), 33–38.

Soloff, P.H., George, A., Nathan, R.S., Schulz, P.M., & Perel, J.M. (1986a). Paradoxical effects of amitriptyline on borderline patients. *American Journal of Psychiatry, 143,* 1603–1605.

Soloff, P., George, A., Nathan, R.S., Schulz, P.M., Ulrich, R.F., & Perel, J.M. (1986b). Progress in pharmacotherapy of borderline disorders: A double-blind study of amitriptyline, haloperidol and placebo. *Archives of General Psychiatry, 43,* 691–697.

Sutherland, S.M., & Davidson, J.R.T. (1994). Pharmacotherapy for post-traumatic stress disorder. *Psychiatric Clinics of North America, 7,* 409–423.

Tyrer, P., Casey, P., & Gall, J. (1983). Relationship between neurosis and personality disorders. *British Journal of Psychiatry, 142,* 404–408.

van Vliet, I.M., den Boer, J.A., & Westenberg, H.G.M. (1994). Psychopharmacological treatment of social phobia: A double-blind, placebo-controlled study with fluvoxamine. *Psychopharmacology, 115,* 128–134.

Versiani, M., Nardi, A.E., Mundim, D., Alves, A.B., Liebowitz, M.R., & Amren, R. (1992). Pharmacotherapy of social phobia: A controlled study with moclobemide and phenelzine. *British Journal of Psychiatry, 161,* 353–360.

Weissman, M.M., Prusoff, B.A., & Klerman, G.L. (1978). Personality and the prediction of long term outcome of depression. *American Journal of Psychiatry, 135,* 797–800.

Wells, K.B., Burnam, A., Rogers, W., Hays, R., & Camp, P. (1992). The course of depression in adult outpatients: Results from the medical outcomes study. *Archives of General Psychiatry, 49,* 788–794.

Zimmerman, M., Coryell, W., Pfohl, B., Corenthal, C., & Stangl, D. (1986). ECT response in depressed patients with and without a *DSM-III* personality disorder. *American Journal of Psychiatry, 143,* 1030–1032.

8

Psychotherapy of Schizophrenia with Comorbidity

ALAN S. BELLACK

JACK J. BLANCHARD

The term *dual diagnosis* has had an inconsistent meaning in the literature on schizophrenia. The illness has characteristically been regarded as an overarching psychobiological condition that dominates the afflicted individual's psychological life and functioning. Documented *premorbid* mental retardation has generally been a criterion for the dual diagnosis label, but adult onset intellectual handicaps have been assumed to reflect the profound impact of the illness on cognitive functioning. Moreover, this use of the dual diagnosis classification has had greater implications for the source of public funding (mental health versus mental retardation agencies) and residential placement than for treatment or prognosis. Affective symptoms and behavioral disturbances such as generalized anxiety, phobias, and depression severe enough to be considered disorders in other individuals have often been discounted as secondary to the central schizophrenia pathology. Schizophrenia patients have also been assumed to lack the insight to experience real phenomenological distress.

Preparation of this manuscript was supported by NIMH Grants MH41577 and MH38636, a NIDA Grant to the first author, and NIMH Grant MH51240 to the second author.

This somewhat dehumanizing perspective has changed in the last 10 years. It has become increasingly apparent that the illness produces terrible pain and distress, and that patients actively attempt to cope with their symptoms and inability to fulfill social roles. Unfortunately, many patients resort to maladaptive coping strategies, including substance use and suicide. Reflecting these trends, the term *dual diagnosis* is now commonly used to categorize schizophrenia patients who meet *DSM-IV* criteria for substance abuse or dependency as well as those who have significant depression. In the latter case, the sobriquet refers primarily to post-psychotic depression and should be distinguished from depressive episodes associated with schizoaffective disorder (see below). In the following sections, the significance of these two types of dual diagnosis is discussed, and some of the assessment and treatment implications of the coexisting conditions are described.

SUBSTANCE ABUSE

Drug and alcohol abuse by schizophrenia patients is one of the most pressing problems facing the mental health system. The lifetime prevalence rate of substance abuse in schizophrenia is close to 50 percent (Regier et al., 1990), and estimates of recent or current substance abuse range from 20 percent to 65 percent (Drake, Osher, & Wallach, 1989; Mueser, Yarnold, & Bellack, 1992). Excessive substance use by schizophrenics has most of the same adverse social, health, economic, and psychiatric consequences as it does for other individuals. Moreover, it has additional serious consequences for these multiply handicapped patients. It increases the risk of symptom exacerbation and relapse, may compromise the efficacy of neuroleptics, and decreases compliance with treatment (Drake et al., 1989, 1990). It often serves as a significant source of conflict in families, a pernicious circumstance for schizophrenia patients who are highly vulnerable to heightened stress. Substance use also has deleterious cognitive effects that are superimposed on an information processing system that is already compromised (Bellack, 1992).

Reasons for Substance Abuse in Schizophrenia

The most prominent explanation for the high rate of substance abuse in psychiatric disorders is self-medication (Khantzian, 1985). It has been suggested that schizophrenia patients prefer to abuse stimulants (e.g., amphetamine, cocaine) to overcome the negative symptoms of schizophrenia (Schneier & Siris, 1987). Many patients also report that alcohol temporarily relieves persistent psychotic symptoms (Freed, 1975). However, studies of substance abusing schizophrenia patients have not documented a consistent relationship between substance use and symptomatology (e.g., Dixon, Haas, Weiden, Sweeney, & Francis, 1991; Negrete, Knapp, Douglas, & Smith, 1986; Sevy, Kay, Opler, & van Praag, 1990). Patients variably describe using drugs or alcohol to get high, relax, or alleviate boredom, and many report that drug use stimulates and energizes them (Dixon et al., 1991; Test, Wallish, Allness, & Ripp, 1989). It appears as if self-medication is only one factor contributing to abuse. Alcohol is the most commonly abused substance in schizophrenia as well as in the general population. Following alcohol, drug choice for schizophrenia patients varies over time and as a function of the demographic characteristics of the sample. For example, Mueser and colleagues (1992) reported that from 1983 to 1986, cannabis was the most commonly abused illicit drug among schizophrenia patients, whereas from 1986 to 1990, cocaine became the most popular drug, a change in pattern similar to that in the general population. For many patients, availability of substances appears to be more relevant than the specific central nervous system (CNS) effects, and polysubstance abuse or changes in drug of choice appear to be the norm. For example, the authors (Mueser et al., 1992) found that 42 percent of schizophrenia patients entering their acute care hospital during a four-year period met (lifetime) *DSM-III-R* criteria for abuse of two or more substances.

The situational context seems to be an important determinant of substance abuse for schizophrenia patients, as it is for other abusers (McCrady, 1993). Most of their illicit drug use (e.g., marijuana, cocaine) occurs in a social setting, as does about half of alcohol abuse (Dixon, Haas, Weiden, Sweeney, & Francis, 1990). These findings suggest that substance use may be associated with social-affiliative needs, including the desire to seem normal and be accepted by peers, as well as help to reduce social anxiety and compensate for social skill deficits. Overall, the data suggest that substance abuse by schizophrenia patients is motivated by the same factors that drive excessive use of harmful substances in less impaired populations: negative affective states, interpersonal conflict, and social pressures (Sandberg & Marlatt, 1991).

Assessment of Substance Abuse in Schizophrenia

DSM Substance Use Disorder Diagnostic Criteria

Criteria for substance *dependence* in the fourth edition of the *Diagnostic and Statistical Manual of Mental Disorders* (*DSM-IV;* American Psychiatric Association [APA], 1994) reflect a maladaptive pattern of use that results in clinically significant impairment or distress as manifested by three (or more) of the following occurring at any time in the same 12-month period: (1) tolerance; (2) withdrawal symptoms; (3) substance taken in larger amounts or over a longer period of time than was intended; (4) persistent desire or unsuccessful attempts to cut down or control use; (5) great deal of time spent to obtain substance or to recover from effects of substance use; (6) social, occupational, or recreational activities given up or reduced due to substance; (7) substance use continued despite knowledge of persistent or recurrent physical or psychological problems caused or exacerbated by use of substance.

The diagnosis of substance *abuse* reflects less severe substance use than that reflected in the *dependence* criteria, yet a diagnosis of substance *abuse* does reflect a maladaptive pattern of substance use. *DSM-IV* criteria for substance abuse require a maladaptive pattern of use that results in clinically significant impairment or distress as manifested by one (or more) of the following occurring at any time in the same 12-month period: (1) recurrent substance use resulting in failure to fulfill role obligations at work, school, or home; (2) recurrent use in situations in which it is physically hazardous; (3) recurrent substance-related legal problems; (4) continued use despite persistent or recurrent social or interpersonal problems caused or exacerbated by the effects of the substance.

Difficulties Specific to Diagnosing
Substance Use Disorders in Schizophrenia

In diagnosing a substance use disorder in an individual also presenting with psychotic symptoms, it is critically important to determine whether the psychotic symptoms are primary or are substance induced. A number of substances can result in psychotic symptoms either during intoxication or following withdrawal. Psychotic symptoms have been documented with excessive use of alcohol (Schuckit, 1982, 1983), cocaine (Tsuang, Simpson, & Kronfol, 1982; Welti & Fishbain, 1985), amphetamines, barbiturates, hallucinogens, marijuana, and opiates (e.g., Tsuang et al., 1982). As reflected in *DSM-IV* (APA, 1994), psychotic symptoms with onset during intoxication can be associated with alcohol, amphetamines, cannabis, cocaine, hallucinogens, inhalants, opioids, phencyclidine, sedatives, hypnotics, or anxiolytics. *DSM-IV* also notes that psychotic symptoms can occur with onset during withdrawal from alcohol, sedatives, hypnotics, or anxiolytics.

A diagnosis of substance-induced psychotic disorder (in *DSM-III-R* referred to as *organic hallucinosis* or *organic delusional disorder*) is appropriate when prominent hallucinations or delusions are present, with evidence from history, physical exam, or lab results that these psychotic symptoms developed during or within one month of intoxication or withdrawal. Evidence suggesting that the symptoms are better accounted for by a psychotic disorder such as schizophrenia might include onset of psychotic symptoms preceding substance use; psychotic symptoms persisting for a period following discontinuation of substance (e.g., one month); psychotic symptoms in excess of what would be expected given the type, dose and duration of substance use; or a clear history of non-substance-induced psychotic disorder.

In addition to differentiating substance-induced and non-substance-induced psychotic symptoms, the diagnostician is also faced with the difficulty of assessing the severity of substance-related problems. Of particular concern are those problems related to social, occupational, or psychological functioning. Specifically, as noted above, *DSM-IV* dependence criteria include a determination that (1) social, occupational, or recreational activities are given up or reduced due to the substance; or (2) substance use is continued despite the user's knowledge of persistent or recurrent physical or psychological problems caused or exacerbated by use of the substance. Similarly, abuse criteria include (1) recurrent substance use resulting in failure to fulfill role obligations at work, school, or home; or (2) continued use despite persistent or recurrent social or interpersonal problems caused or exacerbated by the effects of the substance. The difficulty in assessing these criteria in schizophrenia is that schizophrenia itself is characterized by such symptoms as grossly disorganized behavior and significant social and occupational impairment. Thus, it may be difficult to ascertain whether social or occupational problems arise from substance use or schizophrenia. Furthermore, changes in these domains may be difficult to detect in an individual with schizophrenia who may already live in social isolation or be unemployed or marginally employed. Similarly, one may encounter difficulty in disentangling the causal factors related to symptomatology. Does substance use cause or exacerbate psychotic symptoms or do these symptoms merely arise as a natural manifestation of the course of schizophrenia?

Further confusing the diagnosis of substance use disorders in schizophrenia are the effects of psychosis and cognitive impairment on the accuracy of self-reports. Diagnoses of substance use disorders are much more difficult in dual-diagnosis patients (Lehman, Myers, & Corty, 1989; Weiss

& Mirin, 1989). The marked cognitive impairment in schizophrenia (e.g., Blanchard & Neale, 1994) can also impede a patient's accurate recall. Drake and colleagues (1990) provide compelling data suggesting the importance of using a multimethod assessment involving diagnostic interviews, review of patient records, and ratings from clinical case managers. When only patient interviews were conducted, Drake and associates found that 26 percent of patients with schizophrenia who had a consensus alcohol use disorder denied or significantly minimized their alcohol-related problems during the interview. Clinical records alone were also an insensitive index of alcohol use disorders. Ratings from clinicians who had frequent contact with the patients proved to be a useful index of problems, even when the patients denied such problems in an interview (this form of rating is discussed below). In all, consensus diagnoses that integrate these various forms of information provide the most accurate assessment of substance-related problems and diagnoses.

Measures to Aid in Assessing Substance Use

Structured Clinical Interview for *DSM-IV* (SCID). The Structured Clinical Interview for *DSM-IV* has recently become available (SCID; First, Spitzer, Gibbon, & Williams, 1995). Although reliability information for the *DSM-IV* version is not available, the SCID for *DSM-III-R* (Spitzer, Williams, Gibbon, & First, 1990b, 1992) has demonstrated adequate reliability. Rater agreement for SCID-derived *DSM-III-R* diagnoses is quite adequate, with Kappas greater than .60 (Williams et al., 1992). Kappas were adequate for current and lifetime diagnoses (in patients) of alcohol abuse/dependence (.75, .73, respectively) and for other drug abuse/dependence (.84, .85, respectively). In examining agreement at a site specializing in the treatment of substance dependence, reliability for specific drug classes was examined. Again, Kappas were above .60 for diagnoses of alcohol, sedative, stimulant, opioid, and cocaine dependence. However, agreement was low for cannabis (Kappa = .22) and polydrug (Kappa = .34) dependence. In summary, these data indicate that the SCID is a reliable instrument.

Because the SCID relies on clinical judgment to increase validity, the training and skills of the interviewer are critical in obtaining reliable diagnoses. As recommended by Spitzer and colleagues (1992), diagnostic training of interviews should include study of *DSM-IV* diagnostic logic (Fauman, 1994, may be useful in this regard), the SCID *User's Guide* (Spitzer, Williams, Gibbon, & First, 1990b), and the use of videotape training materials for the SCID available from the Spitzer group. In addition, training is greatly enhanced when trainees have opportunities to observe and be supervised by a skilled SCID interviewer during administration of the SCID.

Clinical Case Manager Ratings. As noted above, Drake and colleagues (Drake et al., 1989, 1990; Drake & Wallach, 1989) have developed a five-point case manager rating scale. Ratings are anchored on the basis of severity of substance-related problems (see Drake et al., 1990). Case manager ratings have been shown to have high interrater agreement (Drake et al., 1989) and to have high agreement with consensus ratings (based on multiple sources of information) of alcohol problems (Drake et al., 1990). The case manager rating scale can provide important information in addition to interview-based assessment (e.g., SCID) in that problems denied in an interview may be picked up by case managers who have been familiar with the patient for some time.

Addiction Severity Index. The Addiction Severity Index (ASI; McLellan et al., 1980, 1992), now in its fifth edition (McLellan et al., 1992), can be used to index addiction-related problems. The ASI is a structured clinical interview designed to assess the severity of addiction-related problems experienced in seven areas: medical, legal, drug use, alcohol use, employment and support, family/social, and *psychiatric status.* For each area, the ASI assesses the number, extent, and duration of problems experienced by the individual in the past 30 days. Additionally, the patient provides subjective ratings of the recent (past 30 days) severity and importance of each problem area. Item severity ratings can be examined to determine specific problems relevant for referral and treatment. Additionally, composite scores for each of the seven problem areas can also be derived.

McLellan (McLellan et al., 1992) has indicated that individuals with a range of educational and background characteristics have been trained to conduct reliable ASI interviews. As with any structured interview, interviewers should have intimate knowledge of the structure and logic of the ASI, and reliability checks should be conducted to guard against rater drift. The reporting period used with the ASI is 30 days. This period has been selected to ensure that those interviewed have accurate recall of recent substance use; asked to report their use over the last 30 days, patients should be able to provide an accurate indication of use-related problems at the time of assessment. Although the ASI has been used in a variety of populations, including psychiatrically ill substance abusers (Lehman, Myers, & Corty, 1989), McLellan (McLellan et al., 1992) does caution that most of the validity and reliability data are based on substance abusers seeking treatment. Of greatest concern may be the validity of ratings obtained with individuals who may be unwilling to provide accurate responses (e.g., court-referred or incarcerated individuals, individuals seeking to avoid treatments).

The ASI has been used extensively in substance abuse research involving a variety of populations and has been translated into nine languages (see McLellan et al., 1992, for a review). The ratings obtained with the ASI have been shown to be reliable and valid for both alcoholics and drug addicts (McLellan et al., 1985, 1992). Additionally, the ASI has proven to be a sensitive indicator of treatment outcome (e.g., Carroll, Power, Bryant, & Rounsaville, 1993; McClellan, Luborsky, Woody, O'Brien, & Druley, 1983).

The Timeline Follow-Back Method. The Timeline Follow-Back (TLFB) method (Sobell & Sobell, 1973, 1992) is used to enhance patient recall in the assessment of alcohol consumption. The TLFB method was developed as a result of treatment goals other than abstinence. With goals such as moderation, there was a need for more precise measures of alcohol consumption to determine treatment outcome. The TLFB method utilizes two memory aids to facilitate recall. First, the TLFB method provides subjects with a calendar and asks them to provide reports of daily drinking over a specified period (typically no longer than 12 months). Key dates such as national holidays and significant personal events (e.g., birthdays, vacations) and newsworthy events (e.g., presidential election) are noted on the daily calendar. The second aid consists of a standard drink-conversion card (e.g., one standard drink = one 12-ounce beer, or one 5-ounce glass of wine, or 1½ ounces of hard liquor). This standardization is intended to teach subjects drink equivalencies and allows for the reporting of more than one type of beverage consumed during a drinking occasion. The TLFB method allows for a summary of the primary dimensions of use, including amount, frequency, pattern, and degree of variability. In addition to amount of drinking per day, the TLFB can also be utilized to obtain a subject's report of days spent in jail, in a hospital, or in a residential treatment facility. As summarized in Sobell and Sobell (1992), the TLFB method has demonstrated good test-retest reliability and good convergence with collateral reports of subjects' drinking; it also corresponds to official records of incarceration or treatment.

Broader Issues in Assessment of Substance Use

Assessment is critical not only in assigning a diagnosis but also in formulating proper treatment. Assessment should provide a functional analysis of an individual patient's use behavior and also a basis for evaluating the efficacy of the chosen treatment intervention. The assessment of substance use should not be considered a single event occurring prior to treatment; rather, assessment is an ongoing process. Continued assessment may suggest that initial treatment formulations require revision as (1) new relevant factors may arise during the course of treatment (e.g., the occurrence of family stress such as marital discord, or other environmental and financial stressors such as loss of housing or employment) or (2) individuals may disclose information they did not provide during the initial phases of assessment.

There are some guidelines regarding the minimal areas of assessment to facilitate treatment planning. The following outline for establishing a thorough functional analysis of substance use is adopted from Sobell, Sobell, and Nirenberg (1988) as well as McCrady (1993):

1. *A substance use profile for each client.* Specifically, patterns of use should be identified, including the different categories of drugs used, their frequency and amount of use, frequency and amount of use in a typical day, and route of administration.
2. *Usual and unusual substance use circumstances and patterns.* Such factors as social context (e.g., use alone or only with friends), time of day, or pattern during the week (e.g., only on weekends) should be recorded.
3. *Mood states and situations preceding and following substance use.* As an example, substance use may occur only when negative affective states such as anxiety or depression are experienced. Subsequent to use, individuals may report an increase of some moods or symptoms (e.g., guilt or psychotic symptoms) or a decrease in others (e.g., anxiety may diminish during the experience of the acute effects of the substance).
4. *History of withdrawal symptoms and tolerance.* A history of withdrawal symptoms will not only serve to determine *DSM-IV* dependence criteria but will also suggest the risk of withdrawal symptoms following future abstinence (e.g., during treatment or hospitalization). Physical dependence may indicate the need for detoxification within an inpatient, partial hospital, or outpatient program.

5. *Medical problems associated with or exacerbated by substance use.* An evaluation of medical complications exacerbated by substance use (e.g., seizure disorders, ulcers) or medical complications caused by substance use, such as impaired hepatic functioning in alcoholism or the possibility of infection with the human immunodeficiency virus (HIV) in individuals using intravenous routes of administration, will be important in understanding the severity of substance use and the full range of stressors faced by the individual. This knowledge is necessary to ensure proper medical intervention.

6. *Identification of possible hurdles client may encounter during treatment for substance use disorder.* For example, a likelihood of withdrawal symptoms or a lack of any prior attempts at abstinence may be risk factors. Similarly, continued contact with peer groups that use substances may also pose difficulties for treatment.

7. *Identification of social and personal resources.* If a patient has support from family members or friends, ambulatory treatment may be a good treatment alternative. Regarding personal resources, an individual's ability to set goals and change behavior in other contexts should again provide support for outpatient treatment. However, if cognitive functioning is impaired (e.g., in the areas of memory, problem solving, or as reflected in persistent thought disorder), a higher level of care might be considered.

8. *Full history of substance use problems and prior treatment or abstinence.* Information regarding number and type of prior treatments, and number of substance-related arrests will be useful to ascertain the extent and severity of substance use problems. Prior treatment information may also assist in identifying methods the individual has found useful, or those methods that have not been successful with the patient.

9. *Reports of thoughts, beliefs, or urges to take substance.* The assessment of cognitive events such as expectancies may serve to identify factors that trigger or maintain substance use.

10. *Positive consequences of substance use.* Knowledge regarding the reinforcing aspect of substance use (e.g., social facilitation, decrease in anxiety, increase in pleasure) will be useful in determining maintaining factors and methods of providing other means of achieving these reinforcers.

11. *Other life problems.* Knowledge of other problems in a patient's life is particularly critical in persons with schizophrenia, as they are likely

facing multiple stressors and problems associated with both substance use and schizophrenia. These factors may include poor or no housing, social isolation, family conflict, and financial difficulties.

Treatment of Substance Abuse in Schizophrenia

Obstacles to Effective Treatment

An extensive body of research on substance abuse and addiction in the general population indicates that critical factors in abstinence and controlled use of addictive substances include high levels of motivation to quit, the ability to exert self-control in the face of temptation (urges), cognitive and behavioral coping skills, and social support or social pressure (Miller, 1989; Rounsaville & Carroll, 1992; Sandberg & Marlatt, 1991). Unfortunately, the schizophrenic abuser often has limitations in each of these areas.

First, several factors can be expected to diminish motivation in schizophrenia patients. Most patients suffer from some degree of generalized avolition and anergia as a function of hypoactivity of the dorsolateral prefrontal cortex (Weinberger, 1987), medication side effects, or other social, psychological, and biological factors that contribute to negative symptoms (Andreason, Flaum, Swayze, Tyrell, & Arndt, 1990). They lack the internal drive and/or executive capacity to initiate the complex behavioral routines required for abstinence. They also frequently lack the positive social pressures from employers and family members that often stimulate efforts to reduce substance use (Osher & Kofoed, 1989). Evidence suggests that schizophrenia patients are hypersensitive to criticism and negative feedback, and they tend to deny or avoid discussion of their shortcomings (Bellack, Mueser, Wade, & Sayers, 1992); thus, they may be even more loath than other substance abusers to admit to problems pertaining to excessive substance use and to seek out help. Finally, self-medication is a powerful incentive for continued use. Persistent psychotic symptoms are among the most terrifying and disruptive aspects of the schizophrenia, leading to anxiety, depression, and withdrawal. It may be impossible to stimulate patients to be concerned about intra- and interpersonal goals, such as decreasing substance use, when they are besieged by hallucinations, confused by delusions, and overwhelmed by minor stresses. In light of these problems, an effective substance use program must (1) limit the demands for self-motivation and self-control, (2) minimize confrontation and criticism, and (3) help reduce the distress engendered by residual symptoms.

The *second* problem faced by schizophrenia patients is lack of the social and problem-solving skills necessary for behavior change. Social skills deficits are a hallmark of schizophrenia (Bellack & Mueser, 1993). Poor social competence contributes to the impoverished quality of life and social isolation experienced by many patients. Social disability is a primary source of stress, and it prevents patients from developing the supportive relationships that could provide a buffering effect. Schizophrenia patients also have substantial deficits in social problem-solving ability. In a recent study, schizophrenia subjects consistently overestimated the effectiveness of poor solutions to problems enacted by others; their own solutions were less suited to the problem situation, were less capable of being implemented, and were less likely to work; and these patients were less able to implement effective problem-solving strategies in conversations (Bellack, Sayers, Mueser, & Bennett, 1994). Schizophrenia patients have previously been shown to be unassertive and to have a variety of nonverbal and paralinguistic deficits (Morrison & Bellack, 1987). Data from Bellack and Mueser (1993) demonstrate that they are also less persistent in defending their point of view and less able to negotiate solutions to conflicts. Consequently, a substance abuse program should include social skills and problem-solving training that will enable patients to (1) develop relationships with nonabusing peers, (2) resist social pressures to imbibe, and (3) find alternative ways to cope with boredom and urges to use substances.

The *third* issue that must be considered in any psychosocial treatment for schizophrenia is the profound and pervasive cognitive impairment that characterizes the disorder. As previously indicated, schizophrenia patients have deficits in a host of specific information processing domains, including diverse aspects of attention and memory, and in executive functions necessary for initiating and carrying out higher-order reasoning and problem-solving processes (Neuchterlein & Dawson, 1984; Seidman, Cassens, Kremen, & Pepple, 1992). They often fail to initiate cognitive and behavioral routines that are in their response repertoire, a phenomenon described as "forgetting to remember." Moreover, they are highly vulnerable to stress, a susceptibility that further impairs their already limited information processing capacity. Given these impairments, it is unlikely that schizophrenia patients can respond to social learning strategies that place a premium on self-control, problem solving, and increasing self-efficacy. An effective substance abuse treatment must place limited demands on higher-level cognitive processes and teach skills that reduce the processing load in the natural environment. For example, schizophrenia patients can be taught stress reduction techniques, such as muscle relaxation, as well as ways to identify and avoid designated stress-provoking and high-risk situations. Diminished information processing capacity must be considered in implementing every aspect of a substance abuse program.

Treatment Needs

The problem of substance abuse in schizophrenia has generated a large literature, but to date there have been no well-controlled trials of an intervention specifically designed to deal with this pernicious combination. Several recent pilot and demonstration projects have yielded mixed results (Drake, McHugo, & Noordsy, 1993; Lehman, Herron, Schwartz, & Myers, 1993). Nevertheless, there is broad agreement on a number of requirements for effective treatment. First is the contention that dually diagnosed patients need a special program that integrates elements of both psychiatric and substance abuse treatment (Lehman et al., 1989). Traditional substance abuse programs are too confrontational and cognitively demanding for most schizophrenia patients, whereas substance abusing schizophrenia patients tend to be disruptive and noncompliant in purely psychiatric programs.

Schizophrenia and substance abuse are not simply additive but tend to exacerbate one another, dramatically complicating the treatment process. Consequently, treatment programs must be multidimensional, long term, and flexible (Test et al., 1989). Osher and Kofoed (1989) have conceptualized treatment as a four-stage process. The patient must first be *engaged* in treatment. Next, the individual must be *persuaded* to "accept long-term abstinence-oriented treatment" (p. 1027). Once these two stages have been achieved, the individual is ready for *active treatment,* which involves learning the skills needed to remain sober. Finally, the patient must be taught *relapse prevention* skills. The latter two stages require a variety of nonconfrontational elements commonly employed in treatment of primary substance abusers, including social skills training, problem-solving training, and a variety of strategies to anticipate and avoid high-risk situations and to cope with urges (Annis & Davis, 1989; Hall, Wasserman, & Havassy, 1991; Marlatt & Gordon, 1985). Some schizophrenia patients may not be able or willing to accept complete abstinence as a goal (Lehman et al., 1993; Test et al., 1989), in the same way that they often are reluctant to accept the possibility that they have an enduring and disabling illness. Hence, the initial treatment contract may need to focus on reducing the adverse consequences of substance use rather than on decreased use per se.

A Treatment Model

The authors are currently conducting pilot testing of a behavioral (skills training) therapy that will (ultimately) serve as a core component of a comprehensive rehabilitation program for schizophrenia patients with substance use problems. The therapy contains a number of elements organized into four segments: (1) social skills and problem-solving training to reduce interpersonal conflict that leads to substance use and that will enable patients to develop nonsubstance using social contacts; (2) coping skills for managing stress and residual psychotic symptoms that contribute to substance use; (3) education about the dangers of substance abuse and the availability of alternative self-help behaviors coupled with goal setting (i.e., for decreased use or abstinence); and (4) behavioral (social learning) treatment to decrease substance use and teach relapse prevention skills (e.g., drug avoidance and refusal skills; coping with urges). Segments 1 and 2 are implemented first and serve to facilitate engagement, making patients more receptive to segments 3 and 4.

The training approach is based on social skills training techniques that have been successfully employed since the 1970s with schizophrenia patients (Bellack, 1992). The content of segments 3 and 4 are adapted from substance abuse programs based on social learning theory that have proven to be effective with less-impaired patients (Annis & Davis, 1989; Hall et al., 1991; Marlatt & Gordon, 1985). The techniques are modified to meet the specific handicaps and needs of schizophrenic patients. The intervention is manualized to facilitate replication and dissemination. It is intended to be implemented as part of a comprehensive, long-term treatment program that includes sophisticated pharmacotherapy, training in activities required for daily living (ADLs), case management, and (where appropriate) family therapy.

A central tenet of the intervention is that limited generalization should be expected from cognitive rehabilitation programs for schizophrenia patients, and that the emphasis of training should be on overlearning of specific skills that are tied to specific situations (Bellack, 1992; Bellack & Mueser, 1993). Successful rehabilitation depends, in part, on minimizing demands on executive functions and other higher-order cognitive processes. The goal should be to develop a relatively automatic response repertoire that can be implemented in response to internal and/or environmental cues without complex reasoning or high levels of motivation.

Treatment Procedures

Segments 1, 2, 4, and the educational component of Segment 3 of the treatment are administered in a small group (six to eight) format, twice a week for 60 to 90 minutes (the goal setting component of segment 3 is administered individually). The group format allows patients to benefit from modeling and role-playing with peers. The small size provides ample opportunity for all patients to get adequate practice, while minimizing demands for sustained attention (i.e., they can rest while peers are role-playing). This group size also allows therapists to control even highly symptomatic patients. Groups are led by two therapists, permitting one therapist to work with one or two patients who are having particular difficulty with a skill while the main group continues to move along. It also allows one therapist to serve as a model and role play partner, while the other one directs the training.

The primary training techniques are instructions, modeling, role-play, and rehearsal. Each skill is broken down into component elements and competence is shaped by reinforcing gradual increments in the quality of performance. Patients have repeated practice opportunities within sessions and are urged to do homework assignments between sessions. Each session begins with a review of skills covered in the previous session. Patients are given written materials and prompt cards to minimize demands on memory. In general, the goal is to minimize demands on self-motivation and higher-level information processing by identifying a minimal number of relatively simple skills necessary to achieve conservative goals in specific situations, reaching a minimally acceptable performance level on each skill, overlearning by repeated practice, and using environmental prompts and supports wherever possible.

Segment 1: Social Skills Training. The goals of the social skills training segment are to enable patients to develop new social relationships and to avoid or reduce interpersonal conflict. It includes units on basic conversational skills, including beginning and ending conversations, asking open-ended questions, giving personal information, and making "I" statements.

A primary reason that traditional assertion skills do not generalize to the community is that patients often experience assertion as anxiety provoking and find it safer to escape from or avoid situations that involve even minor confrontations. However, avoidance and escape may themselves result in increased conflict and stress as, for example, when frustrated relatives escalate their level of criticism and hostility (Hahlweg et al., 1989). Consequently, the focus is on skills that serve to decrease conflict and arousal, including compromise, apology, and making requests. Patients are also taught how to make graceful exits from stressful or unpleasant situations that they cannot handle effectively.

The underlying assumption is that patients can be taught not to automatically avoid and escape from difficult situations if (1) they learn how to appraise what the interpersonal partner wants and might do, and (2) they have some response options they can use to deal with the situation (e.g., to gather more information, to leave gracefully, to apologize). Consequently, clinicians provide problem-solving training that focuses on teaching patients how to make accurate judgments about a partner's goals and the potential response consequences associated with different affective displays. The intent is to teach patients a specific and relatively narrow skill: how to determine what an interpersonal partner wants and what he or she is likely to do next. The teaching includes a combination of instruction and feedback applied first to audiovisual stimuli and then in role-playing.

Segment 2: Symptom Coping Techniques. Persistent psychotic symptoms are among the most distressing and disruptive aspects of the illness, leading to depression, withdrawal, and substance abuse. This domain has largely been viewed as the purview of neuroleptics, yet recent studies indicate that many patients whose symptoms are not eliminated by medication have learned to cope with these phenomena by using distraction, self-verbalization, and other nonmedical strategies (Wiedl & Schottner, 1991). Some of these ad hoc strategies are appropriate and effective, but some create problems in and of themselves (e.g., screaming back at voices), and some patients fail to discover effective strategies. This observation has led to increased recognition of the importance of teaching patients how to manage their symptoms more effectively (Strauss, 1989; Tarrier, 1992).

In a preliminary study, Tarrier (Tarrier et al., 1993) reported positive results for a coping skills training program that taught patients how to use a diverse set of cognitive, behavioral, sensory, and physiological strategies. The intervention used behavioral techniques (e.g., modeling, role-play, imaginal rehearsal, homework) and was tailored to the preferences and needs of each individual patient. The coping technique training described here is based on the program developed by Tarrier and associates.

As schizophrenia patients often are very reluctant to admit to having psychotic symptoms, coping training is introduced in segment 2, after patients have had some successful experiences and have developed a sense of trust for the therapists and group members in segment 1. The group format of the intervention facilitates the training as patients can suggest strategies to one another, share concerns and successes, provide mutual support, and learn from observation of their peers.

Segment 3: Education and Goal Setting. Perhaps the most critical aspect of reducing substance abuse with any population is getting each individual to recognize that he or she has a problem and needs to do something about it (Hall et al., 1991; Miller, 1989). Prochaska and DiClemente (1982) have hypothesized that this recognition and the decision to reduce consumption is a process rather than an event; the inclination to change evolves gradually over time, during which motivation to change behavior waxes and wanes. Characteristically, there are many false starts and failures before durable change occurs. This process has not been studied in schizophrenia, but schizophrenia patients appear to be at least as reluctant to admit having a problem as other abusers, and have at least as much difficulty making a commitment to change (Lehman et al., 1993). The education and goal setting components of the intervention are designed to enhance motivation to change.

Education about the negative consequences of substance use serves to increase the perceived value of behavior change, disabuse patients of myths that facilitate consumption, and provide information that makes change easier. The educational component is administered in one to two group sessions, modeled after the educational training used in other substance abuse programs (Heather, 1989). Emphasis is placed on providing information that is personally relevant to group members rather than presenting a general admonition about the dangers of substance use. Patients are prompted to relate personal experiences with psychoactive substances in an effort to alter the perceived risk/benefit ratio of substance use. The training proper is adjusted to the attention and learning capacity of patients and makes extensive use of audiovisual materials and handouts.

Abstinence is generally viewed as the most appropriate goal for non-schizophrenic drug abusers, and some clinicians have suggested that it is the most appropriate goal for schizophrenia patients as well (Osher & Kofoed, 1989). Nevertheless, abstinence is not a viable goal for all patients who enter treatment (Lehman et al., 1993; Test et al., 1989). There also is increasing evidence with nonschizophrenia populations that outcomes are better when patients select their own goals than when goals are imposed by programs (Miller, 1992; Rounsaville & Carroll, 1992). Consequently, the program described here promotes abstinence but does not require it as a precondition for participation. Moreover, experience has shown that some schizophrenia patients profit from substance abuse training without *ever* formally admitting that they have a problem and want to reduce usage. As long as they actively participate in the education and training, they can acquire skills and information that may be of use to them at some time in the future. In addition, patients may become more amenable to making changes if they have first acquired some skills and developed an increased sense of efficacy.

Goal setting is done in individual sessions after completion of the educational component. This strategy is based on Miller's (1989) *motivational interviewing* approach. The therapist gently but persistently applies pressure in an effort to help the patient see the negative consequences of substance use for him or her, as well as indicating that change is possible. The discussion is nonconfrontative and noncritical, emphasizing concrete risks and benefits for the individual patient rather than abstract or societal factors. Goals are written down in a formal contract that is signed by both parties and the patient is given a copy to keep. The goal is reviewed biweekly in brief individual sessions before or after group sessions for the duration of the intervention; changes are entertained, success is reinforced, and failures (lapses) are responded to with problem solving and encouragement.

Segment 4: Substance Use and Relapse Prevention Training. A number of behavioral treatment programs have been developed for treating addictive behaviors (Annis & Davis, 1989; Carroll, Rounsaville, & Gawin, 1991; Marlatt & Gordon, 1985). The programs differ in specifics, but they each emphasize the use of social learning principles to teach a variety of cognitive and behavioral skills. The authors employ a number of these procedures that are especially germane for the problems faced by schizophrenia patients and that they are likely to be able to learn and implement effectively. These include identifying and avoiding high-risk situations, resisting social pressure, problem solving to identify alternatives to substance use, and coping with urges and negative affect. Treatment in this segment builds on skills taught earlier (e.g., social skills and symptom coping skills) and employs the same basic social learning strategies: instruction, modeling, role-play, and feedback.

High-risk situations. Substance use appears to be under stimulus control (i.e., is associated with specific internal and external cues), and most patients have a number of high-risk situations in which they have considerable difficulty exerting control. Each patient is helped to identify the three or four most risky situations for him or her through group discussion. Then a variation of the problem-solving strategy that is employed in segment 1 is used to teach patients how to anticipate these situations and help them identify specific ways to avoid each high-risk situation. The goal here is to identify specific risks and solutions rather than teach a generic strategy that patients can use to deal with any new situation they might encounter.

Resisting social pressure. The unit on resisting social pressure employs the same techniques that were used for social skills training. Patients are helped to identify specific people and specific situations that might be difficult for them to resist. Effective refusal and escape skills are taught, and patients are presented with gradually increasing levels of demand and increasing realism. Patients are taught to discriminate playful teasing from ridicule and hostility, and to choose between remaining in the situation without imbibing and leaving the situation.

Coping with urges. Training for this skill capitalizes on the symptom coping training conducted in segment 2. Emphasis is placed on distraction, avoidance, and tension reduction. The therapists lead the group in identifying behaviors that are incompatible with substance use, analogous to the process employed to identify symptom coping strategies. Members are encouraged to share their own strategies as well as make suggestions to one another. Patients are helped to identify three or four key techniques that meet their needs, and they are led through real or simulated rehearsal whenever possible.

DEPRESSION

Affective symptoms are commonplace in schizophrenia (Siris, 1991). Anhedonia, anergia and alogia, dysphoria, hopelessness and demoralization, somatic concerns, disturbances of sleep and appetite, and interpersonal difficulties are evident at different points in the course of illness for most patients. The lifetime prevalence of suicide among schizophrenia patients is as high as 10 percent to 15 percent, and suicide is the leading cause of death among young male patients (Caldwell & Gottesman, 1990). Although suicide sometimes is tied to delusions or command hallucinations, it appears to be more commonly associated with hopelessness and depression. Depressive symptoms also appear to be the most reliable prodromal markers of impending relapse (Herz & Melville, 1980), although it is not clear whether these symptoms actively contribute to decompensation or simply reflect an evolving process. Depressive symptoms are thought to contribute to noncompliance with treatment and to be major sources of conflict between patients and their families (Hogarty et al., 1995).

Depressive symptoms may co-occur with psychotic symptoms in several different temporal patterns. Some patients with schizophrenialike illnesses experience major depressive episodes during periods of psychotic remission or when they otherwise fail to meet *DSM* or *International Classification of Diseases* (*ICD*) criteria for schizophrenia. For the most part, these individuals are more appropriately diagnosed as having schizoaffective disorder or bipolar disorder than schizophrenia (see later section). A second group suffer from a relatively chronic dysphoric mood, manifesting notable depression across phases of the schizophrenic illness. A third pattern entails prodromal depressive symptoms which, as indicated earlier, may serve as a stressor that contributes to breakdown or be a correlate of an incipient psychotic process.

A fourth pattern, which has been of greatest interest to clinicians and researchers is referred to as post-psychotic depression. As reported in a series of studies, between 25 percent and 60 percent of carefully diagnosed schizophrenia patients meet criteria for major depression in the months after recovery from acute psychotic episodes (Hogarty et al., 1995; Siris, Bermanzohn, Mason, & Shuwall, 1994), and many others suffer from subsyndromal depression. Although there is some suggestion that these depressive episodes are tied to recovery from psychotic episodes and are relatively short-lived, a 4.5-year follow-up by Harrow, Yonan, Sands, and Marengo (1994) found that syndromal depression may appear long after acute psychotic symptoms have remitted and that it may be enduring.

Unfortunately, depressionlike symptoms are not pathognomonic of a specific syndrome, phenomenology, or pathophysiology. To the contrary, they present a diagnostic, etiologic, and therapeutic dilemma. Many schizophrenia patients clearly experience true depression in response to the torment associated with psychotic symptoms or the despair that results from their repeated psychotic episodes and inability to achieve their life goals. This phenomenon is thought to be a major factor in postpsychotic depression, as patients become aware of their continued vulnerability. Schizophrenia patients have sometimes been assumed to lack sufficient insight or self-reflection to experience true hopelessness and depression. To the contrary, as evidenced by the data on suicide rates, the illness is undeniably a source of tremendous pain and suffering for most patients during at least some periods of their lives.

Depressivelike symptoms may also result from two entirely different factors: negative or deficit symptoms and extrapyramidal side effects (EPS) of antipsychotic medication. *Negative symptoms* make up one of three relatively orthogonal symptom domains that are common in schizophrenia (the others are delusions and hallucinations, and formal thought disorder/disorganization). The negative syndrome includes a variety of symptoms that are also associated with depression, including anhedonia, avolition, asociality, alogia, and flattened affect. Primary negative symptoms, also referred to as the deficit or defect state, create an enduring pattern that is associated with poor premorbid functioning, poor response to neuroleptics, and severe social impairment (Carpenter, Heinrichs, & Wagman, 1988). Numerous neuroimaging studies have reported structural and metabolic anomalies in patients with high levels of negative symptoms, especially in the frontal cortex (Wolkin et al., 1992). Although *secondary* negative symptoms may, in fact, actually be a manifestation of depression in some patients, primary negative symptoms are not phasic and are not accompanied by guilt, hopelessness, or other manifestations of intrapsychic pain that characterize true depression.

Neuroleptic drugs are assumed to work by decreasing the availability of dopamine or by blocking dopamine receptors in the frontal cortex (van Kammen & Kelley, 1991). However, dopaminergic systems are widely distributed throughout the brain and the action of neuroleptics are not specific to the system that is involved in the production of psychotic symptoms. Consequently, these medications have significant side effects that result from interference with normal dopaminergic activity in other brain regions, including the motor control areas of the extrapyramidal nervous system. One of the most disruptive extrapyramidal side effects is *akinesia* (or bradykinesia), a pervasive pattern of motoric slowing and reduction in spontaneous movements that resembles the lack of interest and energy seen in severely depressed patients (Casey, 1991; Harrow et al., 1994). Akinesia (along with other EPS side effects) appears within weeks after introduction of neuroleptics and typically declines with their discontinuation or with the introduction of supplementary anticholinergic medications. However, injectable forms of neuroleptics can be detected for as long as six months after drug discontinuation, confounding the differentiation of akinesia from depression. The differential diagnosis is especially difficult in patients who cannot or will not disclose their affect state, and when neuroleptics cannot be withdrawn.

A third factor that might be either a fundamental aspect of schizophrenia or a neuroleptic side effect also warrants brief mention: downregulation of dopaminergic reward systems. Dopamine plays a major role in the experience of reward or reinforcement (Carlsson, 1995). Schizophrenia may be associated with an endogenous downregulation of the portion of the dopaminergic system that controls the mediation of reward, especially in patients with pronounced deficit symptoms. Alternatively, the reward system may be suppressed by neuroleptics (Harrow et al., 1994). In either case, failure to experience reward or reinforcement from the environment could result in anhedonia or a depressionlike dysphoric state.

Assessment of Depression in Schizophrenia

Comorbid Depression and DSM-IV *Diagnostic Criteria*

In the assessment of depression in schizophrenia, one of the major diagnostic determinations concerns the distinction between schizophrenia and schizoaffective disorder. The validity for the distinction between schizophrenia and schizoaffective disorder has been addressed in several studies (e.g., Kendler, McGuire, Gruenberg, & Walsh, 1995; Maier et al., 1993). Kendler and colleagues (1995) found that although schizoaffective and schizophrenia probands had equivalent levels of positive symptoms, schizoaffective probands had significantly fewer negative symptoms, more affective symptoms, and a better course and outcome than did schizophrenia probands. Additionally, differences were found in the patterns of psychopathology in the families of schizophrenic and schizoaffective probands. Specifically, relatives of probands with schizophrenia and schizoaffective disorder had similar risks for schizophrenia; however, relatives of schizoaffective probands had greater risk for affective disorders than did relatives of schizophrenia probands (Kendler et al., 1995). In addition to determining an appropriate diagnosis, the assessment of depression may also be important in selecting appropriate use of adjunctive medications (e.g., Hogarty et al., 1995).

The *DSM-IV* criteria for schizoaffective disorder include a period of illness in which, at some time, there was a major depressive episode, a manic episode, or a mixed episode (i.e., a period in which criteria for both depressive and manic episode were met) concurrent with criteria A symptoms of schizophrenia (i.e., delusions, hallucinations, disorganized speech, grossly disorganized behavior or catatonic behavior, and negative symptoms including affective flattening, alogia, or avolition). The major depressive episode must include depressed mood. Thus, loss of interest or pleasure is not deemed sufficient in determining a major depressive episode according to *DSM-IV*, based on the frequent occurrence of loss of pleasure or interest in the nonaffective psychotic disorders. During the period of illness, delusions and hallucinations must occur in the absence of prominent mood symptoms for at least two weeks. These criteria are intended to rule out mood disorder with psychotic features. Other symptoms that might normally be counted toward a mood episode (e.g., difficulty sleeping, difficulty concentrating) are not allowed if they are the result of schizophrenia (e.g., a patient has difficulty sleeping because of hallucinations, psychotic disorganization impairs concentration, or there is weight loss because of delusions concerning poisoning).

Finally, symptoms that meet criteria for a mood episode must be present for a substantial portion of the total duration of the active and residual periods of the illness. These criteria are often the most difficult to assess accurately. First, doing so requires a detailed and accurate evaluation of *both* the active and residual symptoms covering the period of psychotic illness. Residual symptoms include negative symptoms (e.g., flat affect, poverty of speech, or avolition) or attenuated positive symptoms such as eccentric behavior, mildly disorganized speech, odd beliefs, or unusual perceptual experiences. Second, the duration of the depressive episode (with the above constraints in mind) must also be fully established. With information obtained concerning the temporal duration and the relationship between affective symptoms and schizophrenia established, a diagnosis can be made. The determination of schizophrenia versus schizoaffective disorder turns on whether the total duration of the mood episode was either "brief relative to the total duration of the active and residual periods" (schizophrenia) or "present for a substantial portion of the duration of the active and residual periods" (schizoaffective). As the *DSM-IV* notes, this distinction requires clinical judgment. Some examples may help clarify *DSM-IV* diagnostic differences between schizophrenia and schizoaffective disorder.

If a patient presents with Criterion A symptoms of schizophrenia for three months without a mood episode, then develops a major depressive episode lasting four months concurrent with symptoms of schizophrenia, and then has one month when the depressive episode remits but symptoms of schizophrenia persist and then fully remit, the appropriate diagnosis would be schizoaffective disorder; the mood episode was present for four of eight months and thus represents a substantial portion of the period of illness. However, the diagnosis may change if this patient were to continue to experience residual symptoms of schizophrenia for the next three years. The diagnosis would become schizophrenia because the total duration of illness is now 44 months and the depressive episode now represents only a brief period relative to the total episode. An additional diagnosis of depressive disorder not otherwise specified would be given to reflect the superimposed mood episode. These examples demonstrate the importance of establishing the temporal relationship of symptoms.

Depression and Negative Symptoms

In the assessment of depression in schizophrenia, one concern may be the clinician's ability to distinguish between the vegetative signs of depression and negative symptoms such as asociality, alogia, avolition-apathy, or blunted affect. However, despite the phenomenological overlap, some investigators have concluded that there is a clear distinction between negative symptoms and depression as evidenced in studies of schizophrenia (e.g., see Pogue-Geile & Zubin, 1988, for a review) and investigations comparing schizophrenics and other patient groups on ratings of depression and negative symptoms (e.g., Lewine, 1990; Pogue-Geile & Harrow, 1984). However, other investigators have identified correlations between ratings of depression and some negative symptoms such as avolition-apathy and anhedonia-asociality (Kitamura & Suga, 1991) or have found a high degree of comorbidity between depressive and negative symptoms (Siris et al., 1988).

The distinction between depression and negative symptoms may be clarified by examining the duration of these symptoms. Negative symptoms may represent enduring deficits (deficit symptoms; Carpenter, Heinrichs, & Wagman, 1988) whereas other negative symptoms may merely be transient and arise from environmental privation, drug effects, or dysphoric mood. Although a number of reliable scales are available for measuring negative symptoms (e.g., see Fenton & McGlashan, 1992) the Schedule for the Deficit Syndrome (SDS; Kirkpatrick, Buchanan, McKenney, Alphs, & Carpenter, 1989) is the only one that explicitly attempts to identify enduring traitlike negative symptoms and exclude negative symptoms that may be secondary to other factors such as depression. One comparative study examining methods of assessing negative symptoms has demonstrated that the SDS may provide ratings of negative (deficit) symptoms that show the greatest temporal stability (Fenton & McGlashan, 1992).

Treatment of Depression in Schizophrenia

There is an extensive literature on the use of individual and group psychotherapy with schizophrenia patients, but no treatment was found that was specifically developed to deal with depression. Generic verbal psychotherapies have proven to have small benefit for schizophrenia patients, and there is little reason to think that such treatments would be successful in alleviating depression (Bellack & Mueser, 1993; Mueser & Bellack, 1995). There is strong empirical support for both cognitive behavior therapy (CBT) and interpersonal therapy (IPT) in treating nonpsychotic populations. However, the data from the National Institute of Mental Health (NIMH) collaborative study suggest that these treatments were less effective with the more severely impaired patients in the sample. By implication, it seems unlikely that the prognosis for either treatment would be positive with schizophrenia patients. As indicated above in the discussion of substance abuse, these patients have significant information processing deficits, including difficulties with memory, problem solving, and complex reasoning. Structural or functional impairments in the dorsolateral prefrontal cortex also limit their ability to draw relationships between past and present experience and initiate effortful cognitive activity. These liabilities make it unlikely that they could successfully engage in the abstract processes involved in both CBT and IPT, or use the procedures spontaneously in the community.

This pessimistic view does not imply that clinicians cannot be of help to depressed schizophrenia patients. Moreover, the high risk for suicide makes it mandatory that some effort be made. Several clinical techniques have been shown to be useful with some patients, albeit without empirical support. A critical issue for many young patients is dealing with repeated relapses and failure to achieve life goals (e.g., to work, marry). Patients must eventually accept the fact that they have a chronic, debilitating illness, and recalibrate their goals and plans without becoming demoralized and hopeless. Schizophrenia patients, like many people adapting to other tragedies in life, often find it helpful to have a supportive relationship as they make this readjustment. Of course, schizophrenia patients also have difficulty developing close relationships and their thought disorder frequently creates distortions that make it difficult for them to accept help. They also rarely seek such help; it has to be made available for them to sample at their own pace. When it works, the process of relationship building is very gradual and often runs a very checkered course. The clinician must be consistent, patient, and willing to operate at the patient's comfort level. Even then, there is no guarantee of success; some patients are never able to develop a trusting relationship with a clinician.

Young schizophrenia patients, like many other young people, tend to have difficulty accepting advice from older individuals. The clinician must avoid becoming an arbiter of behavior and beliefs that may be bizarre and socially undesirable. It is necessary to develop a balance between honesty and responsibility on the one hand (e.g., pointing out risks or dangerous behaviors), and tolerance of the consequences of the illness on the other (e.g., not trying to talk the patient out of delusional beliefs). Schizophrenia patients seem to be hypersensitive to criticism; consequently, it is particularly important that the clinician learn to point out other ways to think about things or other solutions to problems without being overtly critical of the patient's choices, or lack thereof (e.g., "Maybe your neighbor really doesn't like you, but I wonder if there could be another reason that he doesn't smile when he sees you").

Another approach involves working with the patient's family members. The impact of family education and communication training on the course of schizophrenia is extensively documented in the literature (Bellack & Mueser, 1993; Mueser & Bellack, 1995). There are no specific data on the effects of these treatments on syndromal depression, but dysphoric affect, demoralization, and goal setting are frequent topics of discussion in these family treatments. In particular, family members are taught to better understand the very deleterious effects of the illness and to modify their own goals and expectations so as to put less pressure on their ill relative. In particular, they are taught that the patient's failure to work or go to school is often a direct result of the illness (e.g., negative symptoms), not a sign of laziness. One of the goals of such education is to reduce the level of conflict and hostility in the household. It is difficult enough for young patients to come to grips with their own limitations and disappointments. They can only experience heightened stress, unhappiness, and a sense of failure if their parents or siblings are openly critical and hostile about their lack of achievement. One additional point in regard to families is that they frequently are in a position to detect changes in their ill relatives before members of the clinical team do so. As depressive symptoms are among the most common prodromal signs, the family should be enlisted to help clinicians identify an increase in dysphoria that may put the patient at greater risk for suicide.

SUMMARY

Schizophrenia is a multihandicapping disorder that produces tremendous pain and suffering for patients and their families. The severity of the illness and its effects are magnified when the patient suffers from other disorders as well. This chapter has provided overviews of the two disorders that co-occur with schizophrenia most frequently: substance abuse and depression. Both conditions may result from the effects of schizophrenia and/or have independent diatheses. They also both present significant diagnostic dilemmas. An additional problem in regard to depression is that depressivelike symptoms may be produced by medication side effects and the negative symptoms of schizophrenia.

Substantial interest has developed in recent years in the treatment of both these conditions. Numerous psychosocial strategies have been promoted for dealing with substance abuse in schizophrenia, but the data to date are far from overwhelming. The authors have provided a summary description of a multicomponent behavioral treatment they are currently investigating with a grant from the National Institute of Drug Abuse (NIDA). At the current time, the only available treatments for depression with any empirical support are pharmacological (primarily tricyclic antidepressants). There does not appear to be much promise for psychotherapies used with less-impaired populations because of the significant cognitive impairments that accompany the disorder. Nevertheless, the risk of suicide is very high in this population, mandating that continued efforts be made to provide support for patients. Suggested here are some strategies that have proven helpful in the clinical setting; also encouraged is the use of family interventions to reduce hostility and stress in the home and to help identify prodromal signs of relapse.

REFERENCES

American Psychiatric Association. (1994). *Diagnostic and statistical manual of mental disorders* (4th ed.). Washington, DC: Author.

Andreasen, N.C., Flaum, M., Swayze, V.W., Tyrell, G., & Arndt, S. (1990). Positive and negative symptoms in schizophrenia: A critical reappraisal. *Archives of General Psychiatry, 47,* 615–621.

Annis, H.M., & Davis, C.S. (1989). Relapse prevention. In R. K. Hester & W. R. Miller (Eds.), *Handbook of alcoholism treatment approaches* (pp. 170–182). New York: Pergamon Press.

Bellack, A.S. (1992). Cognitive rehabilitation for schizophrenia: Is it possible? Is it necessary? *Schizophrenia Bulletin, 18,* 43–50.

Bellack, A.S., & Mueser, K.T. (1993). Psychosocial treatment for schizophrenia. *Schizophrenia Bulletin, 19,* 317–336.

Bellack, A.S., Mueser, K.T., Wade, J., & Sayers, S. (1992). The ability of schizophrenics to perceive and cope with negative affect. *British Journal of Psychiatry, 160,* 473–480.

Bellack, A.S., Sayers, M., Mueser, K.T., & Bennett, M. (1994). An evaluation of social problem solving in schizophrenia. *Journal of Abnormal Psychology, 103,* 371–378.

Blanchard, J.J., & Neale, J.M. (1994). The neuropsychological signature of schizophrenia: Generalized or differential deficit? *American Journal of Psychiatry, 151,* 40–48.

Caldwell, C.B., & Gottesman, I.I. (1990). Schizophrenics kill themselves too: A review of risk factors for suicide. *Schizophrenia Bulletin, 16,* 571–589.

Carlsson, A. (1995, December) *Cortical and subcortical pathways possibly involved in the deficit pathology of schizophrenia.* Paper presented at the 34th Annual Meeting of the American College of Neuropsychopharmacology, San Juan, Puerto Rico.

Carpenter, W.T., Heinrichs, D.W., & Wagman, A.M.I. (1988). Deficit and nondeficit forms of schizophrenia: The concept. *American Journal of Psychiatry, 145,* 578–583.

Carroll, K.M., Power, M-E., Bryant, K., & Rounsaville, B. (1993). One-year follow-up status of treatment-seeking cocaine abusers: Psychopathology and dependence severity as predictors of outcome. *Journal of Nervous and Mental Disease, 181,* 71–79.

Carroll, K.M., Rounsaville, B.J., & Gawin, F.H. (1991). A comparative trial of psychotherapies for ambulatory cocaine abusers: Relapse prevention and interpersonal psychotherapy. *American Journal of Drug and Alcohol Abuse, 17,* 229–247.

Casey, D.E. (1991). Neuroleptic drug-induced extrapyramidal syndromes and tardive dyskinesia. *Schizophrenia Research, 4,* 109–120.

Dixon, L., Haas, G., Weiden, P.J., Sweeney, J., & Francis, A.J. (1990). Acute effects of drug abuse in schizophrenic patients: Clinical observations and patients' self-reports. *Schizophrenia Bulletin, 16,* 69–79.

Dixon, L., Haas, G., Weiden, P.J., Sweeney, J., & Francis, A.J. (1991). Drug abuse in schizophrenic patients: Clinical correlates and reasons for use. *American Journal of Psychiatry, 148,* 224–230.

Drake, R.E., & Wallach, M.A. (1989). Substance abuse among the chronic mentally ill. *Hospital and Community Psychiatry, 40,* 1041–1046.

Drake, R.E., McHugo, G.J., & Noordsy, D.L. (1993). Treatment of alcoholism among schizophrenic outpatients: 4-year outcomes. *American Journal of Psychiatry, 150,* 328–329.

Drake, R.E., Osher, F.C., & Wallach, M.A. (1989). Alcohol use and abuse in schizophrenia: A prospective community study. *Journal of Nervous and Mental Disease, 177,* 408–414.

Drake, R.E., Osher, F.C., Noordsy, D.L., Hurlbut, S.C., Teague, G.B., & Beaudett, M.S. (1990). Diagnosis of alcohol use disorders in schizophrenia. *Schizophrenia Bulletin, 16,* 57–67.

Fauman, M. A. (1994). *Study guide to* DSM-IV. Washington, DC: American Psychiatric Association.

Fenton, W.S., & McGlashan, T.H. (1992). Testing systems for assessment of negative symptoms in schizophrenia. *Archives of General Psychiatry, 49,* 179–184.

First, M.B., Spitzer, R.L., Gibbon, M., & Williams, J.B.W. (1995). *Structured Clinical Interview for* DSM-IV *Axis I Disorders—Patient Edition (SCID–I/P, Version 2.0).* New York: New York State Psychiatric Institute, Biometrics Research Department.

Freed, E.X. (1975). Alcoholism and schizophrenia: The search for perspectives. *Journal of Studies on Alcohol, 36,* 853–881.

Hahlweg, K., Goldstein, M.D., Neuchterlein, K.H., et al. (1989). Expressed emotion and patient-relative interaction in families of recent onset schizophrenics. *Journal of Consulting and Clinical Psychology, 57,* 11–18.

Hall, S.M., Wasserman, D.A., & Havassy, B.E. (1991). Relapse prevention. In R.W. Pickens, C.G. Leukefeld, & C.R. Schuster (Eds.), *Improving drug abuse treatment* (pp. 279–292). NIDA Research Monograph No. 106. Rockville, MD: National Institute on Drug Abuse.

Harrow, M., Yonan, C.A., Sands, J.R., & Marengo, J. (1994). Depression in schizophrenia: Are neuroleptics, akinesia, or anhedonia involved? *Schizophrenia Bulletin, 20,* 327–338.

Heather, N. (1989). Brief intervention strategies. In R. K. Hester & W. R. Miller (Eds.), *Handbook of alcoholism treatment approaches* (pp. 93–116). New York: Pergamon Press.

Herz, M.I., & Melville, C. (1980). Relapse in schizophrenia. *American Journal of Psychiatry, 137,* 801–805.

Hogarty, G.E., McEvoy, J.P., Ulrich, R.F., DiBarry, A.L., Bartone, P., Cooley, S., Hammill, K., Carter, M., Munetz, M.R., & Perel, J. (1995). Pharmacotherapy of impaired affect in recovering schizophrenic patients. *Archives of General Psychiatry, 52,* 29–41.

Kendler, K.S., McGuire, M., Gruenberg, A.M., & Walsh, D. (1995). Examining the validity of *DSM-III-R* schizoaffective disorder and its putative subtypes in the Roscommon Family Study. *American Journal of Psychiatry, 152,* 755–764.

Khantzian, E.J. (1985). The self-medication hypothesis of addictive disorders: Focus on heroin and cocaine dependence. *American Journal of Psychiatry, 142,* 1259–1264.

Kirkpatrick, B., Buchanan, R.W., McKenney, P.D., Alphs, L.D., & Carpenter, W.T. (1989). The Schedule for the Deficit Syndrome: An instrument for research in schizophrenia. *Psychiatry Research, 30,* 119–123.

Kitamura, T., & Suga, R. (1991). Depressive and negative symptoms in major psychiatric disorders. *Comprehensive Psychiatry, 32,* 88–94.

Lehman, A.F., Herron, J.D., Schwartz, R.P., & Myers, C.P. (1993). Rehabilitation for adults with severe mental illness and substance use disorders. A clinical trial. *Journal of Nervous and Mental Disease, 181,* 86–90.

Lehman, A.F., Myers, P., & Corty, E. (1989). Assessment and classification of patients with psychiatric and substance abuse syndromes. *Hospital and Community Psychiatry, 40,* 1019–1025.

Lewine, R.R.J. (1990). A discriminant validity study of negative symptoms with a special focus on depression and antipsychotic medication. *American Journal of Psychiatry, 147,* 1463–1466.

Maier, W., Lichtermann, D., Minges, J., Hallmayer, J., Heun, R., Benkert, O., & Levinson, D.F. (1993). Continuity and discontinuity of affective disorders and schizophrenia. *Archives of General Psychiatry, 50,* 871–883.

Marlatt, G.A., & Gordon, J.R. (1985). *Relapse prevention: Maintenance strategies in the treatment of addictive behaviors.* New York: Guilford Press.

McCrady, B.S. (1993). Alcoholism. In D.H. Barlow (Ed.), *Clinical handbook of psychological disorders* (2nd ed., pp. 362–395). New York: Guilford Press.

McLellan, A.T. (1990). Measurement issues in the evaluation of experimental treatment interventions. *NIDA Research Monograph, 117,* 18–30.

McLellan, A.T., Kushner, H., Metzger, D., Peters, R., Smith, I., Grissom, G., Pettinati, H., & Argeriou, M. (1992). The fifth edition of the Addiction Severity Index. *Journal of Substance Abuse Treatment, 9,* 199–213.

McLellan, A.T., Luborsky, L., Cacciola, J., Griffith, J., Evans, F., Barr, H.L., & O'Brien, C.P. (1985). New data from the Addiction Severity Index. Reliability and validity in three centers. *Journal of Nervous and Mental Disease, 173,* 412–423.

McLellan, A.T., Luborsky, L., Woody, G.E., & O'Brien, C.P. (1980). An improved diagnostic evaluation instrument for substance abuse patients: The Addiction Severity Index. *Journal of Nervous and Mental Disease, 168,* 26–33.

McLellan, A.T., Luborsky, L., Woody, G.E., O'Brien, C.P., & Druley, K.A. (1983). Predicting response to alcohol and drug abuse treatments: Role of psychiatric severity. *Archives of General Psychiatry, 40,* 620–625.

Miller, W.R. (1989). Increasing motivation to change. In R.K. Hester & W.R. Miller (Eds.), *Handbook of alcoholism treatment approaches* (pp. 67–80). New York: Pergamon Press.

Miller, W.R. (1992). The effectiveness of treatment for substance abuse: Reasons for optimism. *Journal of Substance Abuse Treatment, 9,* 93–102.

Morrison, R.L., & Bellack, A.S. (1987). The social functioning of schizophrenic patients: Clinical and research issues. *Schizophrenia Bulletin, 13,* 715–726.

Mueser, K.T., & Bellack, A.S. (1995). Psychotherapy for schizophrenia. In S.R. Hirsch & D.R. Weinberger (Eds.), *Schizophrenia* (pp. 626–648). Oxford: Blackwell Science.

Mueser, K.T., Yarnold, P.R., & Bellack, A.S. (1992). Diagnostic and demographic correlates of substance abuse in schizophrenia and major affective disorder. *Acta Psychiatrica Scandinavica, 85,* 48–55.

Negrete, J.C., Knapp, W.P., Douglas, D.E., & Smith, W.B. (1986). Cannabis affects the severity of schizophrenic symptoms: Results of a clinical survey. *Psychological Medicine, 16,* 515–520.

Neuchterlein, K.H., & Dawson, M.E. (1984). Information processing and attentional functioning in the developmental course of schizophrenic disorders. *Schizophrenia Bulletin, 10,* 160–203.

Osher, F.C., & Kofoed, L.L. (1989). Treatment of patients with psychiatric and psychoactive substance abuse disorder. *Hospital and Community Psychiatry,* *40,* 1025–1030.

Pogue-Geile, M.F., & Harrow, M. (1984). Negative and positive symptoms in schizophrenia and depression: A follow-up. *Schizophrenia Bulletin, 10,* 371–387.

Pogue-Geile, M.F., & Zubin, J. (1988). Negative symptomatology and schizophrenia: A conceptual and empirical review. *International Journal of Mental Health, 16,* 3–45.

Prochaska, J.O., & DiClemente, C.C. (1982). Transtheoretical therapy: Toward a more integrative model of change. *Psychotherapy: Theory, Research, and Practice, 19,* 276–288.

Regier, D.A., Farmer, M.E., Rae, D.S., Locke, B.Z., Keith, S.J., Judd, L.L., & Goodwin, F.K. (1990). Comorbidity of mental disorders with alcohol and other drug abuse. *Journal of the American Medical Association, 264,* 2511–2518.

Rounsaville, B.J., & Carroll, K.M. (1992). Individual psychotherapy for drug abusers. In J.H. Lowinson, P. Ruiz, R.B. Millman, & J.G. Langrod (Eds.), *Substance abuse: A comprehensive textbook* (2nd ed., pp. 496–507). Baltimore: Williams & Wilkins.

Sandberg, G.G., & Marlatt, G.A. (1991). Relapse prevention. In D.A. Ciraulo & R.I. Shader (Eds.), *Clinical manual of chemical dependence* (pp. 377–399). Washington, DC: American Psychiatric Press.

Schneier, F.R., & Siris, S.G. (1987). A review of psychoactive substance use and abuse in schizophrenia: Patterns of drug choice. *Journal of Nervous and Mental Disease, 175,* 641–650.

Schuckit, M.A. (1982). The history of psychotic symptoms in alcoholics. *Journal of Clinical Psychiatry, 43,* 53–57.

Schuckit, M.A. (1983). Alcoholism and other psychiatric disorders. *Hospital and Community Psychiatry, 34,* 1022–1027.

Seidman, L.J., Cassens, G.P., Kremen, W.S., & Pepple, J.R. (1992). Neuropsychology of schizophrenia. In R. F. White (Ed.), *Clinical syndromes in adult neuropsychology: The practitioner's handbook* (pp. 381–449). New York: Elsevier.

Sevy, S., Kay, S.R., Opler, L.A., & van Praag, H.M. (1990). Significance of cocaine history in schizophrenia. *Journal of Nervous and Mental Disease, 178,* 642–648.

Siris, S.G. (1991). Diagnosis of secondary depression in schizophrenia: Implications for *DSM-IV. Schizophrenia Bulletin, 17,* 75–95.

Siris, S.G., Adan, F., Cohen, M., Mandeli, J., Aronson, J., & Casey, E. (1988). Postpsychotic depression and negative symptoms: An investigation of syndromal overlap. *American Journal of Psychiatry, 145,* 1532–1537.

Siris, S.G., Bermanzohn, P.C., Mason, S.E., & Shuwall, M.A. (1994). Maintenance imipramine therapy for secondary depression in schizophrenia. *Archives General Psychiatry, 51,* 109–115.

Sobell, L.C., & Sobell, M.B. (1973). A self-feedback technique to monitor drinking behavior in alcoholics. *Behaviour Research and Therapy, 11,* 237–238.

Sobell, L.C., & Sobell, M.B. (1992). Timeline follow-back: A technique for assessing self-reported ethanol consumption. In J. Allen & R.Z. Litten (Eds.), *Measuring alcohol consumption: Psychosocial and biological methods* (pp. 41–72). Totowa, NJ: Humana Press.

Sobell, L.C., Sobell, M.B., Leo, G.I., & Cancilla, A. (1988). Reliability of time-line method: Assessing normal drinkers' reports of recent drinking and a comparative evaluation across several populations. *British Journal of Addiction, 83,* 393–402.

Sobell, L.C., Sobell, M.B., & Nirenberg, T.D. (1988). Behavioral assessment and treatment planning with alcohol and drug abusers: A review with an emphasis on clinical application. *Clinical Psychology Review, 8,* 19–54.

Spitzer, R.L., Williams, J.B.W., Gibbon, M., & First, M.B. (1990a). *Structured Clinical Interview for* DSM-III-R. Washington, DC: American Psychiatric Press.

Spitzer, R.L., Williams, J.B.W., Gibbon, M., & First, M.B. (1990b). *SCID: User's Guide for the Structured Clinical Interview for* DSM-III-R. Washington, DC: American Psychiatric Press.

Spitzer, R.L., Williams, J.B.W., Gibbon, M., & First, M.B. (1992). The Structured Clinical Interview for *DSM-III-R* (SCID). I: History, rationale, and description. *Archives of General Psychiatry, 49,* 624–629.

Strauss, J.S. (1989). Subjective experiences of schizophrenia: Toward a new dynamic psychiatry II. *Schizophrenia Bulletin, 15,* 179–187.

Tarrier, N., Beckett, R., Harwood, S., Baker, A., Yusupoff, L., & Ugarteburu, I. (1993). A trial of two cognitive-behavioral methods of treating drug-resistant residual psychotic symptoms in schizophrenic patients: I. Outcome. *British Journal of Psychiatry, 162,* 524–532.

Tarrier, N. (1992). Management and modification of residual positive psychotic symptoms. In M. Birchwood & N. Tarrier (Eds.), *Innovations in the psychological management of schizophrenia: Assessment, treatment, and services* (pp. 147–169). Chichester: Wiley.

Test, M.A., Wallisch, L.S., Allness, D.J., & Ripp, K. (1989). Substance use in young adults with schizophrenic disorders. *Schizophrenia Bulletin, 15,* 465–476.

Tsuang, M.T., Simpson, J.C., & Kronfol, Z. (1982). Subtypes of drug abuse with psychosis: Demographic characteristics, clinical features, and family history. *Archives of General Psychiatry, 39,* 141–147.

van Kammen, D.P., & Kelley, M. (1991). Dopamine and norepinephrine in schizophrenia: An integrative perspective. *Schizophrenia Research, 4,* 173–191.

Weinberger, D.R. (1987). Implications of normal brain development for the pathogenesis of schizophrenia. *Archives of General Psychiatry, 44,* 660–669.

Weiss, R.D., & Mirin, S.M. (1989). The dual diagnosis alcoholic: Evaluation and treatment. *Psychiatric Annals, 19,* 261–265.

Welti, C.V., & Fishbain, D.A. (1985). Cocaine-induced psychosis and sudden death in recreational cocaine users. *Journal of Forensic Sciences, 30,* 873–880.

Wiedl, K.H., & Schottner, B. (1991). Coping with symptoms of schizophrenia. *Schizophrenia Bulletin, 17,* 525–538.

Williams, J.B.W., Gibbon, M., First, M.B., Spitzer, R.L., Davies, M., Borus, J., Howes, M.J., Kane, J., Pope, H.G., Rounsaville, B., & Wittchen, H.U. (1992). The Structured Clinical Interview for *DSM-III-R* (SCID). II: Multisite test-retest reliability. *Archives of General Psychiatry, 49,* 630–636.

Wolkin, A., Sanfilipo, M., Wolf, A.P., Angrist, B., Brodie, J.D., & Rotrosen, J. (1992). Negative symptoms and hypofrontality in chronic schizophrenia. *Archives of General Psychiatry, 49,* 959–965.

9

Drug Treatment of Schizophrenia with Comorbidity

SAMUEL G. SIRIS
PAUL C. BERMANZOHN
RICHARD J. KESSLER
RICHARD PITCH

Schizophrenia is well known to be a heterogeneous disorder, but there is still no agreement on how that heterogeneity ought best be organized—specifically, for the purposes of treatment. The current *Diagnostic and Statistical Manual of Mental Disorders* (*DSM-IV*) (American Psychiatric Association [APA], 1994) specifies the following standard diagnostic categories: paranoid, disorganized, catatonic, undifferentiated, and residual; these, however, have never been particularly useful subgroupings for informing psychopharmacologic treatment strategies. This chapter, therefore, approaches the issue of medication management in schizophrenia from the perspective of *comorbidity*, or, as these features might alternatively be conceptualized, *associated syndromes* in the course of schizophrenia.

For the most part, these associated syndromes appear, and take on clinical importance, over the longitudinal course of the schizophrenic disorder. Their implications for treatment are therefore likely to assume importance not only during florid psychotic episodes but also during chronic maintenance phases of treatment. At these times, specifically psychotic symptomatology may be stable, residual, or in remission, although behavioral or communication peculiarities or negative symptom features may still be evident.

MOOD SYNDROMES

Prominent among the associated syndromes that may occur in the course of schizophrenia are a variety of syndromes that, but for the existence of the schizophrenic state, would be unmistakably diagnosable as one of several primary mood syndromes. These can be organized into depressionlike syndromes, anxietylike syndromes, and obsessive compulsivelike syndromes. Each of these is considered in terms of its phenomenology and/or differential diagnosis and its relevant psychopharmacologic approaches.

Depressionlike Syndromes

A differential diagnosis of depressionlike syndromes in the course of schizophrenia includes medical or organic conditions that can present a phenocopy of depression, the prodrome of a new psychotic episode, disappointment reactions that can be either acute (situational) or chronic (demoralization), and the extrapyramidal side effects of either akinesia or akathisia. Additionally, the so-called negative symptom syndrome of schizophrenia can frequently mimic depression, and there is the controversial hypothesis that neuroleptic medications can specifically lead to depression as a side effect. A final question involves the frequency with which a "true" depression may occur in the course of schizophrenia. Each of these different diagnoses has different implications for medication management.

Medical or Organic Conditions

Many medical conditions are associated with stigmata that can present similarly to those of depression (Bartels & Drake, 1988). These include anemia, cancer, endocrine disorders, infections, and neurological conditions. Therefore, any schizophrenic patient presenting with a syndrome of depression warrants a medical evaluation. Furthermore, a number of medications used to treat medical conditions are associated with possible side effects that constitute depression. Several antihypertensive and other cardiac medications, including alphamethyl dopa, beta blockers, and possibly calcium channel blockers, are in this category. Vulnerable individuals may also experience sedative hypnotics, sulfonamides, and indomethacin as depressogenic. Other medications have been associated with the generation of depression at the time of their discontinuation. These include cortico-steroids and psychostimulants. The medication management of each of these situations, of course, involves the management of the medical condition from which the patient suffers, with attention to the potential depressogenic effects of the various pharmacologic compounds involved.

Other substances also need to be considered as potentially playing a role as a cause of depression. These include both the use and discontinuation of substances of abuse or common use. Alcohol is probably the most commonly used recreational substance, and both its use and its discontinuation can be associated with depression. Marijuana is another common substance in this category. Cocaine and other stimulants can lead to depression either at the time of acute withdrawal or in association with chronic use. Often overlooked substances of common discontinuation are caffeine and nicotine. Indeed, many inpatient psychiatric units acutely discontinue the use of these pharmacologic compounds as a matter of policy. Similarly, outpatients may abruptly give up smoking or caffeinated coffee and not mention this unless they are specifically asked. A delicate balance of one health effect against another may be required in such situations.

Prodrome of Psychosis

Insomnia, indecisiveness, impaired concentration, reduced energy, and guilty preoccupations have often been reported as components of the early manifestations of psychotic relapse, and blue mood can occur at this stage of illness as well (Docherty, vanKammen, Siris, & Marder, 1978; Green, Nuechterlein, Ventura, & Mintz, 1990; Hirsch et al., 1989). A diagnosis of psychotic prodrome is made definitively only by observing the patient. Therefore, the first step in the treatment of any newly diagnosed case of depression in schizophrenia is to follow up on the patient closely and intervene quickly to treat a psychotic episode if that emerges. If psychosis is going to occur, it will become evident within a few days, or at most a week or two following the onset of depressionlike symptomatology.

Disappointment Reactions

Transient disappointment reactions are most easily identified because they are just that: transient. Usually a logical stressor can be identified, although the psychological and communication difficulties that schizophrenic patients may manifest can render the stressor obscure. At any rate, the same initial watchful waiting, with support, that is appropriate for dealing with the possibility of psychosis prodrome will provide the needed opportunity for a transient disappointment reaction to resolve. Chronic disappointment reactions, in the form of a demoralization syndrome (Klein, 1974), do not resolve on their own in a short period of time. Schizophrenic patients, indeed, often have a considerable amount to be demoralized about, so this situation is important to recognize. There is no specific appropriate psychopharmacological treatment for demoralization, but other pharmacologically treatable forms of depression need to be ruled out before diagnosing it (despite the patient's possible protests that the whole problem is psychological). Demoralization, in its own right, may be important to identify because specific psychosocial interventions may be indicated. Specifically, a subjective sense of incompetence has been described as being central to demoralization rather than a reduction in motivation which is more typical of depression (de Figueiredo, 1993).

Akinesia

Akinesia is an extrapyramidal neuroleptic side effect that can so closely resemble depression that at times it can be an absolute phenocopy (Bermanzohn & Siris, 1992; Rifkin, Quitkin, & Klein, 1975; Siris, 1987; Van Putten & May, 1978). Akinesia, of course, is often easily diagnosable by manifestations of muscle stiffness or reduced large muscle movements such as limited arm swing, shuffling gait, or bent posture. Less readily recognizable manifestations may include reductions of small muscle movements, such as those of the larynx or face, which can result in monotonous speech or lack of changes in facial expression. But the form of akinesia that is most easily mistaken for depression, and that can occur in the absence of any muscle stiffness or lack of muscle movement, is the form that is manifested by a lack of initiation or maintenance of motor activity. Behaviorally, this situation presents as a lack of spontaneity. Such patients may sit "like a bump on a log" or "as if their starter motor is broken." They can respond to social advances by others but apparently have grossly reduced initiative on their own. The patients themselves, of course, do not recognize the origin of this circumstance as being extrapyramidal. Doing little, they find their lives uninteresting, boring, and/or pleasureless, blame themselves for being lazy, and see their situation as hopeless and helpless. Such akinetic patients can also show prominent blue mood, completing a depressive syndrome, although it can be unclear whether the blue mood is secondary to the situation or a primary component of the akinesia itself. It is crucial to recognize this form of akinesia, or "akinetic depression" (Van Putten & May, 1978), because it is readily responsive to antiparkinsonian medication, generally resolving within a few days to a week when adequate doses of antiparkinsonian drugs are employed. Adequate doses drugs are required, however. Indeed, as there can be as much as a 10-fold variation in the metabolic rate of antiparkinsonian medications (Tune & Coyle, 1980), it is sometimes necessary to increase the doses of these drugs gradually until anticholinergic side effects are encountered (or until the akinesia clears) to be certain that the trial was adequate. Nonetheless, treating akinesia aggressively is often well worth the effort because the positive results can be dramatic, in terms of both the patients' mood and their functional capacities.

Akathisia

The other common extrapyramidal neuroleptic side effect that can easily present as a phenocopy of depression is akathisia. As a state of motor restlessness, akathisia is the opposite of akinesia because with akathisia, patients act as if "their starter motor won't turn off." Similar to akinesia, however, akathisia often represents a substantially dysphoric state (Van Putten, 1975). Sometimes the motor aspects of the akathisia are subtle and the restlessness relatively minor, but the dysphoria can still be prominent. Perhaps because of the propensity for motor activity, akathisia can be a dangerous, depressionlike state in schizophrenia because it has been associated with suicide (Shear, Frances, & Weiden, 1983). Unfortunately, akathisia responds only sporadically to antiparkinsonian medications. It may, however, resolve with adjunctive benzodiazepine or propanolol treatment (Fleischhaker, Roth, & Kane, 1990).

Negative Symptoms of Schizophrenia

Negative symptoms of schizophrenia also can present a situation of substantial phenomenologic overlap with depression (Bermanzohn & Siris, 1992; Carpenter, Heinrichs, & Alphs, 1985; Siris et al., 1988). The most important features common to these two conditions are lack of energy and reduced pleasure. On the other hand, the features that best distinguish these two states would be depressed mood (indicating depression) and blunted affect (indicating negative symptoms). Often, however, these two features are not sufficiently unequivocal clinically to make this distinction clear. From a mechanistic perspective, negative symptoms are thought to represent aspects of a hypodopaminergic state, a dopamine drought as it were, in distinction to the dopamine storm that is considered to occur in psychosis (Davis, Kahn, Ko, & Davidson, 1991). It is therefore easy to see how excessive doses of neuroleptic medications, which block dopamine neurotransmission, could exacerbate such a condition. By the same token, low-dose neuroleptic maintenance strategies may have been successful in terms of the patients' psychosocial functioning based on this mechanism. This negative symptom consideration may constitute yet one more aspect to the uncertainty, both clinical and theoretical, about whether neuroleptic drugs can cause depression as a side effect.

Neuroleptic-Induced Dysphoria

There is controversy as to whether neuroleptic medications produce the side effect of dysphoria beside that properly subsumed under the heading of akinesia or akathisia. An explanation for this effect would be readily available, as rat experiments have shown that dopaminergic pathways that can be blocked by neuroleptic administration are involved in the experience of reward or pleasure (Wise, 1982). Although several early anecdotal reports appear to support this notion (DeAlarcon & Carney, 1969; Galdi, 1983; Johnson, 1981), and one recent major study has shown results congruent with this hypothesis (Harrow, Yonan, Sands, & Marengo, 1994), most of the more recent more highly controlled studies have failed to find confirming evidence (Barnes, Curson, Liddle, & Patel, 1989; Hirsch et al., 1989; Siris, 1991a). These include studies that have tracked depressive symptomatology over the course of neuroleptic-treated psychotic episodes (Green et al., 1990; Hirsch et al., 1989), studies in which schizophrenic patients on neuroleptics are compared with those not receiving neuroleptics (Hirsch et al., 1989; Hogarty & Munetz, 1984), and studies in which patients on higher versus lower neuroleptic doses are compared, or higher versus lower blood levels of the neuroleptic are compared (Barnes et al., 1989; Roy, 1984; Siris, Strahan, Mandeli, Cooper, & Casey, 1988).

Syndromal Depression in Schizophrenia and the Use of Antidepressants

Reviews of the literature have indicated that depressive syndromes occur in approximately one-quarter of schizophrenic patients at times when they are not floridly psychotic (McGlashan & Carpenter, 1976; Siris, 1991a). Questions have consequently been raised about the therapeutic utility of using antidepressant medication in this condition. Early work seemed to establish that antidepressants used as the *only* drug in schizophrenia were not helpful and probably contributed to an exacerbation of psychosis (Siris, vanKammen, & Docherty, 1978). However, a different story seems to emerge from careful double-blind studies of antidepressants used adjunctively to neuroleptics in patients who are clearly depressed and otherwise relatively stable (Hogarty et al., 1995; Siris, 1991a). Particularly this appears to be the case among outpatients, and the strongest positive effects have been noted when vigorous efforts have been made beforehand to rule out the confound of neuroleptic induced akinesia (Siris, Morgan, Fagerstrom, Rifkin, & Cooper, 1987). It may be useful to increase the dosage of an adjunctive antidepressant more slowly than would be the case in primary depressions, but full therapeutic doses of antidepressants should ultimately be tried, and for adequate durations of treatment (nine weeks or more) to get optimal effects. The target symptoms of this treatment are blue mood, low energy level, and similar symptoms classically associated with the depression syndrome (Siris et al., 1987). Among those depressed schizophrenic patients who respond favorably to an adjunctive antidepressant initially, the one study that has addressed the point indicates that continuation and maintenance treatment with the adjunctive antidepressant are beneficial (Siris, Bermanzohn, Mason, & Shuwall, 1994). Indeed, in that study, not only was the risk of recurrent depression lower in patients maintained on the adjunctive antidepressant than among those randomized to adjunctive placebo, but the risk of psychotic exacerbation was actually lower in the adjunctive antidepressant group as well. On the other hand, adjunctive treatment with an antidepressant medication for schizophrenic patients who are flagrantly psychotic as well as depressed has not been shown to be beneficial (Kramer et al., 1989). Therefore, the current evidence indicates that the first choice treatment for acute episodes of schizoaffective depression, for example, would be with a neuroleptic alone, not the combination of a neuroleptic and an antidepressant (Siris, 1993b).

Anxiety Syndromes

Research about depressionlike syndromes in the course of schizophrenia has sparked and informed investigations of anxietylike syndromes as well. Anxiety syndromes may have been difficult to recognize in schizophrenic patients for several reasons. First, until the *DSM-III-R* in 1987, most of the anxiety disorders were excluded from diagnosis if the patient also met criteria for schizophrenia. This is a hierarchical bias in diagnosis that may continue to lead the clinician's attention away from anxiety syndromes in schizophrenic patients. Second, the field has had a tendency to explain away anxiety as a natural and expected response to frightening psychotic experiences, much as the field originally tended to understand postpsychotic depression simply as the patient's reasonable grief at recognizing his illness and its impact after recovery from an episode of acute psychosis. Third, patients with schizophrenia are likely to report associated anxiety symptoms in a distorted or even delusional way. For these reasons, the clinician must look for anxiety syndromes specifically in order to identify them.

The differential diagnosis of anxietylike syndromes in the course of schizophrenia includes situational anxiety, anxiety as a prodrome or component of psychosis, panic, agoraphobia, social phobia, akathisia, medical conditions, and substance-related anxiety.

Situational Anxiety

Situational anxiety can arise when a person faces a possibility of harm that he or she may not be able to avoid. From a cognitive processing model (Beck & Emery, 1985), pathological anxiety usually arises when a person tends either to overestimate the degree of danger and probability of harm or to underestimate his or her ability to cope with the perceived threats. Schizophrenic patients may be at increased risk for this kind of anxiety because of their misperceptions of danger and/or an appreciation of their impaired coping strategies. Frequently, when they are unable to filter out stimuli as insignificant, they may experience ideas of reference and persecution and become hypervigilant and anxious. Conversely, when schizophrenic patients filter out too much, or too badly, they may exercise poor judgment and get themselves into truly dangerous situations. They may eventually learn more global avoidance behaviors to reduce this risk. In all these cases, reality testing and cognitive retraining may help reduce the anxiety and the real dangers these patients experience.

Prodromal Anxiety

Like depression, anxiety is sometimes an early manifestation of a psychotic relapse (Docherty et al., 1978). Patients may report a free-floating anxiety or a hypervigilance that they cannot explain before going on to develop frank psychotic symptoms. To that end, some authors have suggested augmentation of neuroleptics with benzodiazepines when such early anxiety presents, to prevent full relapse of psychosis; these results, however, are variable (for reviews of this literature, see Pies, 1984; Siris, 1993b). Anxiety and agitation can also arise as a component of increased psychosis. Patients may become hypervigilant as a natural response to delusions of persecution or broadcasting, or become fearful of losing control to dangerous command hallucinations. Theoretically, though, anxiety may represent not only a response to these primary psychotic processes but as part and parcel of the process itself. Such a stress-diathesis model is supported by neurochemical evidence that a gamma aminobuteric acid (GABA)-dopamine mechanism mediates the response to stress in schizophrenia (Breier, Wolkowitz, & Pickar, 1989). Treatment of this kind of anxiety is generally with antipsychotic medication with or without the addition of benzodiazepines.

Panic and Agoraphobia

Panic attacks may occur in at least one quarter of schizophrenic patients (Cutler, 1994), but may remain unidentified when clinicians fail to look for them specifically. Panic itself is a very distressing symptom that leads to heavy use of mental health services (Boyd, 1986). It is associated with significant morbidity and mortality, including impairment in social and occupational functioning and suicide. Because the patient with schizophrenia is already at risk for these complications, it seems prudent to look for and treat this associated syndrome.

The physical symptoms associated with panic attacks may make them easier to recognize than other anxiety syndromes in schizophrenic patients. The nature of the panic attacks, as well as the associated anticipatory anxiety and avoidance behaviors, seems to be virtually identical to those symptoms reported by patients without schizophrenia (Cutler, 1994). Cutler also points out, however, that schizophrenic patients frequently present their symptoms with a psychotic overlay, explaining them with delusional material, and that panic attacks in these patients can be associated with an increase in delusions and hallucinations. Relevant to that observation, Sandberg and Siris offer a case report of a patient who labeled his panic attacks as "paranoid attacks" (Sandberg & Siris, 1987).

Agoraphobia may be harder to recognize in schizophrenic patients and its prevalence is not as well studied. It should, however, be considered in the differential diagnosis of social withdrawal and avoidance, along with depression, negative symptoms, akinesia, and social phobia.

Most reports describing the treatment response of paniclike symptomatology in schizophrenia have focused on the benzodiazepines, which can often be a useful adjunct in doses similar to those used for patients without comorbid schizophrenia. Interestingly, improvement in panic might be associated with reduction of positive and negative symptoms of schizophrenia as well (Kahn, Puertollano, Schane, & Klein, 1988). There are two additional reports in which imipramine reduced panic attacks in this population (Siris, Aronson, & Sellew, 1989; Yergani, Balon, & Pohl, 1989). Because tricyclic antidepressants have been shown to be effective in the treatment of panic disorder in nonschizophrenic patients, it is possible that imipramine and other antidepressants could also be helpful in treating schizophrenic patients with panic attacks. Double-blind, placebo-controlled trials are still needed for these classes of medication. Further investigation into the effectiveness of cognitive-behavioral therapy for panic and agoraphobia in this population is also needed.

Social Anxiety

Patients with schizophrenia may have difficulty negotiating the intricate and subtle rules of social interaction (Siris, 1991b), a difficulty that provokes and is maintained by anxiety in social situations. Social isolation in schizophrenia has often been attributed to deficits in social skills, but social anxiety may also be a significant contributor to this problem (Penn, Hope, Spaulding, & Kucera, 1994). To that end, Penn and associates suggest that social skills training for a subgroup of schizophrenic patients with significant social anxiety may need to incorporate interventions modeled on treatment for social phobics—for example, in vivo exposure and desensitization to feared situations. The authors are not aware of any studies of medication trials (as with selective serotonin reuptake inhibitors or monoamine oxidase inhibitors) that have been done in patients with comorbid social phobia and schizophrenia.

Akathisia

Akathisia is an extrapyramidal syndrome produced by antipsychotic and possibly other medications and can present as a phenocopy of anxiety (Van Putten, 1975). Patients experience a sense of muscular tension or motor restlessness, they appear fidgety and sometimes pace or march in place. This motor symptom is often hard to distinguish from psychic anxiety, psychotic agitation, or agitated depression. As previously noted, akathisia often does not respond well to antiparkinsonian agents and a trial of propanolol or a benzodiazepine often may be more effective (Fleischhaker et al., 1990). Alternatively, the antipsychotic medication should be lowered or changed.

Medical Conditions and Substance-Related Anxiety

A large number of medical conditions from which schizophrenic patients may suffer may produce anxiety syndromes. These include cardiovascular conditions (e.g., arrhythmias, ischemic heart disease), metabolic disturbances (e.g., hypoglycemia, hypocalcemia, hypoxia), endocrine disorder (e.g., hyperthyroidism, Cushings syndrome), and tumors (e.g., pheochromocytoma). Clinical leads must be followed so these medical conditions can be treated. Additionally, many medications used to treat medical conditions can produce anxiety as a side effect (e.g., prednisone, theophylline, pseudoephedrine). Frequently, psychotropic medications also can be anxiogenic (e.g., selective serotonin reuptake inhibitors, neuroleptics).

Recreational substances commonly produce anxiety with short-term or chronic use, abuse, or discontinuation. Chronic alcohol use and alcohol withdrawal, cocaine intoxication, excessive caffeine use, and nicotine withdrawal are frequent examples. Schizophrenic patients are at increased risk for substance abuse as well as interactions from polypharmacy, which should be considered in the differential diagnosis and treatment of anxiety in this population.

Obsessive Compulsive Syndromes

Although obsessive compulsive (OC) symptoms have been described in schizophrenia for many years, their significance has been debated and their treatment has only begun to be studied. Earlier it was thought that OC symptoms served as a defense against psychotic decompensation. Based on case reports (Stengel, 1945) and retrospective chart reviews (Rosen, 1957), some clinicians suggested that OC symptoms attenuated the schizophrenic illness and made for a less virulent course. More recent systematic studies, however, have found the contrary. Fenton and McGlashan (1986) followed up 23 OC-schizophrenic patients an average of 15 years after an index admission in the Chestnut Lodge Follow-up Study and found that OC symptoms were associated with a global decline in function. Berman and associates (1995a) questioned the therapists of 108 chronic schizophrenia patients about the presence of OC symptoms and the patients' functioning and found that those with OC were judged to have a lower capacity for age-appropriate function, confirming Fenton and McGlashan's (1986) findings.

Phenomenology of OC in Schizophrenia

Because obsessive compulsive disorder may have at its core an absurd or pathological belief (e.g., "I am contaminated and will die unless I can wash off all the germs"), differentiating such phenomena from schizophrenic psychosis may be difficult. Insel and Akiskal (1986) described several patients with OCD in whom insight into the absurd or pathological nature of their obsessive thoughts varied widely across a spectrum of belief. Those patients at the extreme end of the spectrum, who had lost all insight and believed their obsessive thoughts, were described as suffering psychotic OCD.

Most cases of OC symptoms in schizophrenia reported in the literature have been of patients in whom the OC symptoms are distinct from the patient's psychotic symptoms and clearly obsessive compulsive in nature (such as ritualistic hand washing). Indeed, in many cases the patient can readily distinguish between the two types of experiences, the OC symptoms being dystonic and actively resisted whereas the psychotic symptoms are believed and actively embraced. Commonly, patients refer to the psychotic symptoms as "my illness" and the OC symptoms as "something else."

However, there are cases in which delusional beliefs may become the focus of an obsession, making a clear distinction difficult both for the patient and the clinician. Such symptoms may be referred to as "obsessive delusions." Other psychotic phenomena may also become the focus of an obsession. Jaspers (1972) raised the possibility of hallucinations becoming the intrusive focus of a patient's attention and called this "compulsive hallucinations." Pies (1984) described the successful treatment of such a case using clomipramine (CMI). Such an intertwining of phenomena complicates the task of distinguishing between psychotic and obsessional phenomena and makes the development of a treatment strategy difficult.

Treatment of OC Symptoms in Schizophrenia

Although such symptoms have been reported for many years, OC symptoms in schizophrenia have achieved only a limited recognition and, perhaps for this reason, few studies have been done of their pharmacological treatment. Five small studies and a number of anecdotal case reports have been published about the pharmacological treatment of OC symptoms in schizophrenia (see later section). Although each involved a somewhat different population and provided varying amounts of information about the sample, the study design, and the results, some tentative conclusions may be drawn from them.

All the organized studies reported to date (as well as several additional multiple case reports) have involved treating OC symptoms in schizophrenic patients with CMI and have been generally positive about the effects of this drug used adjunctively in patients with both schizophrenia and OC symptoms. Several case reports of using selective serotonin reuptake inhibitors (SSRIs) have also appeared in the literature.

Clomipramine. In an early study of CMI for OCD, Yaryura-Tobias and colleagues (1976) openly treated ten outpatients with schizophrenia and OC symptoms. Even though neuroleptics could be used ad libitem, four of the ten patients experienced an exacerbation of psychosis. The six remaining patients who were able to tolerate the eight-week trial experienced a reduction in anxiety, particularly anxiety associated with rituals. No other changes were found. Based on the psychotic exacerbation found in four patients, the authors concluded that CMI should be given to patients with psychosis "with caution, concomitant with neuroleptic medication, and only where the severity of OC symptoms makes the treatment imperative" (p. 545). However, as there was no control group, it is impossible to say whether relapses to psychosis occurred at greater than a spontaneous rate. Pulman, Yassa, and Ananth (1984) reported on an informal open trial in which they gave CMI to six chronic, hospitalized schizophrenic patients, three of whom had no resistance to their OC symptoms. Four patients had an improvement in their OC symptoms and one experienced an exacerbation of psychosis. Unfortunately, the doses and duration of treatment were left unspecified, and conditions were uncontrolled, making this report difficult to interpret. Stroebel, Szarek, and Glueck (1984) documented giving CMI openly to 17 outpatients with OC symptoms and schizophrenia as part of a larger report on their experience using CMI for OCD. Other medications were not held constant, and the duration of treatment was not specified, described only as lasting up to 757 days. Seven patients (41 percent) showed improvement in their OC symptoms, and although at least one patient was not on neuroleptic medication at some time during the trial, four had a worsening of psychosis. A lack of system in the report of these data as well as a lack of symptom scales to rate symptom severity limits the utility of this report. Zohar, Kaplan, and Benjamin (1993) openly administered CMI to five patients, three with a diagnosis of schizophrenia and two diagnosed with schizoaffective disorder, for a period lasting longer than six weeks. The patients were then taken off CMI, later placed back onto it, and systematically rated during the course of these changes. In all five patients, OC symptoms diminished. Four of the five patients also experienced a reduction of psychotic symptoms, whereas one patient had an exacerbation of psychotic symptoms.

The best-controlled study reported thus far of the treatment of OC symptoms in schizophrenia is a pilot study done by Berman and colleagues (1995b) in which they gave CMI to six stable outpatients in a double-blind crossover trial. Under double-blind conditions, patients were given either placebo or active CMI first, then switched to the other agent. This design allowed patients to act as their own controls. Patients taking low-potency neuroleptics, such as chlorpromazine or thioridazine, were excluded because the researchers feared that the anticholinergic effects of the CMI might be additive with those of the neuroleptic. Patients improved significantly more on CMI than on placebo. All six patients also had a reduction in psychotic symptoms. On the other hand, Bark and Lindenmayer (1992) reported on a schizophrenic patient in whom a course of CMI failed to improve OC symptoms and was associated with a significant exacerbation of psychosis.

Selective Serotonin Reuptake Inhibitors (SSRIs). The selective serotonin reuptake inhibitors, which may be effective in the treatment of OCD without schizophrenia (Freeman, Trimble, Deakin, Stokes, & Ashford, 1994; Goodman et al., 1990; Greist, Jefferson, Kobak, Katzelnick, & Serlin, 1995), have also been added to neuroleptics to treat OC symptoms in schizophrenia in several case reports, but no systematic trial has yet been reported. Hwang and Opler (1994) reported giving fluoxetine to a 44-year-old male with chronic schizophrenia and compulsive rituals who had significant improvement in the rituals lasting over two years. Several cases of OC symptoms thought to have been induced by clozapine (see below) have also been treated with SSRIs with good results. Lindenmayer, Vakharia, and Kanofsky (1990), however, reported exacerbation of agitation and psychotic symptoms, with no improvement of OC symptoms in a chronically hospitalized schizophrenic patient treated with fluoxetine.

Clozapine and OC Symptoms. A number of cases have been reported of patients with schizophrenia developing new or exacerbated OC symptoms during treatment with clozapine (Baker et al., 1992; Patel & Tandon, 1993; Patil, 1992). The investigators attributed their patients' development or worsening of OC symptoms to clozapine's blockade of 5HT-2 receptors. Three cases have been reported in which patients who developed new or exacerbated OC symptoms while in treatment with clozapine, had their OC symptoms treated with adjunctive SSRIs. Patel and Tandon (1993) used fluoxetine to treat the increased OC symptoms in their two clozapine-treated schizophrenic patients. They reported that there was a reduction of the OC symptoms and that the fluoxetine treatment was not associated with an increase in psychotic symptoms. Similarly, Allen and Tejera (1994) reported on the successful treatment with sertraline of one schizophrenic patient who developed OC symptoms while treated with clozapine. That patient experienced a reduction of OC symptoms without any exacerbation of psychosis or significant side effects.

Psychopharmacological Recommendations
Concerning OC in Schizophrenia

Given the current state of knowledge regarding the pharmacotherapy of OC symptoms in schizophrenia, and with the limitations of the few studies done thus far, several tentative recommendations may be made: (1) Treatment of OC symptoms in schizophrenia may be undertaken when the severity of this psychopathology justifies the risks. The patients should be otherwise psychiatrically stable on a maintenance neuroleptic and free of florid psychosis. Although the use of antidepressants in stable patients with chronic schizophrenia may be safe (Siris et al., 1994; Siris, Morgan, Fagerstrom, Rifkin, & Cooper, 1987), there is some evidence that using antidepressant agents in acutely psychotic schizophrenic patients may be less likely to be effective (Kramer et al., 1989). (2) Antiobsessional agents may be selected based on their pharmacokinetics and their profile of side effects, and how these medication effects might be expected to interact with those of the patient's neuroleptic drug (Siris, 1993a). (3) Patients receiving clozapine as their maintenance neuroleptic should be carefully assessed to determine, if possible, whether their OC symptoms preceded the start of clozapine therapy. If the OC symptoms appear to have started only with the institution of clozapine treatment, consideration might be given to switching to another neuroleptic agent. This would require a careful weighing of the benefits derived from clozapine against the morbidity caused by the OC symptoms. If clozapine is to be continued, SSRIs might be the antiobsessional treatment of choice. CMI is highly anticholinergic, as is clozapine. The additive effect of using both agents together might cause an unacceptable level of side effects. It is possible, however, that the addition of an SSRI to the regimen of at least some schizophrenic patients may be associated with an increased risk of agitation (Lindenmayer et al., 1990).

SUBSTANCE ABUSE

Substance abuse itself is by no means a homogeneous issue. Various substances may be used or abused by various routes for various durations in various doses. Substances may have acute effects, chronic effects, and effects at their points of discontinuation. Substances have direct biological (i.e., pharmacologic) effects on the brain, direct effects on the body, and interactive effects with psychiatric (as well as nonpsychiatric) medications; they also affect the metabolism of other prescribed medications. They have effects that are psychological and effects that are social. Additionally, they can lead to important interpersonal, financial, and legal consequences. All these issues are included under the concept of *comorbidity of substance abuse.*

Substance Abuse and Psychosis

Generally, the most significant concern is that substance abuse will lead to either increased frequency or severity of psychotic symptomatology or increased difficulty in engaging the patient in treatment (Galanter, Castaneda, & Ferman, 1988). Complicating these issues is the observation that schizophrenic patients may be more likely to abuse psychostimulant compounds preferentially (Breakey, Goodell, Lorenz, & McHugh, 1974; McLellan & Druley, 1977; Richard, Liskow, & Perry, 1985; Schneier & Siris, 1987). These are compounds that have been found, in other contexts, particularly likely to be psychotogenic (Angrist & vanKammen, 1984; Lieberman, Kane, & Alvir, 1987; Lieberman, Kane, Sarantakos, et al., 1987). The approach to treating substance abuse in schizophrenia is therefore two-pronged: preventing or limiting the substance abuse, and treating the effects of the substances once they have been used (Siris, 1990).

Neuroleptic Agents

Fortunately, neuroleptic agents appear to be useful in the treatment of psychotic exacerbations occasioned by substances of abuse, although this is an issue that, for the most part, has been documented in nonschizophrenic populations (Dubin, Weiss, & Dorn, 1986; Ellison & Jacobs, 1986; Slaby & Swift, 1987). The dosage range that appears to be effective is apparently similar to that used for antipsychotic results in other situations. If patients are kept free of additional substance use, the substance or substances of abuse are likely to pass out of their systems relatively rapidly, within a matter of one to several days. Therefore, patients should be observed particularly closely during this interval because the required doses of antipsychotic medications might vary rapidly—even more quickly than steady-state levels can be established. On the other hand, if what is being treated turns out to be not the acute effects of a psychotogenic compound so much as a fresh episode of psychosis triggered by exposure to the substance, then the course of antipsychotic treatment would more closely parallel that of an acute psychotic exacerbation. If the patient is already on a neuroleptic medication at the time of the substance-induced exacerbation, a determination will need to be made of whether any change in dose is actually necessary, so long as the patient gets medical and psychological support and is kept free from the offending substance. In the acutely intoxicated state, the patient's medical and behavioral toxicities are usually best handled in the most conservative manner possible, and the treating team needs to remain alert to the possibility of withdrawal states; these include the possibility of an organic psychosis as a component of a withdrawal state (Dubin et al., 1986; Ellison & Jacobs, 1986; Slaby & Swift, 1987). Along with blood tests for the presence of abused substances, a blood test for the neuroleptic may be useful, as a patient who abuses substances may be prone to play games with the prescribed medications.

Many substances of abuse predispose to orthostatic hypotension, tachycardia, and/or anticholinergic effects. Therefore, high-potency neuroleptic agents are generally preferable to low-potency neuroleptics in this circumstance, because the latter can exert additive effects in these domains (Dubin et al., 1986; Slaby & Swift, 1987). An additional caution in the instance of cocaine exposure is that neuroleptics can exacerbate cocaine-induced hypothermia (Kosten & Kleber, 1988).

Prophylaxis

Some clinicians suggest that neuroleptic medications may be used in prophylaxis against the use of psychostimulant substances, as they would be expected to counteract the effects of these agents (Gawin & Kleber, 1986; Pollack, Brotman, & Rosenbaum, 1989). This is, however, a hypothesis that has by no means been proven. The possibility exists that the reverse effect may actually occur if patients attempt to use illicit psychostimulants to override unwanted neuroleptic effects, such as sedation or extrapyramidal reactions (e.g., akinesia or akathisia discussed above). Indeed, one of the hypotheses concerning substance abuse in schizophrenia is that it can represent street corner psychopharmacology approaches to self-medication (Millman & Sbriglio, 1986; Richard et al., 1985; Schneier & Siris, 1987; Siris, 1990). Such a sequence of events could then argue for a minimalization of doses of maintenance neuroleptic agents as a strategy to counteract substance abuse. Obviously, in such a circumstance, there is no substitute for a meaningful and frank relationship between the patient and clinician in which such issues can be discussed so that the most effective strategies can be formulated (Siris, 1990; Siris & Docherty, 1990). When issues of neuroleptic compliance are the stumbling block, long-acting parenteral preparations should be considered, with the clinician bearing in mind that their long half-lives result in their steady state not being achieved for as much as six months or more; thus, doses that initially seem correct can possibly accumulate into relative overmedication with time (Marder et al., 1986).

Antiparkinsonian Medication

The above-described self-medication hypothesis may also contribute to some of the putative cases of abuse of antiparkinsonian medications. Their abuse potential has been presumed to result from their anticholinergic properties (Dilsaver, 1988; Fisch, 1987; Tandon & Greden, 1989), but it is possible that patients, especially patients with subtle akinesia, may be ingesting these agents in order to feel normal in circumstances where their doctors should have recognized the problem and been legitimately prescribing these agents. Patients may also be self-medicating other associated mood syndromes, such as depression or anxiety states noted earlier in this chapter. Therefore, these states should be inquired for by the treating clinician, and where they are present, their appropriate treatment may reduce or eliminate the patient's pattern of substance abuse. Such an approach, however, has not been systematically tested and reported in schizophrenic patients, so its pursuit would have to be evaluated empirically, on a case-by-case basis. Three cases of noncompliance with antiparkinsonian medications have been reported (Bermanzohn & Siris, 1994), but no systematic studies of this problem have been done.

Disulfiram and Methadone

For cases of alcoholism or narcotic abuse, the parameters of use for disulfiram and methadone are similar for schizophrenic patients maintained on neuroleptic medications and for the nonschizophrenic population. However, at the time of initiation, patients with schizophrenia require close monitoring because it has occasionally, but not consistently, been reported that schizophrenic-like psychoses may be triggered by disulfiram (Galanter, Castaneda, & Ferman, 1988; Siris, 1990) and that methadone may alter neuroleptic requirements in schizophrenia (McKenna, 1982; Verebey, Volavka, & Clouet, 1978).

Nicotine and Caffeine

Finally, any discussion of substances in schizophrenia is incomplete without mention of nicotine and caffeine. Occasionally, large amounts of one or both of these substances may be consumed by patients and the possibility of abuse considered. Sometimes this situation represents an attempt at self-medication, especially for akinesia; if that is the case, it should be dealt with accordingly. This is not to say, however, that caffeine should necessarily be eliminated. Often, caffeine seems to be an important part of patients' getting started in the morning or keeping going during the day, and its moderate use for these purposes should be allowed if not encouraged. Many patients may have a similar reaction to nicotine, and, although smoking is clearly associated with a number of serious medical problems, its advantages and disadvantages may have to be weighed on a case-by-case basis (Lavin, Siris, & Mason, 1996; Lohr & Flynn, 1992). In schizophrenia, however, aggressive treatment of akinesia as a neuroleptic side effect, or mood states as associated syndromes, may reduce patients' tendencies to self-medicate by smoking. Smoke-free or caffeine-free units may also create situations of withdrawal from these substances for newly admitted patients; clinicians will need to remain alert to these situations.

MENTAL RETARDATION

People who are mentally retarded, according to *DSM-IV* (APA, 1994), represent roughly 1 percent of the general population but manifest psychiatric disorders at a rate of approximately 40 percent (Einfeld, 1992). Yet only in the past two decades have these "dually diagnosed" patients (Ruedrich & Menolascino, 1984) become the subject of growing psychiatric interest. The removal of mental retardation, in *DSM-III-R* (APA, 1987), from the category of Axis I psychiatric disorders to the status of a developmental disorder on Axis II, represented a landmark in the study of comorbidity in mental retardation. (*Developmental disorder* is a more inclusive term than mental retardation. The *pervasive developmental disorders,* such as autistic or childhood disintegrative disorder, are often but not always associated with mental retardation. They are recorded on Axis I.) This action expressed the principle that psychopathology in this group should be conceived of as something additional to and not synonymous with mental retardation. Nevertheless, although mentally retarded patients present with the full spectrum of psychiatric disorders seen in normal intelligence populations, diagnostic and treatment challenges are especially intense. Many mentally retarded patients present with symptoms that do not readily conform to standard patterns (Einfeld, 1992). They often have poor communication skills and lack the ability to self-reflect or the abstract ideation to describe subtle subjective experiences. Current diagnostic systems and standardized assessment instruments may be difficult to apply to patients with mental retardation and, as clinical psychiatric research with this population is still a rarity, guidelines for psychopharmacologic treatment are sorely wanting.

Currently, there is general consensus on a 3 percent rate of prevalence of schizophrenia among those with mental retardation (Reid, 1993) and agreement that its symptomatology and natural course are similar to that in a population with normal intelligence. Age of onset, sex ratio, and cultural background also seem no different (Reid, 1982). Schizophrenia has been found to occur in mentally retarded patients with a wide range of non-specific chromosomal abnormalities (Reid, 1989), and two large studies (Menolascino, Levitas, & Greiner, 1986; Pary, 1993) have reported that, for the mentally retarded population, paranoid schizophrenia was the most common diagnosis in acute psychiatric admissions.

Diagnostic Principles and Strategies

The first general principle in assessing psychopathology among individuals with mental retardation is that "the only symptom that can be directly attributed to the mental retardation is the intellectual limitation itself. All other symptoms have some other cause" (Einfeld, 1992, p. 50). Assuming such an attitude helps to limit the effect of *diagnostic overshadowing,* a decision-making bias by which the diagnostic significance of abnormal behavior is overshadowed by the finding of subnormal intelligence. This process has, in fact, been demonstrated experimentally to occur in the assessment of schizophrenic symptoms in patients with mental retardation (Reiss, Levitan, & Szyszko, 1982). Bias in the opposite direction, toward the overdiagnosis of schizophrenia, has also been documented (Aman, 1985). Psychiatrists' unfamiliarity with the mentally retarded population is surely a cause. Confusing an openly verbalized fantasy life with delusions, for example, is a common error. Knowledge of some of the behavioral phenotypes of developmental disorders, such as hand flapping and gaze avoidance in fragile X syndrome or hyperphagia in Prader-Willi syndrome, can be of help. Also, *primitive behaviors,* such as intense orality, temper tantrums or public masturbation and fetishism, may seem less bizarre when one considers the mental age of the patient as well as the environmental conditions to which he or she might be responding. A comprehensive assessment over time is perhaps the best antidote for many of these diagnostic challenges.

Because the criteria for the diagnosis of schizophrenia lack the more objective vegetative nucleus seen in affective disorders and represent essentially self-reports of subjective experience, a limited vocabulary, concrete thinking, speech impediments, or receptive or expressive aphasias can hinder the diagnostic process. Drawing information from a wide variety of sources is especially important; these include parents, house managers, activity therapists or job coaches, and other clinicians. Nonclinical daily caregivers need to be educated to the signs and symptoms of mental illness so as to better organize their observations and descriptions. This is especially important because patients often extend their denial of their developmental disability to their psychiatric illness as well. Also, mentally retarded individuals have been shown to demonstrate an increased tendency toward *yea-saying* (Sigelman, Budd, Spanhel, & Schoenrock, 1981). Because the criteria for schizophrenia contain primarily language-based phenomenology, many believe the diagnosis cannot be made with any degree of certainty in a patient with an IQ of less than 45. For others, however, regardless of the IQ level, a deterioration in functioning, including bizarre behavior, persistent withdrawal, echolalia and blunted affect (Menolascino, Ruedrich, Golden, & Wilson, 1985) as well as a positive family history, strongly suggests the diagnosis.

Taking into account attentional difficulties, clinical interviews are best done in multiple short sessions. A history of institutionalization, test failure, and adverse drug reactions may increase the mentally retarded patient's anxiety level. Seeing the patient initially with a caregiver may help reduce this anxiety and also aid in establishing an alliance between the psychiatrist and the caregiver; it can help establish the psychiatrist as an ally. Observing interactions between the patient and caregiver informs the psychiatrist of the level of verbal communication with the patient that will be most fruitful.

Clinical Presentation

There is nothing particularly remarkable about the symptom presentation of schizophrenia in the mentally retarded population. These patients present with the same clinical phenomena as nonretarded patients (Meadows et al., 1991).

Case Example. A 29-year-old mildly retarded man who was working as a clerk in an electronics factory had become increasingly interested in a female co-worker. After receiving an anonymous gift, he became panic stricken that it might have been from someone of the same sex. Subsequently, he began to hallucinate accusations that he was a homosexual and then became convinced that someone was investigating him and was about to claim publicly that his credentials were fraudulent. This persecutory investigation, he felt, was proceeding because a group of foreign agents believed he possessed some important military secrets.

Although, in general, their cognitive limitations and limited range of life experiences tend to rob their delusional symptoms of richness and detail, patients with mental retardation and schizophrenia may occasionally describe delusions of influence with great vividness (Reid, 1993). Auditory hallucinations are common, and visual and tactile hallucinations have also been described (Hucker, Day, George, & Roth, 1979). Especially as their intelligence declines, these patients' delusions and hallucinations tend to appear naive, wish fulfilling, and featureless, or be poorly systematized or sustained.

Case Example. A 33-year-old mildly retarded man with a significant speech impediment began to worry about his job security at a time of cutbacks. He developed the delusion that he was practicing broadcasting to studio audiences through his stereo equipment as preparation for a new job.

Delusions may appear strikingly silly or nonsensical, but they should not be dismissed as hysterical, attention seeking, or evidence of malingering.

Case Example. A 28-year-old moderately retarded man claimed that he was a horse. He occasionally whinnied and showed off his teeth, which he stated were especially white because of all the carrots he had eaten. Later he became terrified of his father, whom he misidentified as a policeman; he believed his father had summoned the rest of the police force to arrest and imprison him.

Behavioral disturbances may seem paramount on presentation, and violence and self-injury, even during hospitalizations, is a frequent problem (Forest & Ogunremi, 1974; Lund, 1985). An increase in the severity or frequency of baseline maladaptive behaviors and deficits may be the first signs of a schizophrenic decompensation (Sovner, 1986). The negative symptoms of schizophrenia, on the other hand, may be difficult to distinguish from the retardation of thought and action characteristic of the patient's developmental disorder. Only a careful developmental history may allow a clinician to make this distinction. Schizophrenic thought disorder has been described in the mentally retarded population as including neologisms, echolalia, perseveration, incoherence, tangentiality, verbigeration, and looseness of associations (Reid, 1972). This disorder, however, may be quite difficult to differentiate from anxiety-induced disorganized thinking, manneristic verbal expression, expressive language disorder, or the language of an autistic patient, especially as cognitive abilities in the retarded have been shown to decline under stress (Campbell & Malone, 1991).

Other behaviors also often found in the mentally retarded can easily be confused with psychotic symptoms. These *pseudopsychotic features* include bizarre behavior, soliloquizing and fantasy play, fearfulness and developmental regression, stereotypic and manneristic behavior, and stress-induced hallucinations (Sovner, 1991). In this patient group, even common neurotic symptoms may seem bizarre and suggest psychosis.

Case Example. A 34-year-old mildly retarded man, with no psychiatric history, presented with a growing fear of the wind. He obsessively examined doors and windows for air leaks and experienced visual illusions of the curtains moving. He listened to the Weather Channel daily for reports of wind velocity. Careful interviewing, however, revealed that he recognized this fear as irrational and knew that the wind couldn't hurt him. Psychotherapy demonstrated a rather traditional psychodynamic picture of this phobia with particularly strong conflicts over aggression that had been intensified by his mother's recent declining health.

Differential Diagnosis

In addition to the usual differential diagnosis for schizophrenia, organic delusional disorders must always be a consideration. Because there is a 25 percent rate of epilepsy in this population, post-ictal psychoses are more likely to be seen among this group. With their adaptive abilities limited, both psychologically and biologically, individuals with mental retardation may be vulnerable to a wide variety of brief reactive psychoses. Acute psychotic reactions secondary to psychological trauma occur and can even become chronic if the original trauma occurred early in development or was particularly intense or prolonged. Toxic psychoses due to prescribed or illicit drug use (Meyers & Pueschel, 1993) are not infrequent. In fact, substance abuse is the most common cause for acute psychotic reactions in mentally retarded patients living unsupervised in the community (Myers, 1986).

Pharmacotherapy

"Psychotropic drugs work in the same manner and are used in the same way regardless of a patient's intelligence" (Szyzmanski & Crocker, 1989, p. 1759). Therefore, the entire array of antipsychotic agents may be utilized for the treatment of schizophrenia in the retarded and, despite a paucity of research, their effectiveness is generally accepted (Lund, 1985). However, the psychiatrist should be aware of the stigma attached to the prescription of these agents in this population. Until the last two decades, drug pre-scribing in both institutional and community settings was characterized by polypharmacy, rapid dose escalation, and inadequate baseline assessment, clinical evaluations, and laboratory monitoring (Campbell & Malone, 1991). Surveys from state and private institutions from 1966–1979 (Hill, Balow, & Bruininks, 1985; Lipman, 1970; Marker, 1975; Sprague, 1977) showed that 30 percent to 60 percent of the mentally retarded individuals in these institutions were receiving phenothiazines with thoridazine, pre-sumably because of its sedative properties—by far the most frequently prescribed. Studies of community settings revealed roughly one third of these percentages, yet in both settings these medications were almost in-variably used for overactive behavior, not psychiatric conditions (Hill et al., 1985). In more recent years, drug-monitoring programs have resulted in the discontinuation of psychotropic agents in as many as 50 percent to 60 percent of the patients, a development that is welcome, considering the many and potentially serious side effects of the antipsychotics.

In an excellent review of research in the use of neuroleptics in mentally retarded individuals, Aman (1989) concluded that most of the reports were uninformative because of significant methodological flaws. However, cer-tain trends do emerge from the literature and clinical experience. Dosages for effective remission of schizophrenic symptoms are probably one-half to two-thirds of those used in a normal population. Because of the difficulty of assessing side effects and therapeutic response and in making clear dif-ferentiations between psychotic symptoms and baseline maladaptive be-havior, titration upward should proceed cautiously. Linaker (1990) found a high correlation between neuroleptic dosage and physician availability, indicating that dose escalation occurred too quickly as a response to be-havior problems. A trend toward the use of more potent antipsychotics (e.g., fluphenazine, haloperidol, and thiothixene) may represent some awareness that sedation slows clinical response, which may compound the problem of a neuroleptic-induced reduction in learning potential (Aman, 1989).

Some recent work with clozapine (Sajatovic, Ramirez, Kenny, & Meltzer, 1994) suggests that it may be particularly useful in mentally retarded schizophrenic patients with aggression, although the antipsychotic effect seemed to be less than optimal. Sajatovic and associates (1994) found no precipitation of seizures in two of his patients with seizure disorders, but their dosages were relatively low. Molindone, because it does not lower the seizure threshold, may be the antipsychotic of choice with patients whose seizure disorder is poorly controlled. There is no evidence that moderate dosages of neuroleptic will precipitate seizures in a mentally retarded population without a history of epilepsy (James, 1986). However, patients on anticonvulsant medication may fail to respond to antipsychotics or decompensate on maintenance treatment because of low plasma concentrations, as carbamazepine, phenytoin, and phenobarbital have been found to lower haloperidol and fluphenazine levels significantly (Jann, Fidone, Hernandez, Amrung, & Davis, 1989). Conversely, upon discontinuation of anticonvulsants, increased levels of neuroleptic and resulting increased extrapyramidal side effects may be anticipated and possibly managed prophylactically.

Susceptibility to extrapyramidal side effects appears to be no different with this population. However, tolerance of these side effects may be reduced in patients who have preexisting motor dysfunction. In addition, recognition of adverse reactions may be made more difficult because of baseline hyperactivity and movement disorders as well as problems in patient reporting. With rare exception (Gualtieri, Schroeder, Hicks, & Quade, 1986), tardive dyskinesia has been found at higher rates in the mentally retarded population and shows the same risk factors (female gender, lower cognitive functioning, increasing age, and cumulative dose) that have been found in the nonretarded schizophrenic population (Cohen, Khan, Zheng, & Chiles, 1991). In addition, Rao, Cowie, and Mathew (1987) found parkinsonism, but not anticholinergic or cumulative anticholinergic dose, to correlate with a higher incidence of tardive dyskinesia. Some studies (Schroeder & Gualtieri, 1985; Szyzmanski & Crocker, 1989) suggest that withdrawal from chronic neuroleptic use can produce a syndrome of behavioral dyscontrol analogous to tardive dyskinesia. Neuroleptic malignant syndrome has been reported in several cases of patients with mental retardation who were receiving neuroleptic medication for schizophrenia (Levenson, 1985; Kuhn & Lippman, 1987; McNally & Calamari, 1988), suggesting that mental retardation may be a risk factor.

As is the case with the initial evaluation process, the assessment of treatment response requires interdisciplinary effort. Patient interviews alone may be inadequate to evaluate the effectiveness of pharmacologic agents or untoward reactions to them. The education and interviewing of caregivers in residential and vocational settings to make them aware of target symptoms and side effects is crucial. For those who spend the bulk of each day in intimate contact with the mentally retarded patient, an appreciation of the impact of a psychotic process on behavior can be instrumental in the caregivers' provision of a supportive environment during the treatment process. An informal quantifying or charting of target symptoms can be helpful in focusing on behaviors most affected by psychotic symptoms.

In summary, the comorbidity of psychiatric syndromes with mental retardation is a fertile field yet mostly unplowed. Nevertheless, the increased incidence of a variety of psychiatric disorders in the mentally retarded population raises fascinating questions about their etiology. The study of these comorbidities should, therefore, yield rich insights into the mechanisms by which biological and psychological vulnerabilities contribute to pathogenesis. In the interim, the diagnosis and treatment of schizophrenia in the mentally retarded population should be conducted within a biopsychosocial framework by an interdisciplinary team, where a careful but aggressive treatment of schizophrenic illness can make a major impact on the mentally retarded person's life and those of his caregivers, peers, and family.

REFERENCES

Allen, L., & Tejera, C. (1994). Treatment of clozapine-induced obsessive-compulsive symptoms with sertraline [Letter to the editor]. *American Journal of Psychiatry, 171,* 1096–1097.

Aman, M.G. (1985). Drugs in mental retardation: Treatment or tragedy? *Australian and New Zealand Journal of Developmental Disabilities, 10,* 215–226.

Aman, M.G. (1989). *Treatment of psychiatric disorders (section 1, mental retardation).* Washington, DC: American Psychiatric Association.

American Psychiatric Association. (1987). *Diagnostic and statistical manual of mental disorders* (3rd ed., rev.). Washington, DC: Author.

American Psychiatric Association. (1994). *Diagnostic and statistical manual of mental disorders* (4th ed.). Washington, DC: Author.

Angrist, B., & vanKammen, D.P. (1984). CNS stimulants as tools in the study of schizophrenia. *Trends in Neurosciences, 7,* 388–390.

Baker, R.W., Chengappa, K.N.R., Baird, J.W., Steingard, S., Christ, M.A.G., & Schooler, N.R. (1992). Emergence of obsessive compulsive symptoms during treatment with clozapine. *Journal of Clinical Psychiatry, 53,* 439–442.

Bark, N., & Lindenmayer, J. (1992). Ineffectiveness of clomipramine for obsessive compulsive symptoms in a patient with schizophrenia [Letter to the editor]. *American Journal of Psychiatry, 149,* 136–137.

Barnes, T.R., Curson, D.A., Liddle, P.F., & Patel, M. (1989). The nature and prevalence of depression in chronic schizophrenic in-patients. *British Journal of Psychiatry, 154,* 486–491.

Bartels, S.J., & Drake, R.E. (1988). Depressive symptoms in schizophrenia: Comprehensive differential diagnosis. *Comprehensive Psychiatry, 29,* 467–483.

Beck, A.T., & Emery, G. (1985). *Anxiety disorders and phobias: A cognitive perspective.* New York: Basic Books.

Berman, I., Kalinowski, A., Berman, S.M., Lengua, J., & Green, A.I. (1995a). Obsessive and compulsive symptoms in chronic schizophrenia. *Comprehensive Psychiatry, 36,* 6–10.

Berman, I., Sapers, B.L., Chang, H.H.J., Losonczy, M.F., Schmidler, J., & Green, A.I. (1995b). Treatment of obsessive compulsive symptoms in schizophrenic patients with clomipramine. *Journal of Clinical Psychopharmacology, 15,* 206–210.

Bermanzohn, P.C., & Siris, S.G. (1992). Akinesia: A syndrome common to parkinsonism, retarded depression, and negative symptoms. *Comprehensive Psychiatry, 33,* 221–232.

Bermanzohn, P.C., & Siris, S.G. (1994). Non-compliance with antiparkinsonian medications in neuroleptic-treated schizophrenic patients: Three cases of an unreported phenomenon. *Journal of Clinical Psychiatry, 55,* 488–491.

Boyd, J.H. (1986). Use of mental health services for the treatment of panic disorder. *American Journal of Psychiatry, 143,* 1569–1574.

Breakey, W.R., Goodell, H., Lorenz, P.C., & McHugh, P.R. (1974). Hallucinogenic drugs as precipitants of schizophrenia. *Hospital and Community Psychiatry, 4,* 255–261.

Breier, A., Wolkowitz, O.M., & Pickar, D. (1989). Stress and schizophrenia. In C. A. Tamminga & S. C. Schultz (Eds.), *Schizophrenia research* (pp. 141–152). New York: Raven Press.

Campbell, M., & Malone, R.P. (1991). Mental retardation and psychiatric disorders. *Hospital and Community Psychiatry, 42,* 374–379.

Carpenter, W.T., Jr., Heinrichs, D.W., & Alphs, L.D. (1985). Treatment of negative symptoms. *Schizophrenia Bulletin, 11,* 440–452.

Cohen, S., Khan, A., Zheng, Y., & Chiles, J. (1991). Tardive dyskinesia in the mentally retarded: Comparison of prevalence, risk factors and topography with a schizophrenic population. *Acta Psychiatrica Scandinavica, 83,* 234–237.

Cutler, J. (1994). Panic attacks and schizophrenia: Assessment and treatment. *Psychiatric Annals, 24,* 473–476.

Davis, K.L., Kahn, R.S., Ko, G., & Davidson, M. (1991). Dopamine in schizophrenia: A review and reconceptualization. *American Journal of Psychiatry, 148,* 1474–1486.

DeAlarcon, R., & Carney, M. W. P. (1969). Severe depressive mood changes following slow-release intramuscular fluphenazine injection. *British Medical Journal, 3,* 564–567.

de Figueiredo, J. M. (1993). Depression and demoralization: Phenomenologic differences and research perspectives. *Comprehensive Psychiatry, 34,* 308–311.

Dilsaver, S. C. (1988). Antimuscarinic agents as substances of abuse: A review. *Journal of Clinical Psychopharmacology, 8,* 14–22.

Docherty, J.P., vanKammen, D.P., Siris, S.G., & Marder, S.R. (1978). Stages of onset of acute schizophrenic psychosis. *American Journal of Psychiatry, 135,* 720–726.

Dubin, W.R., Weiss, K.J., & Dorn, J.M. (1986). Pharmacotherapy of psychiatric emergencies. *Journal of Clinical Psychopharmacology, 6,* 210–222.

Einfeld, S.L. (1992). Clinical assessment of psychiatric symptoms in mentally retarded individuals. *Australian and New Zealand Journal of Psychiatry, 26,* 48–63.

Ellison, J.M., & Jacobs, D. (1986). Emergency psychopharmacology: A review and update. *Annals of Emergency Medicine, 15,* 962–968.

Fenton, W.S., & McGlashan, T.H. (1986). The prognostic significance of obsessive-compulsive symptoms in schizophrenia. *American Journal of Psychiatry, 143,* 437–441.

Fisch, R.Z. (1987). Trihexyphenidyl abuse: Therapeutic implications for negative symptoms of schizophrenia. *Acta Psychiatrica Scandinavica, 75,* 91–94.

Fleischhaker, W.W., Roth, S.D., & Kane, J.M. (1990). The pharmacologic treatment of neuroleptic-induced akathisia. *Journal of Clinical Psychopharmacology, 10,* 12–21.

Forest, A.D., & Ogunremi, O.O. (1974). The prevalence of psychiatric illness in a hospital for the mentally handicapped. *Health Bulletin, 32,* 198–202.

Freeman, C.P.L., Trimble, M.R., Deakin, J.F., Stokes, T.M., & Ashford, J.J. (1994). Fluvoxamine versus clomipramine in the treatment of obsessive compulsive disorder: A multicenter, randomized, double-blind, parallel group comparison. *Journal of Clinical Psychiatry, 55,* 301–305.

Galanter, M., Castaneda, R., & Ferman, J. (1988). Substance abuse among general psychiatric patients: Place of presentation, diagnosis, and treatment. *American Journal of Drug and Alcohol Abuse, 14,* 211–235.

Galdi, J. (1983). The causality of depression in schizophrenia. *British Journal of Psychiatry, 142,* 621–625.

Gawin, F., & Kleber, H. (1986). Pharmacologic treatments of cocaine abuse. *Psychiatric Clinics of North America, 9,* 573–583.

Goodman, W.K., Price, L.H., Delgado, P.L., Palumbo, J., Krystal, J. H., Nagy, L.M., Rasmussen, S.A., Heninger, G.R., & Charney, D.S. (1990). Specificity of serotonin reuptake inhibitors in the treatment of obsessive-compulsive disorder. *Archives of General Psychiatry, 47,* 577–585.

Green, M.F., Nuechterlein, K.H., Ventura, J., & Mintz, J. (1990). The temporal relationship between depressive and psychotic symptoms in recent-onset schizophrenia. *American Journal of Psychiatry, 147,* 179–182.

Greist, J.H., Jefferson, J.W., Kobak, K.A., Katzelnick, D.J., & Serlin, R.C. (1995). Efficacy and tolerability of serotonin transport inhibitors in obsessive-compulsive disorder. *Archives of General Psychiatry, 1,* 53–60.

Gualtieri, C.T., Schroeder, S.R., Hicks, R.E., & Quade, D. (1986). Tardive dyskinesia in young mentally retarded individuals. *Archives of General Psychiatry, 43,* 335–340.

Harrow, M., Yonan, C.A., Sands, J.R., & Marengo, J. (1994). Depression in schizophrenia: Are neuroleptics, akinesia, or anhedonia involved? *Schizophrenia Bulletin, 20,* 327–338.

Hill, B.K., Balow, E.A., & Bruininks, R.H. (1985). A national study of prescribed drugs in institutions and community residential facilities for mentally retarded people. *Psychopharmacology Bulletin, 21,* 279–284.

Hirsch, S.R., Jolley, A.G., Barnes, T.R.E., Liddle, P.F., Curson, D.A., Patel, A., York, A., Bercu, S., & Patel, M. (1989). Dysphoric and depressive symptoms in chronic schizophrenia. *Schizophrenia Research, 2,* 259–264.

Hogarty, G.E., McEvoy, J.P., Ulrich, R.F., DiBarry, A.L., Bartone, P., Cooley, S., Hammill, K., Carter, M., Munetz, M.R., & Perel, J. (1995). Pharmacotherapy of impaired affect in recovering schizophrenic patients. *Archives of General Psychiatry, 52,* 29–41.

Hogarty, G.E., & Munetz, M.R. (1984). Pharmacogenic depression among outpatient schizophrenic patients: a failure to substantiate. *Journal of Clinical Psychopharmacology, 4,* 17–24.

Hucker, S.J., Day, K.A., George, S., & Roth, M. (1979). Psychosis in mentally handicapped adults. In F.E. James & R.P. Snaith (Eds.), *Psychiatric illness and mental handicap* (pp. 27–35). London: Gaskill.

Hwang, M.Y., & Opler, L.A. (1994). Schizophrenia with obsessive-compulsive features: Assessment and treatment. *Psychiatric Annals, 24,* 468–472.

Insel, T.R., & Akiskal, H.S. (1986). OCD with psychotic features: A phenomenologic analysis. *American Journal of Psychiatry, 143,* 1527–1533.

James, D.G. (1986). Neuroleptics and epilepsy in mentally handicapped patients. *Journal of Mental Deficiency Research, 30,* 185–189.

Jann, M.W., Fidone, G.S., Hernandez, J.M., Amrung, S., & Davis, C.M. (1989). Clinical implications of increased antipsychotic plasma concentrations upon anticonvulsant cessation. *Psychiatry Research, 28,* 153–159.

Jaspers, K. (1972). Compulsion phenomena. In J. Hoenig & M.W. Hamilton (Eds.), *General psychopathology* (pp. 133–137). Chicago: University of Chicago Press.

Johnson, D.A.W. (1981). Depressions in schizophrenia: Some observations on prevalence, etiology, and treatment. *Acta Psychiatrica Scandinavica, 63* (Suppl 291), 137–144.

Kahn, J.P., Puertollano, M.A., Schane, M.D., & Klein, D.F. (1988). Adjunctive alprazolam for schizophrenia with panic anxiety: clinical observation and pathogenetic implications. *American Journal of Psychiatry, 145,* 742–744.

Klein, D.F. (1974). Endogenomorphic depression: A conceptual and terminological revision. *Archives of General Psychiatry, 31,* 447–454.

Kosten, T.R., & Kleber, H.D. (1988). Rapid death during cocaine abuse: Variant of the neuroleptic malignant syndrome? *American Journal of Drug and Alcohol Abuse, 14,* 335–346.

Kramer, M.S., Vogel, W.H., DiJohnson, C., Dewey, D.A., Sheves, P., Cavicchia, S., Litle, P., Schmidt, R., & Kimes, I. (1989). Antidepressants in "depressed" schizophrenic inpatients: A controlled trial. *Archives of General Psychiatry, 46,* 922–928.

Kuhn, W.F., & Lippman, S.B. (1987). Neuroleptic malignant syndrome as a possible postoperative complication. *General Hospital Psychiatry, 9,* 179–181.

Lavin, M.R., Siris, S.G., & Mason, S.E. (1996). What is the clinical importance of cigarette smoking in schizophrenia? *American Journal on Addictions, 5,* 189–208.

Levenson, J.L. (1985). Neuroleptic malignant syndrome. *American Journal of Psychiatry, 142,* 1137–1145.

Lieberman, J.A., Kane, J.M., & Alvir, J. (1987). Provocative tests with psychostimulant drugs in schizophrenia. *Psychopharmacology, 91,* 415–433.

Lieberman, J.A., Kane, J.M., Sarantakos, S., Gadaletta, D., Woerner, M., Alvir, J., & Ramos-Lorenzi, J. (1987). Prediction of relapse in schizophrenia. *Archives of General Psychiatry,* 597–603.

Linaker, O.M. (1990). Frequency of and determinants for psychotropic drug use in an institution for the mentally retarded. *British Journal of Psychiatry, 15,* 525–530.

Lindenmayer, J., Vakharia, M., & Kanofsky, D. (1990). Fluoxetine in chronic schizophrenia [Letter to the editor]. *Journal of Clinical Psychopharmacology, 76.*

Lipman, R.S. (1970). The use of psychopharmacologic agents in residential facilities for the retarded. In F.S. Menolascino (Ed.), *Psychiatric approaches to mental retardation* (pp. 387–398). New York: Basic Books.

Lohr, J.B., & Flynn, K. (1992). Smoking and schizophrenia. *Schizophrenia Research, 8,* 93–102.

Lund, J. (1985). The prevalence of psychiatric morbidity in mentally retarded adults. *Acta Psychiatrica Scandinavica, 72,* 563–570.

Marder, S.R., Hawes, E.M., Van Putten, T., Hubbard, J.W., McKay, G., Mintz, J., May, P.R.A., & Mindha, K.K. (1986). Fluphenazine plasma levels in patients receiving low and conventional doses of fluphenazine decanoate. *Psychopharmacology, 88,* 480–483.

Marker, G. (1975). *The use of phenothiazines (major tranquilizers) on mentally retarded persons—a review of the research literature.* Unpublished manuscript.

McGlashan, T.H., & Carpenter, W.J., Jr. (1976). Postpsychotic depression in schizophrenia. *Archives of General Psychiatry, 33,* 231–239.

McKenna, G.J. (1982). Methadone and opiate drugs: Psychotropic effect and self-medication. *Annals of New York Academy of Science, 398,* 44–53.

McLellan, A.T., & Druley, K.A. (1977). Non-random relation between drugs of abuse and psychiatric diagnosis. *Journal of Psychiatric Research, 13,* 179–184.

McNally, R.J., & Calamari, J.E. (1988). Neuroleptic malignant syndrome in a man with mental retardation. *Mental Retardation, 26,* 385–386.

Meadows, G., Turner, T., Campbell, L., Lewis, S.W., Reveley, M.A., & Murray, R.M. (1991). Assessing schizophrenia in adults with mental retardation. *British Journal of Psychiatry, 158,* 103–105.

Menolascino, F.A., Ruedrich, S.L., Golden, C.J., & Wilson, T.E. (1985). Diagnosis and pharmacotherapy of schizophrenia in the retarded. *Psychopharmacology Bulletin, 21,* 316–322.

Menolascino, F.J., Levitas, A., & Greiner, C. (1986). The nature and types of mental illness in the mentally retarded. *Psychopharmacology Bulletin, 22,* 1060–1071.

Meyers, B.A., & Pueschel, S.M. (1993). Differentiating schizophrenia from other mental and behavioral disorders in persons with developmental disabilities. *The Habilitative Mental Healthcare Newsletter, 12,* 94–98.

Millman, R.B., & Sbriglio, R. (1986). Patterns of use and psychopathology in chronic marijuana users. *Psychiatric Clinics of North America, 9,* 533–545.

Myers, B.A. (1986). Psychopathology in hospitalized developmentally disabled individuals. *Comprehensive Psychiatry, 27,* 115–126.

Pary, R.J. (1993). Acute psychiatric hospital admissions of adults and elderly adults with mental retardation. *American Journal on Mental Retardation, 98,* 434–436.

Patel, B., & Tandon, R. (1993). Development of obsessive compulsive symptoms during clozapine treatment [Letter to the editor]. *American Journal of Psychiatry, 5,* 83.

Patil, V.J. (1992). Development of transient obsessive compulsive symptoms during treatment with clozapine (letter). *American Journal of Psychiatry, 149,* 272.

Penn, D.L., Hope, D.A., Spaulding, W., & Kucera, J. (1994). Social anxiety in schizophrenia. *Schizophrenia Research, 11,* 277–284.

Pies, R. (1984). Distinguishing obsessional from psychotic phenomena. *Journal of Clinical Psychopharmacology, 4,* 345–347.

Pollack, M.H., Brotman, A.W., & Rosenbaum, J.F. (1989). Cocaine abuse and treatment. *Comprehensive Psychiatry, 30,* 31–44.

Pulman, J., Yassa, R., & Ananth, J. (1984). Clomipramine treatment of repetitive behavior. *Canadian Journal of Psychiatry, 29,* 254–255.

Rao, J.M., Cowie, V.A., & Mathew, B. (1987). Tardive dyskinesia in neuroleptic medicated mentally handicapped subjects. *Acta Psychiatrica Scandinavica, 76,* 507–513.

Reid, A.H. (1972). Psychoses in adult mental defectives: Schizophrenic and paranoid psychoses. *British Journal of Psychiatry, 120,* 213–218.

Reid, A.H. (1982). *The psychiatry of mental handicap.* Oxford: Blackwell Scientific Publications.

Reid, A.H. (1989). Schizophrenia in mental retardation: Clinical features. *Research in Developmental Disabilities, 10,* 241–249.

Reid, A.H. (1993). Schizophrenic and paranoid syndromes in persons with mental retardation: Assessment and diagnosis. In R.J. Fletcher & A. Dosen (Eds.), *Mental health aspects of mental retardation* (pp. 98–110). New York: Lexington Books.

Reiss, S., Levitan, G.W., & Szyszko, J. (1982). Emotional disturbance and mental retardation: Diagnostic overshadowing. *American Journal of Mental Deficiency, 86,* 567–574.

Richard, M.L., Liskow, B.I., & Perry, P.J. (1985). Recent psychostimulant abuse in hospitalized schizophrenics. *Journal of Clinical Psychiatry, 46,* 79–83.

Rifkin, A., Quitkin, F., & Klein, D.F. (1975). Akinesia: A poorly recognized drug-induced extrapyramidal behavioral disorder. *Archives of General Psychiatry, 32,* 672–674.

Rosen, I. (1957). The clinical significance of obsessions in schizophrenia. *Journal of Mental Science, 103,* 773–788.

Roy, A. (1984). Do neuroleptics cause depression? *Biological Psychiatry, 19,* 777–781.

Ruedrich, S., & Menolascino, F.J. (1984). Dual diagnosis of mental retardation and mental illness: An overview. In F.J. Menolascino & J.A. Starks (Eds.), *Handbook of mental illness in the mentally retarded* (pp. 45–81). New York: Plenum Press.

Sajatovic, M., Ramirez, L.F., Kenny, J.T., & Meltzer, H.Y. (1994). The use of clozapine in borderline-intellectual-functioning and mentally retarded schizophrenic patients. *Comprehensive Psychiatry, 35,* 29–33.

Sandberg, L., & Siris, S.G. (1987). "Panic disorder" in schizophrenia: A case report. *Journal of Nervous and Mental Disease, 175,* 627–628.

Schneier, F.R., & Siris, S.G. (1987). A review of psychoactive substance use and abuse in schizophrenia: Patterns of drug choice. *Journal of Nervous and Mental Disease, 175,* 641–650.

Schroeder, S.R., & Gualtieri, C.T. (1985). Behavioral interactions induced by chronic neuroleptic therapy in persons with mental retardation. *Psychopharmacology Bulletin, 21,* 310–315.

Shear, K., Frances, A., & Weiden, P. (1983). Suicide associated with akathisia and depot fluphenazine treatment. *Journal of Clinical Psychopharmacology, 3,* 235–236.

Sigelman, C., Budd, E.C., Spanhel, C.L., & Schoenrock, C.J. (1981). When in doubt, say yes: Acquiescence in interviews with mentally retarded persons. *Mental Retardation, 19,* 53–58.

Siris, S.G. (1987). Akinesia and post-psychotic depression: A difficult differential diagnosis. *Journal of Clinical Psychiatry, 48,* 240–243.

Siris, S.G. (1990). Pharmacological treatment of substance-abusing schizophrenic patients. *Schizophrenia Bulletin, 16,* 111–122.

Siris, S.G. (1991a). Diagnosis of secondary depression in schizophrenia: Implications for *DSM-IV. Schizophrenia Bulletin, 17,* 75–98.

Siris, S.G. (1991b). Is life a Wisconsin card sorting test? [Letter to the editor]. *American Journal of Psychiatry, 148,* 1413–1414.

Siris, S.G. (1993a). Adjunctive medications in the maintenance treatment of schizophrenia and their conceptual implications. *British Journal of Psychiatry, 163* (Suppl 22), 66–78.

Siris, S.G. (1993b). The treatment of schizoaffective disorder. In D.L. Dunner (Ed.), *Current psychiatric therapy* (pp. 160–165). Philadelphia: W.B. Saunders Co.

Siris, S.G., Adan, F., Cohen, M., Mandeli, J., Aronson, A., & Casey, E. (1988). Post-psychotic depression and negative symptoms: An investigation of syndromal overlap. *American Journal of Psychiatry, 145,* 1532–1537.

Siris, S.G., Aronson, A., & Sellew, A.P. (1989). Imipramine-responsive panic-like symptomatology in schizophrenia. *Biological Psychiatry, 25,* 485–488.

Siris, S.G., Bermanzohn, P.C., Mason, S.E., & Shuwall, M.A. (1994). Maintenance imipramine therapy for secondary depression in schizophrenia: A controlled trial. *Archives of General Psychiatry, 51,* 109–115.

Siris, S.G., & Docherty, J.P. (1990). Psychosocial management of substance abuse in schizophrenia. In M.I. Herz, J.P. Docherty, & S.K. Klein (Eds.), *Handbook of schizophrenia: Vol. 4, Psychosocial therapies* (pp. 339–354). New York: Elsevier.

Siris, S.G., Morgan, V., Fagerstrom, R., Rifkin, A., & Cooper, T.B. (1987). Adjunctive imipramine in the treatment of post-psychotic depression: A controlled trial. *Archives of General Psychiatry, 44,* 533–539.

Siris, S.G., Strahan, A., Mandeli, J., Cooper, T.B., & Casey, E. (1988). Fluphenazine decanoate dose and severity of depression in patients with postpsychotic depression. *Schizophrenia Research, 1,* 31–35.

Siris, S.G., vanKammen, D.P., & Docherty, J.P. (1978). The use of antidepressant medication in schizophrenia: A review of the literature. *Archives of General Psychiatry, 35,* 1368–1377.

Slaby, A.E., & Swift, R. (1987). Diagnosing and managing drug-induced psychiatric emergencies. *Psychiatric Medicine, 3,* 233–251.

Sovner, R. (1986). Limiting factors in the use of *DSM-III* criteria with mentally ill/mentally retarded persons. *Psychopharmacology Bulletin, 22,* 1055–1059.

Sovner, R. (1991). Does my client have a mental illness? In P. Miller (Ed.), *Research to practice in mental retardation: Biomedical aspects* (pp. 199–202). Baltimore: University Park Press.

Sprague, R.L. (1977). Overview of psychopharmacology for the retarded in the United States. In P. Mittler (Ed.), *Research to practice in mental retardation: Biomedical aspects* (pp. 199–202). Baltimore: University Park Press.

Stengel, E. (1945). A study on some clinical aspects of the relationship between obsessional neurosis and psychotic reaction types. *Journal of Mental Science, 91,* 166–187.

Stroebel, C.F., Szarek, B.I., & Glueck, B.C. (1984). Use of clomipramine in treatment of obsessive-compulsive symptomatology. *Journal of Clinical Psychopharmacology, 4,* 98–100.

Szyzmanski, L.S., & Crocker, A.C. (1989). Mental retardation. In H.J. Kaplan & B.J. Sadock (Eds.), *Comprehensive textbook of psychiatry* (pp. 1728–1771). Baltimore: Williams & Wilkins.

Tandon, R., & Greden, J.F. (1989). Cholinergic hyperactivity and negative schizophrenic symptoms. *Archives of General Psychiatry, 46,* 745–753.

Tune, L., & Coyle, J.T. (1980). Serum levels of anticholinergic drugs in the treatment of acute extrapyramidal side effects. *Archives of General Psychiatry, 37,* 293–297.

Van Putten, T. (1975). The many faces of akathisia. *Comprehensive Psychiatry, 16,* 43–47.

Van Putten, T., & May, P.R.A. (1978). "Akinetic depression" in schizophrenia. *Archives of General Psychiatry, 35,* 1101–1107.

Verebey, K., Volavka, J., & Clouet, D. (1978). Endorphines in psychiatry: An overview and a hypothesis. *Archives of General Psychiatry, 35,* 877–888.

Wise, R.A. (1982). Neuroleptics and operant behaviour: The anhedonia hypothesis. *Behavioral and Brain Sciences, 5,* 39–87.

Yaryura-Tobias, J.A., Neziroglu, M.A., & Bergman, L. (1976). Clomipramine for obsessive-compulsive neurosis: An organic approach. *Current Therapeutic Research, 20,* 541–548.

Yergani, V.K., Balon, R., & Pohl, R. (1989). Schizophrenia, panic attacks, and antidepressants [Letter to the editor]. *American Journal of Psychiatry, 146,* 279.

Zohar, J., Kaplan, Z., & Benjamin, J. (1993). Clomipramine treatment of obsessive compulsive symptomatology in schizophrenic patients. *Journal of Clinical Psychiatry, 54,* 385–388.

10

Psychotherapy of Substance Abuse with Comorbidity

ARTHUR T. HORVATH

The standard psychotherapeutic treatments of patients with substance abuse can be identified in two ways. From the perspective of what is most common, most substance abuse treatment in the United States is provided by counselors who use a combination of disease and Twelve Step (e.g., Alcoholics Anonymous) treatment models (National Academy of Sciences, 1990a). From the perspective of effectiveness, however, the treatments with the most empirical support are primarily cognitive behavioral, even though they are not widely offered in the United States (Miller et al., 1995). Most substance abuse counselors presumably have insufficient training to provide cognitive-behavioral treatment (CBT), and they and their institutions typically do not embrace CBT models.

Some psychotherapists nevertheless treat substance abuse and other behavioral disorders using empirically supported treatment methods. Based on national estimates, about one fifth to two thirds of their substance abuse cases will also have comorbid mental health diagnoses (see Chapter 2). This chapter focuses on (1) the screening and assessment for substance dependence and abuse (SDA, as defined by *DSM-IV*) and (2) the outpatient psychotherapeutic treatment of patients who are discovered to have both SDA and an anxiety or mood disorder (A/MD). The treatment options recommended are primarily cognitive behavioral, although the information

253

presented may also be useful for providers working from a disease or Twelve Step perspective. The reader is assumed to be familiar with standard screening, assessment, and treatment of A/MD, but not of SDA. Treatment of comorbid SDA and schizophrenia (or other major mental illness) is covered in Chapters 8 and 9, and medication treatment of comorbid SDA and A/MD, in Chapter 11. The reference list for this chapter—Chapter 10—includes phone numbers for the less-well-known publishers.

SCREENING

The purpose of screening patients for SDA is to discover whether assessment of SDA is needed: One cannot assess a problem if its existence is unknown. The extent of screening will depend on the setting. In the typical outpatient mental health setting, screening can be accomplished with intake forms and interview follow-up.

An intake questionnaire, one that every new patient completes for review during the intake interview, could include the following questions:

1–4. What is your pattern of (smoking/use of tobacco products), (drinking), (other drug use), (coffee drinking/use of caffeinated products)? When was your last smoke/drink/use? (For consistency, it is useful to identify the standard drink of alcohol, which is the amount of alcohol in a 12-ounce beer, or a 4- to 5-ounce glass of wine, or a shot of liquor. Although the concentrations of alcohol are different, each beverage, in the amount noted, contains about the same amount of pure alcohol.)

5. What is your pattern of eating?

6. Are there any other substances that have a significant role in your life? What is your pattern of using them?

7. Are there any activities that consistently occupy much of your time, possibly with some negative results? What is your pattern of doing them?

Some version of the first three or four questions would be appropriate in most settings. Question four—the item about caffeine—is especially relevant for anxiety patients. Any question could be eliminated if asked in an interview or if reviewed in the context of the patient's daily activities. Having the patient complete an activity schedule (an hourly list of what occurs each day) for several weeks or more can provide important clinical data, including data relevant to the above questions. The intake questionnaire is assumed to include a question about prescription medication, so that the use of potentially addictive medications can be explored.

Another screening approach is to ask about health- and lifestyle-risk factors, which include addictive behavior. One advantage of this approach is that it can be less threatening than more direct questions. Skinner (1994) has developed software that screens for addictive behavior and other health-risk factors; it also assesses the patient's level of motivation to change.

The above screening questions aim at identifying addictive behavior in general rather than substance dependence and abuse alone. Addictive behavior includes both the repetitive (compulsive) use of substances (substance problems) and the repetitive engagement in activities (activity problems; e.g., gambling, promiscuous sexuality, overspending, relationships), such that the costs of the behavior exceed the benefits. The behavior can range from mild to severe, as measured by the costs incurred. A diagnosis based on addictive behavior is usually made only when the costs of the behavior are moderate or severe. However, even mild addictive behavior may be clinically relevant. For instance, getting drunk several times per year may not meet *DSM-IV* criteria for alcohol abuse but may be highly relevant because of the context in which it occurs (e.g., sexual encounters).

A broader focus (all addictive behavior) is desirable for screening purposes because addictive behaviors tend to cluster: Drinkers tend to be smokers, users of one illicit drug tend to use others, sexual addicts tend to have substance problems, and so on. Consequently, the identification of one addictive behavior may be the clue that leads to the identification of others. For treatment planning purposes, even nondiagnosable addictive behavior may be a necessary focus of treatment, and the consideration of all the patient's addictive behavior can lead to a more realistic treatment plan. Throughout most of this chapter, the term *addictive behavior* can be substituted for *substance dependence and abuse* without loss of meaning.

Throughout all phases of treatment, it is critical for rapport, and for the accuracy of patient report, that the provider maintain a nonjudgmental and empathic attitude (Horvath, 1994). During screening, it is better for the clinician not to convey expectations about so-called proper levels of use. If the patient presents vague answers ("I drink a little beer on the weekends"), an appropriate response is a low-end/high-end question ("Is a 'little' closer to 8 beers, or 48 beers?"), or a high-end question ("How often do you drink four 12-packs or more in a weekend?"). Patients with lower use are unlikely to be offended, and those with higher use may be more open ("Gee, I never drink more than four or five 6-packs").

An interview follow-up for positive answers to screening questions can also begin to identify connections between SDA and other symptoms (e.g., What effect does drinking have on your level of tension?) and set the stage for proposing a more in depth evaluation of both. Use of interview follow-up may also be necessary at other times in treatment. For instance, well into treatment, a patient who deliberately withheld information about his daily marijuana smoking remarked that he happened to have a "joint with some friends on Saturday." For reasons elaborated below, the clinician's response was, "How much fun was it?" which led to an initial interview assessment of his marijuana use.

Patients who voluntarily seek treatment, and who are not intoxicated, give mostly accurate reports of their substance use. Intoxicated patients are much less reliable. However, even highly trained observers may not be able to identify an intoxicated patient who has well-developed tolerance for a substance (explaining why law enforcement officers use elaborate field sobriety tests). The psychotherapist should be alert only for blatant signs of use (e.g., alcohol on the breath, highly delayed responding to questions, slurred speech, unsteady gait), and he or she should otherwise rely on physical testing and collateral reports if firm evidence of sobriety is desired. The Final Call Breathalyzer is an inexpensive, one-time-use alcohol breathalyzer that has about a one-year shelf life (U.S. Alcohol Testing, 1-800-753-4625). It or similar products are accurate enough for screening purposes and would be suitable in almost any setting. In most cases, any patient who tests positive should return to complete the assessment when he or she is alcohol-free.

Equivocal screening results can be followed by patient self-monitoring, which may last the length of treatment. Some mild problems may resolve by this intervention alone.

ASSESSMENT

If screening has suggested SDA (or other clinically relevant addictive behavior), then the purpose of assessment is to discover the behavioral information necessary to include that SDA in an effective treatment plan. As with screening, the extent of assessment will depend on the setting, and most important, on the patient's level of motivation. The author assumes (and the assessment can confirm) that the patient is suitable and motivated for outpatient treatment and is unlikely to need intensive medical services for substance withdrawal. Given these assumptions, the modal patient will have drinking problems and anxiety or mood disorder.

The patient's level of motivation to resolve his or her substance dependence or abuse may be the most significant predictor of outcome. Although the patient is usually not ambivalent about overcoming anxiety or mood disorder, he or she may have substantial ambivalence about resolving SDA. Consequently, assessing patient motivation is critical to developing a realistic treatment plan.

Prochaska, DiClemente, and Norcross (1992) have proposed a motivational classification system, the *stages of change,* that has become widely accepted: Precontemplation (unwilling to consider change); Contemplation (willing to consider change); Determination (planning to change in the next 30 days); Action (moderation or abstinence has begun); Maintenance (moderation or abstinence has been achieved for six months and relapse prevention is the focus); and Termination (special relapse prevention efforts are no longer required). Instruments for assessing these stages have been developed, but in the clinical setting, interviewing may be sufficient for obtaining an estimate of the level of motivation (e.g., "How willing are you to consider reducing or stopping your cocaine use?").

Another way to assess motivation is the cost-benefit analysis (Horvath, 1993), which is a functional analysis of the perceived consequences of SDA. The cost-benefit analysis usually begins by focusing on the (typically immediate) perceived benefits of SDA ("What do you like about using/ drinking?"). The costs of SDA are taken up only after the benefits have been thoroughly considered. This aspect of the cost-benefit analysis can significantly enhance rapport. Patients appreciate explicit acknowledgment that SDA has been chosen not for the problems it causes, but for the perceived benefits it confers (or used to confer). For this reason, beginning the assessment with the cost-benefit analysis—benefits first—is often desirable. The costs of SDA typically have a delayed onset and can include physical dependence; facilitation of other addictive behavior; and medical/physical, sexual, neuropsychological, financial, legal, relationship, vocational, and psychological consequences—especially loss of self-respect. The patient's conclusions about the cost-benefit analysis are an indicator of motivation ("I guess pot really causes a lot more harm than good for me").

The benefits of SDA are crucial for treatment planning because the patient usually needs to learn new methods to achieve them (e.g., learning how to feel comfortable socializing without being high). The cost-benefit analysis can reveal connections between the SDA and A/MD, highlighting both how SDA may be a self-medication for A/MD, and how A/MD increases because of SDA. The patient's confidence about learning new methods to achieve positive substance effects is also an indirect assessment of his or her motivation. Low confidence suggests low motivation to change, but it also points to the value of skill and confidence building as an early phase of treatment.

A comprehensive assessment of the SDA could also include (1) diagnosis (abuse or dependence); (2) quantities and frequencies of current and past use; (3) completion of the remainder of the functional analysis (understanding the antecedents [high-risk situations] that trigger the behavior); (4) goals for treatment (from the patient, and from significant others); and (5) assets the patient will have to rely on to accomplish change.

Family history of SDA has been a prominent aspect of traditional SDA assessment, for the purposes of determining the level of genetic risk, and of persuading the patient of the diagnosis of *alcoholic* or *addict*. If the patient has already developed SDA, however, this information is of little practical significance: The problem has already manifested itself, and the patient's acceptance of labels does not necessarily enhance outcomes. Family history is nevertheless useful for many other clinical purposes (including understanding the patient's early learning environment) and should be gathered as appropriate.

Neuropsychological screening is a neglected aspect of SDA assessment. Sobell, Toneatto, and Sobell (1994) recommend use of the Trail Making Test and the Digit Symbol subtest of the WAIS-R as an inexpensive, ten-minute screening. Positive findings can be referred to a neuropsychologist for review. Because many patients may have mild substance-related neuropsychological deficits that are unremediable, the only practical result of a positive finding may be the therapist's effort to lower the speed and complexity of treatment and to increase the clarity of support materials. If patients have substantial withdrawal symptoms, significant cognitive effort is best postponed for several weeks. Careful attention to how the patient is grasping the material that is being presented and consequent appropriate adjustments that should be made are needed in all psychological treatments.

The quantity of alcohol or other sedatives a patient consumes is a predictor of withdrawal severity. Abrupt cessation (withdrawal) from alcohol or other sedatives can, infrequently, be a life-threatening experience. The safest course is to advise all patients to obtain medical supervision of withdrawal. Nevertheless, some patients will elect to experience unsupervised withdrawal. They, and significant others, can be advised to visit an emergency room if symptoms become severe.

Although there are many instruments specific to each of the above assessment targets, in clinical practice the simplicity of a primary, comprehensive instrument, supplemented as needed, is desirable. For alcohol, the Alcohol Use Inventory (Horn, Wanberg, & Foster, 1987) has good psychometrics, easy availability, and low price. When nonalcohol substance use is prominent, the choice is less obvious, and a collection of single-focus instruments—and more extensive interviewing—may be necessary. Comprehensive options include the Addiction Severity Index (McLellan et al., 1990) and the ASIST (Addiction Research Foundation, 1984). Miller, Westerberg, and Waldron (1995) have reviewed instruments for assessing alcohol use, and Sobell and colleagues (1994) have reviewed tools for assessing alcohol and other drug use. A single source for many of the instruments covered in these reviews is the catalog of the Addiction Research Foundation (1995).

Regardless of the instruments used, discussion of the results with the patient allows for an additional confirmation of the validity of the findings. The practice of confirming and clarifying assessment results follows from the collaborative nature of cognitive-behavioral treatment. Even more extensive collaboration will be needed if treatment planning and the treatment that follows are to be successful.

TREATMENT PLANNING: GENERAL CONSIDERATIONS

The potential complexity of applying the foregoing information, combined with the issues of screening and assessing for A/MD, make it easy to overlook the fact that patients seek treatment with goals of their own. The purpose of treatment planning is to establish mutually agreed on treatment goals and methods, but this will be impossible if a substantial effort is not made to understand the patient's goals. Comorbid patients will have even greater difficulty than others in understanding and articulating their feelings, thoughts, and goals; and a major (and potentially time-consuming) step in treatment can be helping them do so. Some patients have such difficulty that they may not progress beyond this phase.

A straightforward approach to treatment planning is to compile patient complaints (arising out of a diligent effort to understand the patient), along with psychotherapist concerns (arising out of screenings, assessments, history, collateral reports, observations over time, etc.), in order to formulate focuses of treatment: a problem list. When these problems are resolved, treatment is successful. The resolution process is likely to involve a mixture of symptom-reduction interventions and modification of presumed underlying causes. In CBT, these presumed underlying causes are irrational beliefs. An extensive presentation on establishing problem lists, hypothesizing underlying irrational beliefs, and establishing treatment plans is found in Persons (1989). Only some aspects of these issues are presented here.

Understanding how the problems (e.g., depression and cocaine use) may be related is a crucial aspect of treatment planning. Many arguments have been offered about whether SDA or A/MD is typically primary (see Chapter 4 for a discussion of primary versus secondary disorder). In the individual case, all possible relationships should be considered. By history, one may clearly be primary (and this may have strong emotional significance to the patient—"I'm not really an 'x'; it just started because of my 'y'"). However, a primary disorder may not be identifiable, and in most cases some level of reciprocal influence in maintaining (as opposed to initiating) each disorder seems likely, or the disorders could be treated independently without complications. This reciprocal influence can be observed in behavioral sequences involving both disorders. For instance, depression can lead the patient to seek momentary relief by the use of cocaine; within hours or days, however, the cocaine use exacerbates the depression, from which further momentary relief is sought by more cocaine use, and so on. Identifying such a sequence is a revelation to some patients, underscoring the difficulty of even establishing treatment goals.

Such behavioral sequences suggest multifaceted intervention. In the example given, it seems reasonable to intervene by attempting to decrease both depression and cocaine use. The joint decisions about how to proceed will depend on many factors, including the patient's level of motivation, frequency of sessions, other treatment goals, the patient's capacity to tolerate discomfort in general and urges to use in particular, immediate pressures at work and at home, and other considerations.

Irrational beliefs arise almost with life itself; but because SDA or its antecedents typically do not begin until adolescence, it seems unlikely that beliefs about SDA would be involved in the deepest irrational beliefs or early maladaptive schemas (Young, Beck, & Weinberger, 1993). Beliefs that maintain SDA are more likely to be associated with underlying assumptions, which maintain, compensate for, or lead to avoidance of the experience of the early maladaptive schema. However, early maladaptive schemas are seen as having a critical role in the treatment of A/MD. In the depression/cocaine example, the schema underlying the depression might be the expectation that a normal degree of emotional support from others is not available, but the underlying assumption of the cocaine use might be that use takes away the pain associated with the schema. Resolving both the depression and cocaine use would involve addressing irrational beliefs at different depths of the matrix of beliefs. The cost-benefit analysis provides one method for rapidly assessing underlying assumptions about substance use.

It is likely that a therapist will encounter patient problems with which the therapist has little experience. These may include problems that few therapists have seen (e.g., an unusual addictive behavior, or an unusual comorbidity combination). In some cases, therapeutic resources for the patient can be identified and the patient will accept referral. However, in many cases the therapist's basic therapeutic expertise (and capacity for learning from diverse sources, including the patient, the literature, and consultation) are reasonable foundations for treatment. For instance, it would seem pointless to attempt to identify a psychotherapist with all the requisite experience to treat a disabled, overweight, lesbian, Hispanic agoraphobic with depression, alcohol dependence, marijuana and cocaine abuse, and a physically abusive girlfriend. These kinds of combinations are not unusual.

Three groups of patients can be identified. The first group, having learned of the probable reciprocal interaction between SDA and A/MD, will elect to abstain from SDA and be successful. Because the base rate for long-term continuous abstinence following substance abuse treatment is about 10 percent, about 10 percent of the group electing to abstain will be successful. For these abstainers, A/MD will be the focus of treatment, and progress is likely to reinforce abstinence. Some patients may request referral to a specialized SDA treatment program prior to A/MD treatment, but such a referral requires careful consideration because of the paucity of empirically based SDA treatment programs.

The second group of patients will desire to resolve their A/MD but not change their SDA. Resolving A/MD under these conditions is possible but unlikely. A trial of (unsuccessful) treatment, with an agreed-on time limit, might persuade the patient to include SDA in the treatment plan. Alternatively, the patient may be willing to make consideration of changing his or her SDA a focus of treatment. Miller and Rollnick (1991) present relevant interventions. Unless these patients eventually elect to change their substance dependence and abuse, their continuation in treatment is doubtful.

The third group, probably by far the largest, will attempt (with varying degrees of motivation and success) to maintain reduced consumption or abstinence while attempting to resolve A/MD and accomplish their other treatment goals. The remainder of the chapter focuses on this group.

Although a goal of abstinence might seem the most straightforward approach, many patients will refuse abstinence. Attempting to force a treatment goal on a patient can lead the individual to terminate treatment. Although in some cases it may be better to insist on certain goals or standards before continuing treatment, many cases can benefit ultimately from a more lenient initial approach, particularly if a long-term (multiyear) view of the case is considered.

Even though refusing permanent abstinence, many patients will abstain temporarily, or dramatically reduce their use. Some patients are willing to abstain for lengthy periods (e.g., up to 12 months), provided there is no suggestion that this condition will necessarily be permanent. The principle of successive approximation suggests that the initial abstinent period might be a week or a month, with an option to renew. Perhaps, because of the patient's recent difficulties in maintaining a long-term perspective, he or she would do well to defer permanent decisions about nearly everything. After a period of abstinence, and a reduction of A/MD, desirable levels of consumption can more prudently be considered. This framing can also be useful for the first group of patients (who initially elect abstinence) because it helps prevent negative emotions arising from the thought, "I can never drink/use again."

Current research on moderation training for alcohol problems suggests a weekly limit of 12 standard drinks for men, and 7 for women (Hester, 1995). Successive approximations to these levels might begin with an initial reduction to 50 percent of baseline consumption, lasting several weeks before the next reduction. Patient moderation training manuals are available and known to be effective for many individuals (Miller & Munoz, 1982; Sanchez-Craig, 1993). No approach to treating alcohol problems is more thoroughly researched than moderation training (Hester, 1995), and its use could be greatly expanded in the United States. Failure to achieve moderation—three months is an adequate trial—can help persuade the patient to consider abstinence.

If the patient uses illegal substances, the therapist can proceed as above, except to clarify that his or her encouragement of reduction of use should not be interpreted as an encouragement of use itself:

> We both know that cocaine use is illegal. For your sake, I hope that you will stop using as fast as you can, immediately if possible. However, I also recognize that the most realistic approach to you seems to be to cut back, and then maybe consider stopping later. I think we are both really headed in the same direction here. We just have a disagreement, for now, about how fast to get there.

This clarification would appear to avoid the appearance of a conspiracy between the therapist and patient regarding illegal activity, and yet it allows them to maintain a therapeutic alliance.

When the therapist and patient reach initial decisions regarding goals and methods for both SDA and A/MD, treatment proceeds. Further data will almost certainly modify the initial treatment plan (perhaps so much that treatment planning again becomes the main focus of sessions). While treatment is occurring, sessions need to be organized to allow multiple focuses, as two or more treatment protocols are interwoven. Agenda setting and following the agenda to the extent the patient can comply are essential:

> You made your drinking goal of 20 drinks this week—Congratulations! You've earned another reward!—and it doesn't sound like there are any hot issues in your life to discuss this week, so I propose we consider your drinking goal for next week and a reward if you make it. Let's discuss how you will handle being offered drinks at the party you want to go to on Saturday night, and then spend the rest of our time continuing to work on how you can feel relaxed and can socialize without alcohol, both at the party and at other times. In our next session, we can come back to the discussion we started last time, about your thinking that your social nervousness may be rooted in how critical your father tended to be—but first, you need more skills for getting through this party. How does all that sound?

A major advantage of CBT is that the underlying assumptions of the treatment of both SDA and A/MD will be identical, and there is less likelihood of patient confusion. Although some patients may benefit from attendance in a Twelve Step group, it seems likely that most (if they elect to attend one) would prefer a support group with a CBT orientation. S.M.A.R.T. Recovery (216-292-0220), Women for Sobriety (215-536-8026), and Rational Recovery (916-621-2667) are abstinence-oriented groups that have a CBT orientation (broadly defined). Moderation Management (313-930-6446) supports moderate drinking for selected individuals. These groups are not yet available in all parts of the country, but their numbers appear to be growing.

Because of the many difficulties these patients have often developed, they may need a wide range of additional support services. The therapist may be in a good position to coordinate these services.

The CBT protocols for A/MD and for alcohol problems (Hester & Miller, 1995) are well defined, researched, and supported; CBT protocols for nonalcohol SDA, however, are not as well developed. Beck, Wright, Newman, and Liese (1993) present an overview of CBT nonalcohol SDA interventions. The most robust finding about nonalcohol SDA outpatient treatment is that longer treatment is better (National Academy of Sciences, 1990b). For all cases, gradual tapering of treatment over one or more years is recommended.

Because of the complexity of these cases, treatment may often progress slowly, if at all. Premature termination is common. The percentage of successful cases is likely to be low. In successful cases, factors in addition to treatment are likely to have a decisive role. Because of the difficulty of conducting outcome research (Carey, 1991), the clinician's artfulness will probably be as important a factor in successful outcome as specific guidance from the research literature.

ANXIETY DISORDERS AND SDA

There may be an even greater paucity of treatment outcome data in this chapter than in other chapters because of the long-standing fractionation of behavioral health care into three components—alcohol, drug, mental health—as exemplified by the three National Institutes in these areas. Nevertheless, behavioral health care is reunifying, and psychotherapists with appropriate alcohol and other drug treatment training are predicted to be its primary practitioners. Until sufficient outcome research is available to provide specific treatment guidance, basic psychotherapeutic skills will need to be the foundation of most treatment for patients with both SDA and A/MD. There is evidence to suggest that simultaneous treatment of both A/MD and SDA can result in better outcomes for some patients, and little evidence appears to suggest that such simultaneous treatment is harmful.

It has long been reported that if the patient can maintain abstinence for several weeks or more, the anxiety disorder seemingly identified on initial assessment will often remit. Nevertheless, even with the remission of the disorder, anxiety symptoms may continue and are common in the post-withdrawal phase, which can last months. These symptoms can be thought of as part of the patient's transition to a more independent (i.e., non-substance-dependent) lifestyle. Correspondingly, if the patient does not abstain, he or she may experience anxiety symptoms as part of both intoxication and withdrawal. Stated differently, distinguishing anxiety from intoxication or withdrawal can be difficult. Consequently, the determination of primary and secondary disorders cannot be made reliably until at least several weeks after abstinence has begun, if then. This distinction may have more implications for medication treatment than for psychotherapy.

Suicide risk is probably even higher in anxiety and SDA than the already high levels associated with anxiety disorders or SDA alone. Up to six weeks or more following a significant interpersonal loss or transition is an especially critical time period.

Graduated exposure to anxiety is a foundation of cognitive-behavioral treatment of anxiety disorders, and graduated exposure to cues and urges for substances (cue exposure) is an emerging foundation for CBT of SDA. The patient can use any success with one problem as a model for success with the other. Otto, Pollack, and Barlow (1995) have written a workbook for patients wishing to taper off antianxiety medication yet remain (or become) panic free.

MOOD DISORDERS AND SDA

As with anxiety disorders, abstinence may resolve the mood disorder in two to six weeks, but depressive symptoms may persist for months. Intoxication and withdrawal symptoms can become intermixed with depressive symptoms, and the relationship between the mood disorder and SDA can be difficult to determine. Suicide risk is similarly high with this type of comorbidity, and careful monitoring, especially at times of interpersonal disruption, is indicated.

Identifying and evaluating automatic thoughts is a foundation of CBT for depression, and identifying and evaluating beliefs about urges is a foundation of the CBT of SDA. The substance user frequently needs to modify his or her beliefs that urges last indefinitely (they are time limited), that urges are harmful (they are uncomfortable but cause no harm), and that urges force action (the patient's power to choose remains available). Additionally, expectations about the positive effects of the substance are often distorted.

REFERENCES

Addiction Research Foundation. (1985). *A structured addictions assessment interview for selecting treatment.* Toronto, Ontario: Author. (800-661-1111)

Addiction Research Foundation. (1995). *Resources: Alcohol and drug treatment.* Toronto, Ontario: Author. (800-661-1111)

Beck, A.T., Wright, F.D., Newman, C.F., & Liese, B.S. (1993). *Cognitive therapy of substance abuse.* New York: Guilford Press.

Carey, K.B. (1991). Research with dual-diagnosis patients: Challenges and recommendations. *The Behavior Therapist, 14*(1), 5–8.

Hester, R.K. (1995). Behavioral self-control training. In W.R. Miller & R.K. Hester (Eds.), *Handbook of effective alcoholism treatment approaches: Effective alternatives* (2nd ed., pp. 148–159). Boston: Allyn & Bacon.

Hester, R.K., & Miller, W.R. (Eds.). (1995). *Handbook of alcoholism treatment approaches: Effective alternatives* (2nd ed.). Boston: Allyn & Bacon.

Horn, J.L., Wanberg, K.W., & Foster, F.M. (1987). *Guide to the Alcohol Use Inventory.* Minneapolis, MN: National Computer Systems. (800-627-7271)

Horvath, A.T. (1993). Enhancing motivation for treatment of addictive behavior: Guidelines for the psychotherapist. *Psychotherapy, 30,* 473–480.

Horvath, A.T. (1994). Comorbidity of addictive behavior and mental disorder: Outpatient practice guidelines for those who prefer not to treat addictive behavior. *Cognitive and Behavioral Practice, 1,* 93–109.

McLellan, A.T., Parikh, G., Bragg, A., Cacciola, J., Fureman, B., & Incmikofki, R. (1990). *Addiction Severity Index administration manual* (5th ed.). Philadelphia: Penn-VA Center for Studies of Addiction. (DeltaMetrics/TRI, 800-238-2433)

Miller, W.R., Brown, J.M., Simpson, T.L., Handmaker, N.S., Bien, T.H., Luckie, L.F., Montgomery, H.A., Hester, R.K., & Tonigan, J.S. (1995). What works? A methodological analysis of the alcohol treatment outcome literature. In W.R. Miller & R.K. Hester (Eds.), *Handbook of alcoholism treatment approaches: Effective alternatives* (2nd ed., pp. 12–44). Boston: Allyn & Bacon.

Miller, W.R., & Munoz, R.F. (1982). *How to control your drinking* (rev. ed.). Albuquerque: University of New Mexico. (CASAA, 505-277-2805)

Miller, W.R., & Rollnick, S. (1991). *Motivational interviewing: Preparing people to change addictive behavior.* New York: Guilford Press.

Miller, W.R., Westerberg, V.S., & Waldron, H.B. (1995). Evaluating alcohol problems in adults and adolescents. In W.R. Miller & R.K. Hester (Eds.), *Handbook of effective alcoholism treatment approaches: Effective alternatives* (2nd ed., pp. 61–88). Boston: Allyn & Bacon.

National Academy of Sciences. (1990a). *Broadening the base of treatment for drug problems.* Washington, DC: National Academy Press.

National Academy of Sciences. (1990b). *Treating drug problems* (Vol. 1). Washington, DC: National Academy Press.

Otto, M.W., Pollack, M.H., & Barlow, D.H. (1995). *Stopping anxiety medication: A workbook for patients wanting to discontinue benzodiazepine treatment for panic disorder.* Albany, NY: Graywind. (518-438-3231; 800-228-0752)

Persons, J.B. (1989). *Cognitive therapy in practice: A case formulation approach.* New York: Norton.

Prochaska, J.O., DiClemente, C.C., & Norcross, J.C. (1992). In search of how people change: Applications to addictive behavior. *American Psychologist, 47,* 1102–1114.

Sanchez-Craig, M. (1993). *Saying when: How to quit drinking or cut down.* Toronto, Ontario: Addiction Research Foundation. (800-661-1111)

Skinner, H.A. (1994). *Computerized lifestyle assessment.* North Tonawanda, NY: Multi-Health Systems. (800-456-3003)

Sobell, L.C., Toneatto, T., & Sobell, M.B. (1994). Behavioral assessment and treatment planning for alcohol, tobacco, and other drug problems: Current status with an emphasis on clinical applications. *Behavior Therapy, 25,* 533–580.

Young, J.E., Beck, A.T., & Weinberger, A. (1993). Depression. In D.H. Barlow (Ed.), *Clinical handbook of psychological disorders* (2nd ed., pp. 240–277). New York: Guilford Press.

11

Pharmacological Treatment of Substance Abuse and Comorbidity

DAVID McDOWELL
EDWARD V. NUNES

Many psychiatric patients are now known to have concomitant drug or alcohol problems. The converse is also true—that patients presenting with drug or alcohol abuse frequently have significant psychopathology (Allen & Frances, 1986; Regier et al., 1990). In substance abuse treatment settings the term *dual diagnosis* has been developed to describe those individuals with one or more psychiatric conditions as well as substance abuse. The term *mentally ill chemical abuser* (MICA) is more commonly used in settings where the principal focus is on psychopathology.

Multiple etiologic relationships between substance abuse and psychopathology have been suggested (Meyer, 1986; Schuckit, 1986), and these may be simplified to three: (1) primary psychopathology with subsequent substance abuse; (2) primary substance abuse with subsequent psychopathology (substance-induced), and (3) simultaneous, independent conditions (First & Gladis, 1993; Nunes et al., 1994).

This work was supported by grants K20DA00154 and P50DA09236 from the National Institute on Drug Abuse.

In primary psychopathology, the *self-medication hypothesis* postulates that underlying psychiatric problems contribute to the development and continuation of substance abuse disorders. This idea derives from the psychoanalytic tradition that substances are used as a means to cope with painful affects (Khantzian, 1985). Alternatively, substance use may be self-treatment for underlying Axis I disorders such as depression or anxiety (Quitkin, Rifkin, Kaplan, & Klein, 1972). According to this model, treating the underlying disorder should reduce the substance use as well. Taken to its extreme, this position results in the cartoon of a patient arriving drunk to psychotherapy sessions in which the therapist never addresses the substance abuse. A more sound approach is to view substance use as either a form of resistance or as ineffective self-treatment, which the patient must give up in order to abet treatment of the underlying condition.

With secondary psychopathology, the psychopathology may be induced by the toxic effects of substances. This model is supported by the consistent finding that psychopathology often remits shortly after abstinence is achieved (DeLeon, Skodol, & Rosenthal, 1973; Rounsaville, Kosten, & Kleber, 1986; Schuckit, 1986; Willis & Osbourne, 1978). If this model is correct, adequate treatment of the substance abuse should cure the presenting psychopathology, whereas attempting to treat the psychopathology may divert attention from the substance abuse, introducing a dangerous resistance in the patient and contributing to denial. This view is part of the tradition of many self-help groups, such as Alcoholics Anonymous. Taken to its extreme this position can suggest that patients not take medications for potentially dangerous conditions such as major depression and bipolar or schizoaffective disorders.

Although this topic can engender considerable controversy among both clinicians and patients, there appears to be support for both models articulated above (primary psychopathology versus primary substance abuse), and the truth for a given patient will often lie somewhere between. Rigid adherence to either view is not in the best interest of patients; instead, a flexible approach is recommended, open to the possibilities that either disorder may be primary or that both may coexist independently (Nunes, McGrath, & Quitkin, 1995).

APPROACH TO THE PATIENT

History

Assessment of patients who present with substance abuse and a psychiatric condition begins with a complete history and physical examination. The history should include four areas: (1) precipitating events leading to presentation; (2) onset and pattern of drug use over the patient's lifetime; (3) positive and negative consequences of drug use for the patient (Does substance use temporarily relieve psychiatric symptoms?); and (4) onset and course of psychiatric comorbidity in relation to course of substance use (Which began first, substance abuse or psychiatric disorder, and does the psychiatric disorder remit or persist during periods of sobriety?). The clinician should also consider the social context in which drugs are used. An adolescent with impulse control problems may take drugs impulsively or to gain peer acceptance. An adult with social phobia may use drugs or alcohol to tolerate social gatherings.

Including members of a patient's social network can often be useful in determining an adequate history and developing a treatment plan. These members can include spouses, family members, friends, employers, social workers, or parole officers. Both patients and network members may resist such involvement, and the clinician must be prepared to overcome the resistance. Patients may initially deny they have any willing network members, when, in fact, nearly everyone has some person in his or her life who can provide help and information (Galanter, 1992).

Substance abusers are sometimes poor historians because of denial, deliberate obfuscation, or poor memory resulting from substance-induced organicity (Hwang & Nunes, 1995). Collateral historians will aid in clarifying the history. On the other hand, both psychiatric diagnosis (Nunes, Goehl, et al., in press; Williams et al., 1992) and self-reported substance use (Magura, Goldsmith, Casriel, Goldstein, & Lipton, 1987) are generally reliable in substance abuse patients, particularly in settings where there are no adverse consequences of accurate reporting. This observation suggests that an open and accepting, rather than a moralistic or disapproving, stance on the part of the clinician is most likely to elicit an accurate history.

Physical and Laboratory Examination

A thorough medical history, with physical and laboratory evaluation, is essential in the patient with dual diagnosis. There are numerous physical consequences of substance use from the direct toxicity of the substances (e.g., substance-induced cognitive impairment, nicotine- or cocaine-related cardiovascular disease, alcoholic liver disease) and the high-risk behaviors associated with intoxication (sexually and parenterally transmitted diseases such as viral hepatitis and acquired immunodeficiency syndrome [AIDS]) as well as harmful consequences of the route of administration, particularly injection drug use, smoking, and freebasing (e.g., chronic lung disease, bacterial endocarditis) (Novick, 1992). In addition to requiring direct evaluation and treatment, many of these diseases may produce fatigue, apathy, cognitive impairment, or anxiety that may mimic psychiatric disorders; therefore, their consideration becomes a critical part of the psychiatric differential diagnosis.

DIFFERENTIAL DIAGNOSIS OF PRIMARY OR INDEPENDENT VERSUS SUBSTANCE-INDUCED PSYCHOPATHOLOGY

As suggested above, the diagnosis of psychopathology in active substance abusers is a challenge and an ongoing source of controversy. The ideal approach, recommended in *DSM-IV* (American Psychiatric Association [APA], 1994), requires persistence of psychopathology during at least a one-month abstinence before the diagnosis of a comorbid disorder such as depression can be made. Although the first effort in diagnostic evaluation should be to treat the substance abuse and achieve abstinence, in practice, abstinence is often difficult to achieve on an outpatient basis, and patients frequently cannot or will not be hospitalized, or can be hospitalized for only a matter of days because of insurance constraints. Further, because psychopathology is known to worsen the severity of substance abuse, as discussed earlier, those very patients with comorbid psychiatric symptoms are often the most difficult to keep abstinent. This creates an unfortunate clinical catch-22 in which a depression, for example, is not diagnosed or treated because of the patient's lack of abstinence, yet for him or her to maintain abstinence may depend on having the depression treated.

The alternative is to attempt the differential diagnosis in an outpatient who may still be actively using substances. Some clinicians hypothesize that features of the history and presentation can indicate whether a comorbid condition is primary or is independent of substance use, warranting specific treatment (Nunes, McGrath, & Quitkin, 1995; Nunes, Goehl, et al., in press; Rounsaville, Anton, Carroll, & Meyer, 1991). These conditions include (1) psychopathology that is chronologically primary (antedates first onset of substance abuse); (2) psychopathology that persists during earlier periods of abstinence; (3) chronic, as opposed to intermittent or transient, psychopathology; (4) emergence of psychopathology during periods of stable substance use, rather than periods of rapidly escalating (or diminishing) use; (5) positive family history of similar psychopathology (as most psychiatric disorders are familial, probably in part because of inherited factors);

and (6) uniqueness of the psychiatric symptoms (for example, agoraphobia, social phobia, and obsessions or compulsions are unique to anxiety disorders and do not usually occur as part of drug toxicity or withdrawal. Likewise, profound suicidal ideation should increase suspicion that a true mood disorder is operating). It is vitally important that the experienced professional exercise clinical judgment after weighing all the evidence.

PHARMACOLOGIC TREATMENTS OF SUBSTANCE ABUSE AND COMORBIDITY

Pharmacotherapy is an important component of the treatment of combined substance use and psychiatric disorders and is the focus of this chapter. However, it cannot be emphasized strongly enough that medication must be part of a comprehensive treatment plan that includes a strong psychotherapeutic and behavioral foundation. Addiction is a disorder of motivation and behavior that requires specific psychological interventions. There are many such techniques, reviewed comprehensively elsewhere (APA, 1995; Galanter & Kleber, 1994; Lowinson, Millman, Ruiz, & Langrod, 1992). In this chapter, psychosocial techniques are discussed only in terms of synergy with specific pharmacotherapies.

Pharmacotherapies for substance use disorders can be divided according to four broad aims: (1) treatment of acute intoxication; (2) treatment of withdrawal; (3) promotion of abstinence or prevention of relapse by blocking the reinforcing effects of drugs, creating or enhancing aversive effects of drugs, or replacing the abused drug with a less toxic agonist; and (4) treatment of comorbid psychiatric conditions. Table 11-1 provides an organizing framework for the chapter by listing pharmacotherapies promoting each of these effects for each class of abused substance. Treatment of (1) intoxication and (2) withdrawal are generic with or without comorbidity, are well described elsewhere (APA, 1995), and are not discussed further here. The remainder of the chapter focuses on the longer-term management of dual diagnosis patients subsumed in aims (3) and (4).

PHARMACOTHERAPIES FOR ALCOHOL USE DISORDERS

Alcohol abuse is a major public health problem, and among alcoholics, psychiatric comorbidity is common and associated with poor prognosis. Fifty-five percent of Americans drink three or more ounces of alcohol per week (*Morbidity and Mortality,* 1989). The lifetime prevalence of alcohol use disorders (abuse or dependence) is 23 percent (Regier et al., 1990). Alcohol-related health conditions are estimated to be the third largest health problem in the country, behind heart disease and cancer (Goodwin, 1992). Alcohol is estimated to be a factor in 50 percent of violent crimes and 25 percent to 30 percent of suicides and accidental deaths (Goodwin, 1992). In the Epidemiologic Catchment Area (ECA) study, the presence of most mood or anxiety disorders in an individual at least doubled the odds that the person would also have an alcohol use disorder (Regier et al., 1990). Psychiatric comorbidity, particularly depression, has been associated with increased severity of drinking (Rounsaville, Dolinsky, Babor, & Meyer, 1987), relapse (Loosen, Dew, & Prange, 1990), and suicide (Murphy, Wetzel, Robins, & McEvoy, 1992). These findings provide a strong impetus for identifying and treating alcoholism and its psychiatric comorbidity.

Disulfiram

Disulfiram is a powerful tool in the management of alcoholism. Taken orally (the usual dose is 250 mg to 500 mg in the morning), disulfiram inhibits acetaldehyde dehydrogenase, resulting in a rapid buildup of acetaldehyde upon ingestion of alcohol. This result creates a very unpleasant reaction, including flushing, nausea, headache, and hypotension. Severe hypotension or shock is rare; it is more likely with excessive dosage or in patients with preexisting cardiopulmonary compromise in whom disulfiram is therefore relatively contraindicated (Gallant, 1991).

Side effects to daily disulfiram, in the absence of alcohol intake, are rare. In one randomized, placebo-controlled study, evaluation of side effects in 158 alcoholic patients who completed the study showed no differences between the placebo and disulfiram groups. Skin reactions, itching, fatigue, or lethargy were no more common in the disulfiram group than in controls (Christensen, Ronstead, & Vaag, 1984). Disulfiram reactions sometimes result from alcohol contained in medications like over-the-counter cough syrups, alcohol used in cooking (although this is usually burned off), or topical perfumes. Patients should be warned to be alert to these.

Disulfiram-induced hepatotoxicity is dangerous but extremely rare. Only about 25 cases have been reported in the world literature (Gallant, 1994). Nevertheless it is prudent to assess liver transaminases periodically (every six months) during disulfiram treatment; patients should be warned that, if symptoms of hepatitis occur, the disulfiram could be involved and a physician should be contacted immediately.

Disulfiram should be considered in any alcoholic patient having difficulty maintaining sobriety during outpatient treatment. One major problem is that patients can easily stop the medication and a few days later begin to

TABLE 11-1

Pharmacotherapies for Substance Use Disorders and Related Psychiatric Comorbidity, by Class of Abused Substance and Pharmacotherapeutic Aim

Class of Substance	Therapeutic Aim	Medication
Alcohol and other sedatives	1. Alleviate withdrawal	• Long acting benzodiazepines or phenobarbital (reduce symptoms; prevent seizures and delirium). • Anti-adrenergic medications, beta-blockers, alpha-1 agonists (does not prevent seizures). • Neuroleptics (sometimes useful in managing withdrawal delirium).
	2. Promote abstinence; prevent relapse	• Disulfiram (renders alcohol aversive via toxic metabolites; best monitored by a significant other). • Naltrexone (reduces relapse risk, perhaps by reducing reinforcing effects of alcohol).
	3. Treat comorbid psychopathology	• Tricyclic antidepressants (treat comorbid depression or panic disorder; may reduce drinking). • Serotonin uptake inhibitors (treat comorbid depression). • Benzodiazepines (relieve panic or other anxiety symptoms; caution due to addictive potential). • Buspirone (treats generalized anxiety; may reduce drinking).
Opiates	1. Manage acute intoxication	• Naloxone (antagonist at opiate receptors; lifesaving for overdoses; precipitates withdrawal; short half-life requires repeated dosage).
	2. Alleviate withdrawal	• Clonidine (reduces sympathetic nervous system arousal; less effect on anxiety, insomnia). • Benzodiazepines (reduce anxiety; enable sleep; less effect on sympathetic arousal). • Long-acting opiate agonists—methadone (effective but require a slow taper). • Clonidine to naltrexone, buprenorphine to naltrexone (rapid; requires close monitoring due to risk of precipitating severe withdrawal).

	3. Promote abstinence; prevent relapse	• Slow-onset, long-acting opiate agonists—methadone, LAAM, buprenorphine (induce cross-tolerance and block effects of illicit opiates; noncompliance produces withdrawal, discouraging recidivism; requires special licensure and program). • Naltrexone (antagonist at opiate receptors; blocks effects of illicit opiates; more successful if monitored by a significant other or combined with contingency contracting).
	4. Treat comorbid psychopathology	• Tricyclic antidepressants (treat comorbid depression or panic disorder; may reduce drug use). • Serotonin uptake inhibitors (treat comorbid depression).
Cocaine and other stimulants	1. Manage acute intoxication	• Benzodiazepines (reduce agitation). • Neuroleptics (manage paranoid psychosis; caution regarding lowered seizure threshold).
	2. Alleviate withdrawal	• Dopamine agonists—amantadine, bromocriptine (small effect, if any; withdrawal usually self-limited, not requiring pharmacotherapy).
	3. Promote abstinence; prevent relapse	• Tricyclic antidepressants—desipramine, imipramine (small effect, if any; effect may be limited to first weeks of abstinence, or to intranasal or depressed cocaine users). • Many other pharmacotherapies have been tested with no clear successes.
	4. Treat comorbid psychopathology	• Tricyclic antidepressants (treat comorbid depression or panic disorder; may reduce cocaine use). • Neuroleptics (treat comorbid schizophrenia; neuroleptic anhedonia may promote stimulant use). • Lithium, other mood stabilizers (treat bipolar I or spectrum disorders).
Nicotine	1. Alleviate withdrawal	• Nicotine replacement with gum or skin patch (concurrent smoking risks nicotine toxicity).
	2. Promote abstinence; prevent relapse	• Nicotine replacement (long-term safety not established; may involve cardiovascular risk).
	3. Treat comorbid psychopathology	• Antidepressants—tricyclics, selective serotonin reuptake inhibitors, or bupropion (smoking cessation may precipitate depression, requiring treatment; effect on prevention of relapse not yet established).

drink. Supervision of disulfiram intake by medical staff or significant others is therefore strongly recommended. Studies in which disulfiram was not found to be effective did not include supervised intake. Supervised disulfiram maintenance has been shown to be significantly superior to voluntary disulfiram in terms of patient retention in treatment and clinical outcome (Sereny, Sharma, & Holt, 1986). Disulfiram compliance can be monitored by inspecting the patient's urine for its metabolite, dithylamine. Administration by spouses or cohabitants of patients, who have received positive reinforcement therapy, results in even more therapeutic gains than for patients receiving it without positive reinforcement (Azrin, Sisson, & Meyers, 1982). If used effectively, disulfiram is not only an aversive agent but a symbol of the patient's commitment to abstinence and treatment. Patients can be instructed to take their daily dose in front of their spouse or loved one, saying "I am taking this as a symbol of my desire to remain abstinent and healthy." If the patient refuses, the spouse is instructed not to argue with the patient but to contact the prescribing physician. At that time, the physician can deal with the patient's resistance.

Patients should be instructed to take their daily dose in the morning when the desire to drink is usually low. Patients are frequently concerned that the drug will take away their control and they will never be able to drink again. These individuals are relieved if told that it takes away their ability to drink for only the next week. This simple instruction is often quite reassuring. In general, PRN disulfiram is not recommended. There are, however, certain individuals for whom this might be applicable. A patient who has been long abstinent but is faced with a particularly stressful situation with an opportunity to drink may be instructed to take a dose before this situation. An example is a businesswoman who has been sober without the aid of antabuse for several years. She is faced with a particularly stressful business retreat where her colleagues and superiors will likely be drinking heavily and, because they are unaware of her alcoholism, will encourage her to drink. Although treatment duration has not been well studied, at least six months of treatment is recommended for the patient attempting to establish abstinence. This periods allows time for patients to learn the coping skills necessary to maintain sobriety.

Although there has been little systematic study of disulfiram in alcoholics with psychiatric comorbidity, clinical experience suggests it is effective in combination with antidepressant medications for alcoholics with mood or anxiety disorders (Nunes et al., 1993; Nunes, Deliyannides, Donovan, & McGrath, in press). Because depressive and anxiety symptoms are often created or worsened by alcohol, establishment of abstinence with disulfiram can help clarify the diagnosis or boost the effectiveness of antidepressant medications. One caveat is that disulfiram has been implicated, in rare cases, in acute onset of psychosis, perhaps because it inhibits dopamine B-hydroxylase activity, raising central dopaminergic tone (Nunes & Quitkin, 1987). Disulfiram should therefore be used with caution in patients with comorbid schizophrenia or mood disorder with a history of psychosis. Chronically psychotic patients may require an increase in their neuroleptic dosage (Gallant, 1994).

Naltrexone

A considerable amount of evidence suggests the hypothesis that opioid antagonists would be useful in treating alcoholism. Opiates and alcohol have similar sedative and euphorigenic effects. There is cross-tolerance between opiates and alcohol in the relief of withdrawal symptoms. In animals, opiate antagonists attenuate alcohol-induced effects. Small doses of opiates increase alcohol consumption in laboratory animals, and opioid antagonists in these same animals will reduce alcohol consumption. Some alcoholics have shown decreased baseline levels of endogenous opiates, and the initial euphoria associated with alcohol is thought to be more reinforcing in this population (Kosten & McCance-Katz, 1995).

Two randomized, placebo-controlled clinical trials in alcohol-dependent patients have indeed suggested that the opioid antagonist naltrexone, taken at 50 mg per day under supervision, significantly reduced drinking compared to placebo (Volpicelli, Alterman, Hyashida, & O'Brien, 1992; O'Malley et al., 1992). Naltrexone appeared to reduce the severity of relapses (i.e., number of drinks) more than their frequency. In other words it can help prevent a lapse from becoming a relapse. The drug may work by attenuating the subjective euphorigenic effects of initial alcohol consumption (Kosten & McCance-Katz, 1995). Psychotherapy administered in the clinical trials had an interesting relationship with naltrexone treatment. The overall outcome was best for those individuals who received relapse prevention/coping skills treatment rather than nonstructured supportive treatment (Volpicelli et al., 1992; O'Malley et al., 1992). Clearly naltrexone needs to be part of a larger and more comprehensive approach. Merely prescribing the drug to patients without other counseling and treatment is unlikely to be successful.

Naltrexone is currently recommended at a dosage of 50 mg per day. Although not sufficiently studied, higher doses may be helpful in some patients. In general, the drug is well tolerated, and side effects are minimal. Periodic monitoring of liver enzymes is recommended because of the remote possibility of hepatotoxicity, which resolves if the drug is discontinued (Arndt, Cacciola, & McLellan, 1986). Dysphoria was not a problem in the controlled trials (O'Malley et al., 1992; Volpicelli et al., 1992), and naltrexone does not appear to reduce the pleasure associated with such activities as running (the runners' high) or sex. Clinical experience at our center suggests that naltrexone is effective at reducing patients' drinking, and is well tolerated in alcoholics with depression (P.J. McGrath, personal communication, 1995) or with schizophrenia or schizoaffective disorder (S. Coomaraswamy, personal communication, 1995).

Antidepressant Medications

An older series of studies, reviewed elsewhere (Ciraulo & Jaffe, 1981; Liskow & Goodwin, 1987), examined various tricyclic antidepressants (TCAs) and monoamine oxidase inhibitors in the treatment of alcoholics. These studies produced no clear evidence of a favorable effect on drinking behavior, but they had significant methodologic weaknesses, including a failure adequately to diagnose depression. Recently, selective serotonin uptake inhibitors (SSRIs) have been suggested for nondepressed alcoholics, based on preclinical evidence that they modestly reduce alcohol intake (Sellers, Higgins, & Sobell, 1992). However, clinical trials to date show no such efficacy (Kranzler et al., 1994). In summary, antidepressants cannot be recommended as effective agents for the reduction of alcohol consumption in *nondepressed* individuals.

In contrast, an emerging body of evidence suggests that for alcoholics with carefully diagnosed depressive syndromes, antidepressant medications are effective in improving mood and in reducing (but usually not eliminating) alcohol consumption. A number of studies have supported this conclusion: (1) an open-label trial of imipramine, followed by placebo-discontinuation, in actively drinking outpatient alcoholics with depressive syndromes that were either chronologically primary, persistent during past abstinences, or chronic (Nunes et al., 1993); (2) a placebo-controlled trial of desipramine in alcoholics with depression that was chronologically secondary but had persisted during a current abstinent period (Mason & Kocsis, 1991); and (3) an open-label trial of fluoxetine in severely depressed alcoholics with suicidal ideation (Cornelius et al., 1993). Tricyclic antidepressants have substantial side effects, such as sedation, which may be of concern in an alcoholic. These drugs are quite lethal in overdose, and dually diagnosed patients are at high risk for suicide. Although more trials of SSRIs are needed, these agents are becoming the treatment of choice in dually diagnosed alcoholics because of their more benign side effect and safety profile. To prevent anxiety reactions or jitteriness, SSRIs should be started at low doses and then gradually titrated up to adequate doses. The most common mistakes in the use of any antidepressant are prescribing too low a dose for too short a period of time and premature discontinuation of the medication once an adequate therapeutic response has occurred.

Anxiolytic Medications

The first priority with an anxious alcoholic is to rule out and treat alcohol withdrawal. It is important to establish the time since the patient's last drink and to examine the patient and take vital signs. Any history of severe alcohol withdrawal, seizures or delirium tremens should be established as these increase the risk of more severe manifestations in the current episode and would warrant more vigorous treatment of withdrawal.

Benzodiazepines are a mainstay in the treatment of alcohol withdrawal, where they reduce minor withdrawal symptoms and protect against the development of seizures and delirium tremens (APA, 1995). However, other than during withdrawal, benzodiazepines should be avoided in alcoholics or used only in special circumstances because of the risk of iatrogenic cross-addiction. Antidepressants, mainly tricyclics or selective serotonin uptake inhibitors, are more effective for most anxiety disorders such as generalized anxiety disorder, panic disorder, or social phobia. There are no published clinical trials of antidepressants in alcoholics with anxiety disorders, other than the observation that a history of panic disorder predicted a favorable response to imipramine in depressed alcoholics (Nunes et al., 1993); and further research in this area is needed. In the meantime, as recommended for depressed alcoholics, less sedating TCAs or SSRIs would be preferred, although moderately soporific agents such as imipramine or traxodone may be chosen if patients have insomnia or if chronically high levels of anxiety are an associated symptom (Nunes, McGrath, & Quitkin, 1995). Despite caveats, there are alcoholic patients with anxiety disorders who require benzodiazepines and judicious use of these agents may be highly effective (Baron, Sands, Ciraulo, & Shader, 1990). Their use is more acceptable if the patient is relatively sober, but it becomes contraindicated in the setting of heavy drinking.

Buspirone is a 5-HT partial agonist, which is indicated for generalized anxiety disorder (GAD). Unlike benzodiazepines, it is not sedating and there may be a delay of several weeks before it begins to work. It has not found wide use as an anxiolytic, although this may be, in part, because higher doses (20 mg twice or three times a day) than those recommended in the *Physicians' Desk Reference* (*PDR*) are often needed. In a placebo-controlled trial with alcoholic dependent patients who had high levels of generalized anxiety after at least a week of sobriety, buspirone was both safe and more effective than placebo in reducing patients' anxiety and improving drinking outcome (Kranzler et al., 1994).

Lithium

An older literature, reviewed elsewhere (Nunes & Quitkin, in press), suggested that lithium was effective in reducing drinking in outpatient alcoholics. However, a large, recent placebo-controlled trial found no such effect of lithium in alcoholics, with or without major depression (Dorus et al., 1989). Thus, lithium cannot be recommended as a treatment for alcoholics, other than for those with lithium-responsive bipolar disorder. Patients with bipolar disorder are at increased risk for alcoholism (Regier et al., 1990), and among patients with bipolar disorder, drinking is particularly likely to worsen during manic episodes.

OPIOIDS

Opioids are those compounds that bind to the family of opiate receptors; they include both naturally occurring alkaloids, such as opium, morphine and codeine, and synthetic and semisynthetic agents, including diacetyl-morphine (heroin), hydromorphone (dilaudid), oxycodone (percodan), propoxyphene (Darvon), meperidine (demerol), methadone and fentanyl. Physical effect includes suppression of the cough reflex, bowel hypomotility, analgesia, and in higher doses, respiratory depression. Subjective effects include indifference to distress and feelings of euphoria and well-being. Although opiates are generally thought to be soporific, some addicts paradoxically report feeling energized. Opiate withdrawal is not medically dangerous, but it can be very unpleasant, with anxiety, dysphoria, flulike aches and pains, and signs and symptoms of autonomic arousal.

Opiates are invaluable tools in the treatment of numerous medical conditions, including the management of acute and chronic pain. The majority of medical patients exposed to opiates do not become addicted. Only a fraction of heroin-exposed servicemen during the Vietnam War remained addicted after returning to the United States (Robins, 1979). However, opiates are highly addictive for vulnerable individuals, and the causes of that vulnerability are not well understood. Current estimates are that at least 750,000 Americans are addicted to heroin, although that figure may be much higher (O'Brien, 1994). Opiate addiction is highly debilitating. A street habit is expensive, causing addicts to drain their financial resources or resort to crime to support their habits. Injection drug use is associated with a host of serious medical problems, including contraction of the human immunodeficiency virus (HIV) and other blood-borne infections.

PHARMACOTHERAPIES FOR OPIATE DEPENDENCE

Methadone and Other Agonist Substitution Therapies

For many patients with chronic relapsing opioid dependence the treatment of choice has been maintenance on the long-acting opioid, methadone. Methadone, taken orally, is slowly absorbed and appears to work by occupying opiate receptors and inducing tolerance, such that the euphoric and reinforcing effects of street opiates are blocked. Its long half-life—24 to 36 hours—permits once daily administration without the development of withdrawal. However, if a patient misses a day's dose, significant withdrawal symptoms develop, a condition that helps to reinforce compliance with treatment. Methadone maintenance has been shown to be highly effective for decreasing opioid dependence, with improvements in health status, decreased mortality, decreased criminal activity and improved social functioning (Ball, Corty, & Myers, 1988).

Methadone maintenance is available only in specially licensed clinics. Federal guidelines limit its use to patients with at least a one-year history of opioid dependence and demonstrated physiologic manifestations of dependence. Daily attendance at a clinic is required so that patients ingest methadone under supervision until they have established a persistent pattern of drug-free urine. Because it is so highly regulated, the methadone delivery system can be quite cumbersome to patients. Negative attitudes toward methadone, usually based on the misconception that it is just a substitute addiction, must also be overcome.

Effectiveness of methadone maintenance requires adequate dosage and concurrent counseling. Doses greater than 80 mg are often needed to resolve withdrawal symptoms and induce abstinence, but the average daily dose across the United States is 40 mg (O'Brien, 1994). The effectiveness of methadone is known to increase with concurrent counseling and available psychosocial and medical services (McLellan, Arndt, Metzger, Woody, & O'Brien, 1993). Discontinuation of methadone once treatment has begun is unfortunately followed by relapse in most patients (Cooper, 1992). To be effective, methadone must be understood as a long-term, perhaps lifelong, treatment.

L-alpha acetylmethadol (LAAM) is a long-acting opiate with action similar to that of methadone; however, it can be taken three times per week, reducing the patient's burden of clinical visits. It has only recently been approved for marketing in the United States and has yet to see wide clinical application. Results of premarketing trials suggest it is effective, but it may be more difficult to regulate at the outset of treatment because of extremely slow absorption and resultant delayed relief of withdrawal symptoms (Kosten & McCance-Katz, 1995).

Buprenorphine is a partial opioid agonist, which binds opiate receptors with high affinity but only partially activates them. It is not yet marketed, but results of premarketing trials suggest it will be a useful alternative to methadone for agonist maintenance. It also appears to produce only relatively mild withdrawal symptoms and thus may be a superior agent for management of opiate withdrawal (Johnson, Fudala, & Jaffe, 1992).

Antagonist Maintenance—Naltrexone

Naltrexone is an orally administered, long-acting opioid antagonist that binds with high affinity to opiate receptors, blocking the euphoric and reinforcing effects of other opiates. It also displaces opiates already resident on receptors and will therefore precipitate withdrawal in dependent individuals. Therefore, clinicians must be sure that prospective patients have been adequately detoxified. The usual dose, 50 mg, blocks the effects of opiates for about 24 hours. The drug may be taken as 50 mg daily, but it is also effective on a three-days-per-week schedule (100 mg on Monday and Wednesday and 150 mg on Fridays).

A major problem with naltrexone is that a patient can easily stop taking it (no withdrawal), and once illicit opiates are resumed, naltrexone cannot be restarted because it will precipitate withdrawal. Concurrent psychosocial treatment, including having significant others or clinic staff supervise naltrexone ingestion is therefore important in increasing a patient's odds of success (Resnick, Schuyten-Resnick, & Washton, 1979). A depot form of the drug is under development and should be enormously helpful as an adjunct or alternative to supervised dosing.

Antidepressant Medications and Anxiolytics

Among opioid addicts, the lifetime prevalence of major depression has been reported at 20 percent to 60 percent (Rounsaville et al., 1986; Weissman et al., 1976), a figure far in excess of the prevalence in the general population (Regier et al., 1990). Depression is associated with a poor prognosis in opiate addicts (DeLeon et al., 1973; Kosten, Rounsaville, & Kleber, 1986; Rounsaville et al., 1986; Willis & Osbourne, 1978). A series of clinical trials, reviewed elsewhere (Nunes et al., 1994), suggests tricyclic antidepressants are effective in treating depression among methadone maintenance patients. Such treatment may also reduce illicit drug use; but this effect is likely modest, and continued drug use needs to be addressed with increased methadone doses or more intensive psychosocial interventions. Opiates are not highly depressogenic or anxiogenic except during withdrawal, so that in patients on stable methadone treatment, there is less concern about substance-induced psychopathology unless the patient is using large quantities of street drugs. Tricyclic antidepressants have been generally well tolerated in methadone patients, although the authors' clinical experience suggests that anticholinergic effects may be problematic. Methadone slows the metabolism of tricyclics (Kosten, Gawin, Morgan, Nelson, & Jatlow, 1990) so that lower doses may be needed, and monitoring of blood levels is prudent.

There are few or no data on the treatment of anxiety disorders in opiate-dependent patients. However, clinical experience suggests that benzodiazepines should be avoided in opioid-dependent patients because of their abuse potential in this population. In addition, knowledge that a given physician will prescribe benzodiazepines may lead to drug-seeking behavior among some patients in this group.

COCAINE

Cocaine is a stimulant that acts by blocking reuptake of norepinephrine, serotonin, and dopamine. It also has local anesthetic and vasoconstrictive as well as euphorigenic effects. General cocaine use has decreased over the past 10 years, although heavy use continues to rise. Estimates from the National Institute on Drug Abuse are that 10 percent to 15 percent of those who initially use cocaine will become problem users. What differentiates those who will go on to become addicted is not understood (Verebey & Gold, 1988).

Subjective effects of cocaine intoxication and use include feelings of confidence and well-being, and magnification of the intensity of normal pleasures. Anxiety is initially decreased and social inhibitions are reduced. Physiologic effects include tachycardia, pupillary dilation, hypertension and hyperactivity. In higher doses paranoia can occur; this clinically is identical to the acute psychosis associated with schizophrenia and mania. There is a postintoxication or withdrawal syndrome that includes exhaustion, hypersomnia, hyperphagia, depressed mood, and intermittent periods of craving for cocaine (Gawin & Kleber, 1986). Recent studies in hospitalized cocaine abusers have shown that these abstinence symptoms are relatively mild for most patients and resolve within a week of their achieving abstinence (Weddington et al., 1990), calling somewhat into question the relevance of these conditions as a target for pharmacotherapy.

Pharmacotherapy for Cocaine Dependence

A large number of agents, mainly antidepressants and dopamine agonists, have been tested as treatments for cocaine abuse, but none have demonstrated clear efficacy. Tricyclic antidepressants, mainly desipramine, have been the most thoroughly studied and have shown some limited promise. Trials of most other pharmacologic agents for cocaine abuse have been more flatly negative. Tricyclics were originally proposed because they reverse the effects of cocaine on the intracranial self-stimulation model, thought to represent cocaine-induced dysregulation and blunting of the brain reward system (Gawin et al., 1989). A recent review of the various placebo-controlled desipramine trials, however, suggests there is probably a small- to medium-size effect on cocaine craving and a marginal effect on cocaine use; this may be restricted to the early weeks of treatment or perhaps limited to intranasal users or depressed users (Nunes, in press).

Tricyclics cannot, therefore, be recommended as a routine treatment for cocaine abuse, although they might be considered in patients who have failed other approaches or who have depressive symptomatology. Depression is common in cocaine abusers, and is associated with poor outcome (Carroll, Power, Bryant, & Rounsaville, 1993). As with alcohol, cocaine induces considerable depressive symptomatology, making differential diagnosis difficult. However, several clinical trials have suggested that depressed cocaine abusers may benefit selectively from tricyclic antidepressants (Nunes et al., 1995; Ziedonis & Kosten, 1991).

The evaluation of anxiety disorders is difficult in cocaine abusers because cocaine is anxiogenic and its use is associated with the induction of panic attacks. In many instances the anxiety will lessen when the substance abuse remits. The clinical principals for differential diagnosis of substance-induced versus independent psychopathology, discussed earlier, can be applied. If an independent anxiety disorder is suspected, then treatment with an antidepressant, either a TCA or an SSRI is warranted. Buspirone also appears to be safe. Caution, as with all substance abusers, should be employed in the consideration of benzodiazepines with this population.

Cocaine, both the intranasal and the smokable form (freebase or crack) has had a devastating effect on the urban poor and homeless population. A large number of these people carry the diagnosis of schizophrenia (Rounsaville et al., 1991). At least part of the symptomatology of the acute psychotic phase of schizophrenia is a manifestation of excessive dopamine neurotransmission. Cocaine increases dopamine neurotransmission and therefore can mimic psychosis or exacerbate an underlying psychotic condition such as schizophrenia. Although formal clinical trials in schizophrenic substance abusers are lacking, experience suggests that neuroleptics are useful in this population. Equally important is prompt attention to the substance dependence. These patients need a great deal of social and therapeutic support, and they may require hospitalization to manage periods of increased cocaine use and psychosis.

NICOTINE

Nicotine has come into focus over the last 15 years as a classically addictive drug. It has subtle stimulantlike effects and is highly reinforcing, apparently because of its action on nicotine receptors in the brain reward system. Fifty-one million people in the United States are nicotine dependent, mostly through cigarette smoking. The adverse public health impact is enormous, contributing to increased incidence of coronary, cerebral, and peripheral vascular disease; chronic obstructive pulmonary disease; and cancer. The nicotine withdrawal syndrome is now well characterized and appears to contribute to difficulty quitting smoking for many individuals (Newhouse & Hughes, 1991).

PHARMACOTHERAPY OF NICOTINE DEPENDENCE

Nicotine Substitution

Nicotine substitution therapies, either through nicotine-containing chewing gum or skin patches, have been extensively evaluated in clinical trials.

They are effective in assisting initial smoking cessation, although subsequent relapse rates are quite high once nicotine replacement is tapered and discontinued (Jarvik & Henningfield, 1988). Long-term nicotine replacement is not currently practiced because of concern about its potential health consequences, although further research on this is probably warranted.

Antidepressant Medications

The nicotine withdrawal syndrome produces much anxiety and depressive symptomatology. Nicotine withdrawal has also been observed to precipitate frank major depression, which resolved when smoking was resumed, and a history of depression predicts failure to quit smoking (Glassman, 1993). Clinical trials of antidepressants as adjuncts to smoking cessation therapy are currently underway. Pending the results of these, it is reasonable to initiate antidepressant medication in smokers with a history of becoming depressed during attempts to quit or who become depressed during a current attempt.

CONCLUSIONS

In summary, the relationship between substance abuse and psychiatric comorbidity is a complex and intertwined one. Differentiating cause and effect is often very difficult. The treating clinician needs to be extremely careful in evaluating these dual problems. In general, it is appropriate to treat both the substance abuse and the psychiatric condition concurrently. It should be emphasized that these disorders always need to be treated in the context of a comprehensive treatment plan. Pharmacology has a major place in the treatment of both substance abuse and psychiatric conditions. It is often a vital and necessary adjunct to an individual's treatment and recovery.

REFERENCES

Allen, M.H., & Frances, R.J. (1986). Varieties of psychopathology found in patients with addictive disorders: A review. In R.E. Meyer (Ed.), *Psychopathology and addictive disorders* (pp. 17–33). New York: Guilford Press.

American Psychiatric Association. (1994). *Diagnostic and statistical manual of mental disorders* (4th ed.). Washington, DC: Author.

American Psychiatric Association. (1995). Practice guidelines for the treatment of patients with substance use disorders: Alcohol, cocaine, opioids. *American Journal of Psychiatry, 152*(11 suppl), 2–59.

Arndt, I.O., Cacciola, J.S., & McLellan, A.T. (1986). A re-evaluation of naltrex-one toxicity in recovering opiate addicts. In L.S. Harris (Ed.), *Problems of drug dependence* (p. 525). NIDA Research Monograph 67. Rockville, MD: National Institute on Drug Abuse.

Azrin, W.H., Sisson, R.W., & Meyers, R. (1982). Alcoholism treatment by disul-firam and community reinforcement therapy. *Journal of Behavior Therapy and Experimental Psychiatry, 13,* 105–112.

Ball, J.C., Corty, E., & Myers, C.P. (1988). *The reduction of intravenous heroin use, non-opiate abuse and crime during methadone maintenance treatment: Further findings.* NIDA Research Monograph 81. Rockville, MD: National Institute on Drug Abuse.

Baron, D.H., Sands, B.F., Ciraulo, D.A., & Shader, R.I. (1990). The diagnosis and treatment of panic disorder in alcoholics: Three cases. *American Journal of Drug and Alcohol Abuse, 16*(3 & 4), 287–295.

Carroll, K.M., Power, M.E., Bryant, K., & Rounsaville, B.J. (1993). One-year follow-up status of treatment-seeking cocaine abusers. Psychopathology and dependence severity as predictors of outcome. *Journal of Nervous and Mental Disorders, 181,* 71–79.

Centers for Disease Control (1989, December 15). *Morbidity and morality.* Atlanta, GA: Author.

Christensen, J.K., Ronstead, P., & Vaag, U.H. (1984). Side effects after disulfiram. *Acta Psychiatrica Scandinavica, 69,* 265–273.

Ciraulo, D.A., & Jaffe, J.H. (1981). Tricyclic antidepressants in the treatment of depression associated with alcoholism. *Journal of Clinical Psychopharma-cology, 1,* 146–150.

Cooper, J.R. (1992). Ineffective use of psychoactive drugs. *Journal of the American Medical Association, 267,* 281–282.

Cornelius, J., Salloum, I.M., Cornelius, M.D., Perel, J.M., Thase, M.E., Ehler, J.G., & Mann, J.J. (1993). Fluoxetine trial in suicidal depressed alcoholics. *Psy-chopharmacology Bulletin, 29,* 195–199.

DeLeon, G., Skodol, A., & Rosenthal, M.S. (1973). Phoenix House: Changes in psychopathological signs of resident addicts. *Archives of General Psychiatry, 28,* 131–135.

Dorus, W., Ostrow, D.G., Anton, R., Cushman, P., Collins, J.F., Schaefer, M., Charles, H.L., Desai, P., Hayashida, M., Malkermeker, U., Willenbring, M., Fiscella, R., & Sather, M.R. (1989). Lithium treatment of depressed and non-depressed alcoholics. *Journal of the American Medical Association, 262,* 1646–1652.

First, M.D., & Gladis, M.M. (1993). Diagnosis and differential diagnosis of psy-chiatric and substance use disorders. In J. Solomon, S. Zimberg, & E. Shol-lar (Eds.), *Dual diagnosis: Evaluation, treatment, training, and program development* (pp. 23–37). New York: Plenum Press.

Galanter, M. (1992). Office management of the substance abuser: The use of learn-ing theory and social networks. In J.H. Lowinson, R. Millman, P. Ruiz, & J.G. Langrod (Eds.), *Substance abuse: A comprehensive textbook* (2nd ed., pp. 543–549). Baltimore: Williams & Wilkins.

Galanter, M., & Kleber, H.D. (Eds.). (1994). *Textbook of substance abuse treatment.* Washington, DC: American Psychiatric Press.

Gallant, D.M. (1991). Recent advances in research and treatment of alcoholism and drug abuse. In A. Geller (Ed.), *ASAM review course manual* (pp. 589–618). Washington, DC: American Psychiatric Press.

Gallant, D.M. (1994). Alcohol. In *Textbook of substance abuse treatment* (pp. 67–90). Washington, DC: American Psychiatric Press.

Gawin, F.H., & Kleber, H.D. (1986). Abstinence symptomatology and psychiatric diagnosis in cocaine abusers. *Archives of General Psychiatry, 43,* 107–113.

Gawin, F.H., Kleber, H.D., Byck, R., Rounsaville, B.J., Kosten, T.R., Jatlow, P.I., & Morgan, C. (1989). Desipramine facilitation of initial cocaine abstinence. *Archives of General Psychiatry, 46,* 117–121.

Glassman, A.H. (1993). Cigarette smoking: Implications for psychiatric illness. *American Journal of Psychiatry, 150,* 546–553.

Goodwin, D.W. (1992). Alcohol: Clinical aspects. In J.H. Lowinson, P. Ruiz, R.B. Millman, & J.G. Langrod (Eds.), *Substance abuse: A comprehensive textbook* (2nd ed.). Baltimore: Williams & Wilkins.

Hwang, M.Y., & Nunes, E.V. (1995). Substance-induced persisting dementia and substance induced persisting amnestic disorders. In G. Gabbard & R.E. Hales (Eds.), *Treatment of psychiatric disorders: The DSM-IV edition* (pp. 555–574). Washington, DC: American Psychiatric Press.

Jarvik, M., & Henningfield, J. (1988). Pharmacological treatment of tobacco dependence. *Pharmacology Biochemistry and Behavior, 30,* 279–294.

Johnson, R.E., Fudala, P.J., & Jaffe, J.H. (1992). A controlled trial of buprenorphine for opioid dependence. *Journal of the American Medical Association, 267,* 2750–2755.

Khantzian, E.J. (1985). The self-medication hypothesis of addictive disorders: Focus on heroin and cocaine dependence. *American Journal of Psychiatry, 142*(11), 1259–1264.

Kosten, T.R., Gawin, F.H., Morgan, C., Nelson, J.C., & Jatlow, P. (1990). Evidence for altered desipramine disposition in methadone-maintained patients treated for cocaine abuse. *American Journal of Drug and Alcohol Abuse, 16,* 329–336.

Kosten, T.R., & McCance-Katz, E. (1995). New pharmacotherapies. *Review of Psychiatry, 14,* 105–126.

Kosten, T.R., Rounsaville, B.J., & Kleber, H.D. (1986). A 2.5 year follow-up of depression, life crises, and treatment effects on abstinence among opioid addicts. *Archives of General Psychiatry, 43,* 733–738.

Kranzler, H.R., Burleson, J.A., DelBoca, F.K., Babor, T.F., Korner, P., Brown, J., & Bohn, M.J. (1994). Buspirone treatment of anxious alcoholics: A placebo-controlled trial. *Archives of General Psychiatry, 51,* 720–731.

Liskow, B.I., & Goodwin, D.W. (1987). Pharmacological treatment of alcohol intoxication, withdrawal and dependence: A critical review. *Journal of Studies of Alcohol, 48,* 356–370.

Loosen, P.T., Dew, B.W., & Prange, A.J. (1990). Long-term predictors of outcome in abstinent alcoholic men. *American Journal of Psychiatry, 147,* 1662–1666.

Lowinson, J.H., Millman, R., Ruiz, P., & Langrod, J.G. (1992). *Substance abuse: A comprehensive textbook* (2nd ed.). Baltimore: Williams & Wilkins.

Magura, S., Goldsmith, D., Casriel, C., Goldstein, P.J., & Lipton, D. (1987). The validity of methadone clients' self-reported drug use. *International Journal of Addictions, 22,* 727–749.

Mason, B.J., & Kocsis, J.H. (1991). Desipramine treatment of alcoholism. *Psychopharmacology Bulletin, 27,* 155–161.

McLellan, A.T., Arndt, I.O., Metzger, D.S., Woody, G.E., & O'Brien, C.P. (1993). The effects of psychosocial services in substance abuse treatment. *Journal of the American Medical Association, 269,* 1953–1959.

Meyer, R.E. (1986). How to understand the relationship between psychopathology and addictive disorders: Another example of the chicken and the egg. In R.E. Meyer (Ed.), *Psychopathology and addictive disorders* (pp. 3–13). New York: Guilford Press.

Murphy, G.E., Wetzel, R.D., Robins, E., & McEvoy, L. (1992). Multiple risk factors predict suicide in alcoholism. *Archives of General Psychiatry, 49,* 459–463.

Newhouse, P., & Hughes, J. (1991). The role of nicotine and nicotinic mechanisms in neuropsychiatric disease (special issue: future directions in tobacco research). *British Journal of Addictions, 86,* 521–525.

Novick, D.M. (1992). The medically ill substance abuser. In J.H. Lowinson, R. Millman, P. Ruiz, & J.G. Langrod (Eds.), *Substance abuse: A comprehensive textbook* (2nd ed., pp. 657–674). Baltimore: Williams & Wilkins.

Nunes, E.V. (in press). *Methodologic recommendations for cocaine abuse clinical trials: A clinician-researcher's perspective.* NIDA Research Monographs. Rockville, MD: National Institute on Drug Abuse.

Nunes, E.V., Deliyannides, D., Donovan, S., & McGrath, P.J. (in press). The management of treatment-resistance in depressed patients with substance use disorders. *Psychiatric Clinics of North America.*

Nunes, E.V., Goehl, L., Seracini, A., Deliyannides, D., Donovan, S., Post, T., Quitkin, F.M., & Williams, J. (in press). Evaluation of depression and panic disorder in methadone patients using a modification of the structured clinical interview for *DSM-III-R:* Test-retest reliability. *American Journal on Addictions.*

Nunes, E.V., McGrath, P.J., & Quitkin, F.M. (1995). Treating anxiety in patients with alcoholism. *Journal of Clinical Psychiatry, 56*(supp 2), 3–9.

Nunes, E.V., McGrath, P.J., Quitkin, F.M., Ocepek-Welikson, K., Stewart, J.W., Keonig, T., Wager, S., & Klein, D.F. (1995). Imipramine treatment of cocaine abuse: Possible boundaries of efficacy. *Drug and Alcohol Dependence, 39,* 185–195.

Nunes, E.V., McGrath, P.J., Quitkin, F.M., Stewart, J.W., Harrison, W., Tricamo, E. & Ocepek-Welikson, K. (1993). Imipramine treatment of alcoholism with comorbid depression. *American Journal of Psychiatry, 150*(6), 963–965.

Nunes, E.V., & Quitkin, F.M. (1987). Disulfiram in bipolar affective disorder. *Journal of Clinical Psychopharmacology, 7,* 284.

Nunes, E.V., & Quitkin, F.M. (in press). *Treatment of depression in drug dependent patients: Effects on mood and drug use.* NIDA Research Monographs. Rockville, MD: National Institute on Drug Abuse.

290 *Treatment Strategies*

Nunes, E.V., Quitkin, F.M., Brady, R., & Koenig, T. (1994). Antidepressant treatment in methadone maintenance patients. *Journal of Addictive Diseases, 13,* 13–24.

O'Brien, C. (1994). Opioids: Antagonists and partial agonists. In M. Gallanter & H. Kleber (Eds.), *Textbook of substance abuse treatment* (pp. 223–238). Washington, DC: American Psychiatric Press.

O'Malley, S.S., Jaffe, A., Chang, G., & Shottenfeld, R.S. (1992). Naltrexone and coping skills therapy for alcohol dependence: A controlled study. *Archives of General Psychiatry, 49,* 881–887.

Quitkin, F.M., Rifkin, A., Kaplan, J., & Klein, D.F. (1972). Phobic anxiety syndrome complicated by drug dependence and addiction: A treatable form of drug abuse. *Archives of General Psychiatry, 27,* 159–162.

Regier, D.A., Farmer, M.E., Rae, D.S., Locke, B.Z., Keith, S.J., Judd, L.L., & Goodwin, F.K. (1990). Comorbidity of mental disorders with alcohol and other drug abuse. *Journal of the American Medical Association, 264,* 2511–2518.

Resnick, R.B., Schuyten-Resnick, E., & Washton, A.M. (1979). Narcotic antagonists in the treatment of opioid dependence: Review and commentary. *Comprehensive Psychiatry, 20,* 116–125.

Robins, L.N. (1979). Addict careers. In R.L. Dupont, A. Goldstein, & J. O'Donnell (Eds.), *Handbook on drug abuse* (pp. 325–336). Washington, DC: U.S. Government Printing Office.

Rounsaville, B.J., Anton, S.F., Carroll, K., & Meyer, R.E. (1991). Psychiatric diagnoses of treatment seeking cocaine abusers. *Archives of General Psychiatry, 48,* 43–51.

Rounsaville, B.J., Dolinsky, Z.S., Babor, T.F., & Meyer, R.E. (1987). Psychopathology as a predictor of treatment outcome in alcoholics. *Archives of General Psychiatry, 44,* 505–513.

Rounsaville, B.J., Kosten, T.R., & Kleber, H.D. (1986). Long-term changes in current psychiatric diagnoses of treated opiate addicts. *Comprehensive Psychiatry, 27,* 480–498.

Schuckit, M.A. (1986). Genetic and clinical implications of alcoholism and affective disorder. *American Journal of Psychiatry, 143,* 140–147.

Sellers, E.M., Higgins, G.A., & Sobell, M.B. (1992). 5-HT and alcohol abuse. *Trends in Pharmacological Science, 13,* 69–75.

Sereny, G., Sharma, V., & Holt, J. (1986). Mandatory supervised Antabuse therapy in an outpatient alcoholism program: A pilot study. *Alcohol and Clinical Experimental Research, 10,* 290–292.

Verebey, K., & Gold, M.S. (1988). From coca leaves to crack: The effects of dose and routes of administration in abuse liability. *Psychiatry Annals, 18,* 513–521.

Volpicelli, J.R., Alterman, A.I., Hyashida, M., & O'Brien, C.P. (1992). Naltrexone in the treatment of alcohol dependence. *Archives of General Psychiatry, 49,* 876–880.

Weddington, W.W., Brown, B.S., Haertzen, C.A., Cone, E.J., Dax, E.M., Herning, R.I., & Michaelson, B.S. (1990). Changes in mood, craving, and sleep during short-term abstinence reported by male cocaine addicts. *Archives of General Psychiatry, 47,* 861–868.

Weissman, M.D., Slobetz, F., Prusoff, B., Mezritz, M.N., & Howart, P. (1976). Clinical depression among narcotic addicts maintained on methadone in the community. *American Journal of Psychiatry, 133,* 1434–1438.

Williams, J.B.W., Gibbon, M., First, M.B., Spitzer, R.L., Davies, M., Borus, J., Howes, M.J., Kane, J., Pope, H.G., Rounsaville, B., & Wittchen, H.U. (1992). The Structured Clinical Interview for *DSM-III-R* (SCID) II. Multisite test-retest reliability. *Archives of General Psychiatry, 49,* 630–636.

Willis, J.H., & Osbourne, A.B. (1978). What happens to heroin addicts? A follow up study. *British Journal of Addictions, 73,* 189–198.

Ziedonis, D.M., & Kosten, T.R. (1991). Pharmacotherapy improves treatment outcome in depressed cocaine addicts. *Journal of Psychoactive Drugs, 23,* 417–425.

PART III
Special Topics

12

Comorbidity and Suicidality

SCOTT WETZLER
WILLIAM C. SANDERSON
DREW M. VELTING
AARON T. BECK

The literature on suicidality clearly demonstrates that patients with psychiatric disorders are at increased risk for suicide and suicide attempts (cf. Hirschfeld & Davidson, 1988). Patients with major depression or dysthymia are well known to have a high rate of completed suicide (Guze & Robins, 1970; Miles, 1977; Pokorny, 1983), but patients with schizophrenia (Appleby, 1992; Miles, 1977; Pokorny, 1983; Tsuang, 1978), substance abuse (Pitts & Winokur, 1966; Pokorny, 1983), and bipolar disorder (Barraclough et al., 1974) have also been found to have high rates of suicide. Psychiatric disorders are also associated with high rates of suicide attempts. For example, even patients who are not thought to be suicidal (e.g., panic disorder patients) are reported to have a surprisingly high rate of past suicide attempts (Weissman, Klerman, Markowitz, & Ouellette, 1989).

The rate of suicide or suicide attempts associated with a given psychiatric disorder appears to vary widely from study to study. In and of itself, the *absolute* rate of reported suicidality may not be meaningful, as a given sample may be highly selected (more or less severe than other samples due to the clinical setting from which the sample is drawn or kind of treatment being sought by the individuals making up the sample). More meaningful is a comparison of the *relative* rates of suicide or suicide attempts among various psychiatric disorders represented in a controlled sample. Pokorny (1983) found that patients with mood disorders and schizophrenia had higher rates of completed suicide than other psychiatric patients (i.e., those with substance abuse or personality disorders). Asnis and colleagues (1993) found that patients with affective disorders and schizophrenia also had higher rates of past suicide attempts than patients with other psychiatric disorders. Thus, affective disorders and schizophrenia appear to place patients at the greatest risk for suicidality.

However, these studies may be misleading as they do not take into account the presence of comorbid psychiatric disorders: In the studies, only one psychiatric diagnosis per patient was considered. As was made clear in Chapter 2, most psychiatric patients meet criteria for multiple diagnoses and we may wonder whether the high rates of suicidality associated with the major psychiatric disorders are solely a function of the principal diagnosis or due to the combination of principal and secondary (or tertiary) diagnoses. In fact, Rich, Young, and Fowler (1986) found that patients who completed suicide had an average of two diagnoses per person, and Henriksson et al. (1993) found that 44 percent of patients who completed suicide had a comorbid Axis I diagnosis.

The literature on comorbidity and suicide is sparse, but in almost all studies, psychiatric comorbidity places patients at increased risk for suicidality. For example, depressed patients with a secondary diagnosis of alcoholism are more likely to complete suicide than are depressed patients without alcoholism (Hirschfeld & Davidson, 1988); panic patients with a secondary depression make more suicide attempts than do panic patients without depression (Rudd, Dahm, & Rajab, 1993; Weissman et al., 1989); schizophrenic patients with a secondary depression are also more suicidal than nondepressed schizophrenic patients (Drake & Cotton, 1986); and patients with almost any psychiatric disorder are likely to be more suicidal if they have a comorbid personality disorder (Hirschfeld & Davidson, 1988; Rich & Runeson, 1992). In the absence of comorbid diagnoses, suicide risk for many people with psychiatric disorders might be quite minimal (cf. Hornig & McNally, 1995).

DATA ON COMORBIDITY AND SUICIDE

To date, no one has formally examined whether psychiatric comorbidity in any form increases suicide risk, whether specific patterns of comorbidity increase suicide risk, or whether the principal psychiatric diagnosis determines level of suicide risk. This omission is surely due to the difficulty of obtaining a large, well-diagnosed sample. In this chapter, the authors report on a sample of 1,778 adult patients who presented for treatment at the Center for Cognitive Therapy, University of Pennsylvania (patients with organic mental disorders and those without an Axis I diagnosis were excluded). All subjects were carefully evaluated for *current* principal, secondary, and tertiary diagnoses by the use of structured clinical interviews for *DSM-III-R* (SCID-I and SCID-II). A history of suicide attempts was also obtained. Although this outpatient psychotherapy sample is highly selected with few severely mentally ill individuals (i.e., few schizophrenic and psychotic patients were included as well as few patients with severe mood disorders), it allows the issue of psychiatric comorbidity and suicide to be examined in some detail.

Table 12-1 presents the rate of patients with a previous history of suicide attempts among the major principal diagnostic groupings as well as the rate of suicide attempters among patients with secondary and tertiary Axis I diagnoses and comorbid Axis II diagnoses. The mean age of this sample was 36.4 years old, and it was predominantly female (57 percent). The number of suicide attempters in this sample was quite low (n = 104, 5.9 percent), and they were mostly female (71 percent). The minimal degree of suicidality is almost certainly due to sample composition, as these outpatients were seeking cognitive therapy, not pharmacotherapy.

The most striking finding is that the presence of a secondary Axis I diagnosis almost doubles the rate of suicide attempts (7.0 percent vs. 3.6 percent). This shows that, in general, comorbid psychiatric disorders do contribute to suicidality, and the presence of a tertiary Axis I diagnosis further contributes to suicidality (8.9 percent). Similarly, the presence of a comorbid Axis II diagnosis also contributes to suicidality (7.5 percent vs. 4.6 percent), although additional Axis II diagnoses do not.

An examination of selective principal Axis II groupings allows one to determine whether the effects of comorbidity on suicide attempts apply to certain disorders and not to others. In this sample, only patients with one of the bipolar disorders (14.1 percent), depressive disorders (8.4 percent), or substance abuse disorders (7.3 percent) had increased frequency of suicide attempts. Patients with anxiety disorders (2.6 percent), adjustment disorders (0 percent), and V code diagnoses (0 percent) were unlikely to have made suicide attempts.

The finding among bipolar patients is consistent with the literature on the frequency of suicide in this group (Fawcett et al., 1987; Barraclough

TABLE 12-1
Percentage of Suicide Attempters by Diagnostic Category
(with and without Comorbidity)

	DEP[1] (n = 843)	BIP[2] (n = 85)	ANX[3] (n = 625)	SUB[4] (n = 41)	ADJ[5] (n = 99)	VCD[6] (n = 39)	OTHER (n = 46)	Total (n = 1778)
Total	8.2	14.1	2.6	7.3	0.0	0.0	4.4	5.9
No 2nd Axis I	5.2	14.3	0.0	0.0	0.0	0.0	7.7	3.6
Any 2nd Axis I	9.9	14.0	3.5	10.7	0.0	0.0	3.0	7.0
No 3rd Axis I	6.3	14.9	2.2	0.0	0.0	0.0	3.7	4.5
Any 3rd Axis I	13.0	11.1	3.3	23.0	0.0	0.0	5.3	8.9
No Axis II	6.3	19.5	2.3	4.4	0.0	0.0	6.7	4.6
Any Axis II	10.7	9.1	3.0	11.1	0.0	0.0	0.0	7.5
No 2nd Axis II	8.9	15.1	2.8	7.9	0.0	0.0	5.1	6.1
Any 2nd Axis II	5.3	8.3	0.0	0.0	0.0	0.0	0.0	3.6

[1]Depressive Disorders
[2]Bipolar Disorders
3Anxiety Disorders
[4]Substance Abuse Disorders
[5]Adjustment Disorders
[6]V Code Diagnoses (other conditions) that may be the focus of clinical attention

et al., 1974). The findings among depressed patients and substance abuse patients are also consistent with the literature (cf. Hirschfeld & Davidson, 1988). There were too few patients with schizophrenia (included among Other disorders) to ascertain their rate of past suicide attempts, which has typically been high in past studies. It is interesting to note the complete absence of suicide attempts among patients with adjustment disorders and V code diagnoses (e.g., relational problems), and the low rate of suicide attempts among the anxiety disorder patients (many of the panic disorder patients in this group were previously described by Beck, Steer, Sanderson, & Skeie, 1991).

Based on these data, it would appear that the presence of secondary psychiatric disorders was associated with a higher rate of past suicide attempts among certain diagnostic groupings, and not with others. For example, none of the substance abuse patients or anxiety disorder patients without comorbid conditions had made a suicide attempt. Only those substance abuse patients (and anxiety disorder patients) with a secondary disorder had made a past suicide attempt. Although some depressed patients without a comorbid disorder had made suicide attempts, the rate was much increased when there was a secondary diagnosis as well. Among bipolar patients, the rate of suicide attempters did not change with or without a secondary diagnosis. Table 12-1 also indicates that tertiary diagnoses further increased the risk of suicide attempts among depressed patients and substance abuse patients.

What can be gleaned from these findings is that bipolar disorder is associated with suicide attempts regardless of comorbidity; that uncomplicated depression is associated with a lower rate of suicide attempts; that depression plus a comorbid disorder greatly increases the rate of suicide attempts; and that uncomplicated cases of anxiety disorder or substance abuse disorder are not associated with suicide attempts, but that substance abuse disorder with comorbidity does have a much increased risk for suicide attempts.

As Table 12-1 further indicates, the adverse effect of Axis II disorders on rate of suicide attempts applied to depressed patients and substance abuse patients but not to bipolar patients or anxiety disorder patients. This finding lends credence to the conclusion that suicidality among depressed or substance abuse patients is related to the presence of comorbidity, and that suicidality among bipolar patients is solely related to the principal Axis I diagnosis.

Given the large sample size, it is possible to examine the rates of suicide attempts among patients with specific depressive disorders and anxiety disorders. The data in Table 12-2 show that patients with major depression, recurrent, had more suicidality than other depressed patients. Although the adverse effect of comorbidity on the rate of suicide attempts applied to depressed patients as a group, it was most pronounced among patients with major depression, single episode or recurrent. The same pattern was found with regard to the effect of a comorbid Axis II diagnosis. Among the two types of major depression, there was a further adverse contribution of a tertiary Axis I diagnosis, but not for a second Axis II diagnosis. This means that a patient with a single episode of major depression is at low risk for

TABLE 12-2
Percentage of Suicide Attempters by Depressive Disorder
(with and without Comorbidity)

	Major Depression, Single Episode (n = 210)	Major Depression, Recurrent (n = 414)	Dysthymia (n = 139)	Depression Not Otherwise Specified (n = 80)	Total (n = 843)
Total	6.7	10.6	5.8	6.3	8.4
No 2nd Axis I	2.8	6.1	4.6	7.9	5.2
Any 2nd Axis I	8.6	12.4	6.3	4.8	9.9
No 3rd Axis I	4.3	7.4	4.9	7.3	6.3
Any 3rd Axis I	11.3	17.6	7.0	0.0	13.0
No Axis II	3.7	8.0	4.5	6.8	6.3
Any Axis II	9.7	13.4	6.9	5.6	10.7
No 2nd Axis II	7.2	11.1	6.1	6.7	8.9
Any 2nd Axis II	3.3	7.3	4.2	0.0	5.3

suicide attempts. Once this depression becomes recurrent or is associated with a comorbid Axis I diagnosis or diagnoses or a comorbid Axis II diagnosis, the risk of suicidality greatly increases.

Among patients with a principal anxiety disorder (see Table 12-3), there was considerable variability in the rates of suicide attempts. Patients with obsessive compulsive disorder (OCD) or social phobia had a significant degree of suicidality, whereas patients with simple phobia, generalized anxiety disorder, or panic disorder did not. In fact, the group of patients with OCD and a comorbid disorder had a fairly high rate of suicide attempters (14.8 percent). This is likely due to the presence of a comorbid depression, a common comorbid pattern. Similarly, an Axis II diagnosis greatly increased the risk of suicide attempts among OCD patients, although not among social phobia patients.

Finally, the sample allows examination also of the specific interrelationships between principal and secondary diagnoses in terms of suicide attempts (see Table 12-4). The assumption had been made that the adverse effect of comorbidity was predominantly due to the presence of a secondary depression, but these results would suggest that almost any comorbid Axis I diagnosis contributes to suicide attempts. Among patients with principal depressions, a secondary depression or secondary substance abuse disorder (included in Any Other Secondary Disorder) increased suicide risk.

TABLE 12-3
Percentage of Suicide Attempters by Anxiety Disorder (with and without Comorbidity)

	Panic Disorder (n = 272)	Generalized Anxiety Disorder (n = 146)	Social Phobia (n = 83)	Obsessive Compulsive Disorder (n = 40)	Simple Phobia (n = 24)	Anxiety, Not Otherwise Specified (n = 48)	Miscellaneous (n = 12)	Total (n = 625)
Total	1.8	0.7	6.0	10.0	0.0	2.1	0.0	2.6
No 2nd Axis I	0.0	0.0	0.0	0.0	0.0	0.0	0.0	0.0
Any 2nd Axis I	2.3	0.9	8.9	14.8	0.0	4.4	0.0	3.5
No 3rd Axis I	0.6	1.1	6.8	6.3	0.0	2.5	0.0	2.2
Any 3rd Axis I	3.7	0.0	4.2	25.0	0.0	0.0	0.0	3.3
No Axis II	1.6	0.0	10.0	6.9	0.0	0.0	0.0	2.3
Any Axis II	2.4	1.4	2.3	18.2	0.0	7.1	0.0	3.0
No 2nd Axis II	2.0	0.8	7.3	10.5	0.0	2.2	0.0	2.8
Any 2nd Axis II	0.0	0.0	0.0	0.0	0.0	0.0	0.0	0.0

TABLE 12-4
Percentage of Suicide Attempters by Type of Comorbid Disorder

	Any Principal Depressive Disorder (n = 843)	Any Principal Anxiety Disorder (n = 625)	Any Other Principal Disorder (n = 310)	Total (n = 1778)
Total	8.4	2.6	5.5	5.9
Any Secondary Depressive Disorder	10.7	3.7	4.0	6.3
Any Secondary Anxiety Disorder	7.9	3.9	6.8	6.4
Any Other Secondary Disorder	13.9	0.0	8.3	9.6
No Secondary Disorder	5.2	0.0	4.5	3.6

Among anxiety disorder patients, a secondary anxiety disorder was as dangerous as was a secondary depression. Among other principal diagnoses, the presence of a secondary depression had the least effect on suicide attempts. Thus, the assumption was wrong. Many types of comorbidity, including disorders not typically associated with suicidality (e.g., substance abuse), contribute to suicide risk.

CLINICAL IMPLICATIONS

Evaluation of suicidality is a critical issue for psychiatrists and psychologists. The role of psychiatric diagnosis in the etiology of suicide is of particular importance. Traditionally, depressed patients were generally accepted as the individuals primarily at risk for suicide. Indeed, suicidality is a symptom of depressive disorders. More recently, clinicians have begun to recognize that patients with other psychiatric disorders (e.g., schizophrenia, bipolar disorder) are also at risk for suicide. There is no longer a clear-cut relationship between suicide and any single psychiatric diagnosis (i.e., depression). Many factors contribute to suicide risk, including the interrelationship of multiple psychiatric disorders.

These findings mean that the clinician cannot overlook the potential for suicide merely because a patient does *not* have a depressive disorder. In fact, the data indicate that patients with bipolar disorder are a greater risk for suicide attempts (and thus would be more likely to complete suicide successfully) than patients with depressive disorders. Barraclough and associates (1974) suggest that suicidality among bipolar patients is greatest as they plunge into the depressive phase of their illness. Apparently, the depressive experience of unipolar patients is not associated with as much risk for suicide.

The data further show that patients with substance abuse disorder may be suicidal, but only when that substance abuse disorder is combined with a secondary psychiatric disorder. Similarly, although anxiety disorder patients as a group are not suicidal, patients with social phobia and OCD patients with a secondary psychiatric disorder are at risk. Thus, patients with certain principal disorders alone may not be suicidal, but when those disorders are combined with a secondary disorder, their suicidality increases dramatically. Such data highlight the importance of evaluating patients for the presence of comorbid Axis I conditions. Making a single diagnosis and then neglecting to evaluate patients for comorbid disorders is a grave clinical error, because patients' suicide potential may also be ignored. Only those patients with principal adjustment disorders, simple phobias, or V code diagnoses appear to be safely protected from suicide attempts.

One of the conclusions that might be drawn from these data is that comorbidity in general worsens suicide risk. Patients with two or three psychiatric disorders are more likely to have made a suicide attempt than patients with an uncomplicated disorder. This should not be surprising, as having two disorders is generally worse than having just one disorder in terms of course, treatment outcome, and relapse potential (as described in many of the previous chapters).

The only condition for which comorbidity did *not* have an adverse influence was bipolar disorder. For patients with this condition, suicidality was significant and independent of any additional diagnosis. Thus, patients with bipolar depression plus alcohol abuse are no more suicidal than patients with uncomplicated bipolar depression. The latter is a serious, quite lethal disorder that needs to be treated with care.

The data set also reveals that comorbid Axis II conditions exert an adverse effect on suicidality as well. In fact, Axis II comorbidity may be even more influential than Axis I comorbidity as it is associated with a slightly higher percentage of suicide attempters. The contribution of Axis II comorbidity to suicidality appears to be limited to patients with either major depression or a substance abuse disorder, not to anxiety disorder patients (except possibly those with OCD and anxiety disorder not otherwise specified). This means that a comorbid personality disorder in the context of major depression (the suicidal substance abuse patients typically had a secondary major depression) significantly increases suicide risk, but that personality disorders associated with other conditions do not.

Such a finding highlights the importance of evaluating personality disorders in the context of major depression. All too often clinicians make the diagnosis of major depression and then fail to evaluate the patient's personality, or they attribute interpersonal difficulties to the depression and not to the underlying personality disorder (Sanderson, Wetzler, Beck, & Betz, 1992). Clinicians often underestimate the impact of personality disorders on severity, course of illness, and response to treatment. In the context of anxiety disorders or adjustment disorders, missing a personality disorder diagnosis does not have the potentially lethal significance that it does in the context of major depression.

It is not enough to determine whether a patient has a personality disorder, because personality disorders vary considerably and they would be expected to have quite different effects on suicidality. For example, borderline personality disorder is defined by suicidal and self-destructive behavior, and all the Cluster B personality disorders are characterized by impulsive, acting-out behavior. Thus, only certain personality disorders might be associated with suicidality.

Although the data in the tables are not presented, borderline personality disorder (10.9 percent) and the other Cluster B disorders (8.3 percent) were *not* associated with increased suicidality in comparison to the other personality disorder clusters (they were associated with more suicidality than patients without a personality disorder [4.6 percent] or those with personality disorder NOS [4.6 percent]). In fact, Cluster A disorders, especially paranoid personality disorder, were associated with the highest percentage of suicide attempters (21.1 percent), although this figure might be unstable as the total number of Cluster A patients was small.

These results suggest that in the context of an Axis I disorder, such as depression, angry and suspicious individuals are at the greatest risk for suicide attempts. Also, borderline patients are at increased risk, but at no more risk than Cluster C patients, who are anxious, fearful, and generally considered more inhibited. On determining that a patient is avoidant or dependent, a clinician should not minimize the suicide risk. Similarly, when a clinician determines that a patient is borderline, it would be a mistake to overestimate the suicide potential. Clinicians should be most cautious with those odd, eccentric patients who do not make good social contact and who may misinterpret interpersonal signals. They are likely to be isolated individuals (a factor also associated with suicidality).

CONCLUSION

By the use of a large data set, it was possible to determine that both Axis I and Axis II comorbidity increases the risk of suicide attempts over and above the suicide risk of an uncomplicated Axis I disorder. Comorbidity matters a great deal in the clinical management of suicidality, especially with regard to certain diagnoses.

The findings presented in this chapter are by no means definitive, especially as the patients represented a highly selected group of patients seeking cognitive therapy. However, the diagnostic evaluations were reliable and based on structured interviews by trained raters. Other assessment methods (e.g., use of self-report tests or different structured interviews) would certainly have found different patterns of comorbidity in the same sample. Finally, this data set only reflects patterns of current comorbidity, not lifetime history of comorbidity, which is often the focus of other studies (e.g., the Epidemiologic Catchment Area study). Nonetheless, relationships were found between current comorbid patterns and lifetime history of suicide attempts.

REFERENCES

Appleby, L. (1992). Suicide in psychiatric patients: Risk and prevention. *British Journal of Psychiatry, 161,* 749–758.

Asnis, G.M., Friedman, T.A., Sanderson, W.C., Kaplan, M.L., van Praag, H.M., Harkavy-Friedman, J.M. (1993). Suicidal behaviors in adult psychiatric outpatients, I: Description and prevalence. *American Journal of Psychiatry, 150,* 108–112.

Barraclough, B.M., Bunch, J., Nelson, B., & Sainsbury, P. (1974). A hundred cases of suicide: Clinical aspects. *British Journal of Psychiatry, 125,* 355–372.

Beck, A.T., Steer, R.A., Sanderson, W.C., & Skeie, T.M. (1991). Panic disorder and suicidal ideation and behavior: Discrepant findings in psychiatric outpatients. *American Journal of Psychiatry, 148,* 1195–1199.

Drake, R.E., & Cotton, P.G. (1986). Depression, hopelessness and suicide in chronic schizophrenia. *British Journal of Psychiatry, 148,* 554–559.

Fawcett, J., Scheftner, W., Clark, D., Hedeker, D., Gibbons, R., Coryell, W. (1987). Clinical predictors of suicide in patients with major affective disorders: A controlled prospective study. *American Journal of Psychiatry, 144*(1), 35–40.

Guze, S.B., & Robins, E. (1970). Suicide and primary affective disorders. *British Journal of Psychiatry, 117,* 437–438.

Henriksson, M.M., Aro, H.M., Marttunen, M.J., Heikkinen, M.E., Isometsa, E.T., Kuoppasalmi, K.I., Lonnquist, J.K. (1993). Mental disorders and comorbidity in suicide. *American Journal of Psychiatry, 150*(6), 935–940.

Hirschfeld, R.M.A., & Davidson, L. (1988). Risk factors for suicide. In A.J. Frances & R.E. Hales (Eds.), *Review of psychiatry* (pp. 307–333). Washington, DC: American Psychiatric Press.

Hornig, C.D., & McNally, R.J. (1995). Panic disorder and suicide attempt: A re-analysis of data from the Epidemiologic Catchment Area study. *British Journal of Psychiatry, 167,* 76–79.

Miles, C. (1977). Conditions predisposing to suicide: a review. *Journal of Nervous and Mental Disease, 164,* 231–246.

Pitts, F.N., & Winokur, G. (1966). Affective disorder VII: Alcoholism and affective disorder. *Journal of Psychiatric Research, 4,* 37–50.

Pokorny, A.D. (1983). Prediction of suicide in psychiatric patients. *Archives of General Psychiatry, 40,* 249–257.

Rich, C.L., Young, D., & Fowler, R.C. (1986). San Diego suicide study, I: Young vs. old subjects. *Archives of General Psychiatry, 43,* 577–582.

Rich, C.L., & Runeson, B.S. (1992). Similarities in diagnostic comorbidity between suicide among young people in Sweden and the United States. *Acta Psychiatrica Scandinavica, 86*(5), 335–339.

Rudd, D.M., Dahm, F.P., & Rajab, H.M. (1993). Diagnostic comorbidity in persons with suicidal ideation and behavior. *American Journal of Psychiatry, 150,* 928–934.

Sanderson, W.C., Wetzler, S., Beck, A.T., & Betz, F. (1992). Prevalence of personality disorders in patients with major depression and dysthymia. *Psychiatry Research, 42,* 93–99.

Tsuang, M.T. (1978). Suicide in schizophrenics, manics, depressives, and surgical controls. *Archives of General Psychiatry, 35,* 153–155.

Weissman, M.M., Klerman, G.L., Markowitz, J.S., & Ouellette, R. (1989). Suicidal ideation and suicide attempts in panic disorder and attacks. *New England Journal of Medicine, 321,* 1209–1214.

13

Comorbidity of Psychiatric Disorders in Children and Adolescents

FRED R. VOLKMAR
JOSEPH L. WOOLSTON

Comorbidity of psychiatric disorders in children and adolescents is the rule rather than the exception. If a child or adolescent has one diagnosis, several others are commonly assigned as well (Achenbach, 1990/1991; Biederman, Newcorn, & Sprich, 1991; Cantwell & Rutter, 1994; Carlson, 1986; Caron & Rutter, 1991; Nottelman & Jensen, 1995). However, because rates of psychopathology in this age group can be relatively high, it is important to establish whether observed rates of comorbidity are greater than would be expected by chance alone. The use of clinical samples to address this issue is limited by issues of referral bias—that is, children with comorbid conditions would presumably be in much greater need of service than children in the general population. Accordingly, additional epidemiological studies are needed to address adequately the issue of comorbidity in children and adolescents (Caron & Rutter, 1991).

Several epidemiological studies have addressed this issue (e.g., Anderson, Williams, McGee, & Silva, 1987; Kashani et al., 1987; Nottelman & Jensen, 1995). Essentially, all such epidemiological studies in children suggest that comorbidity is indeed very common, is not confined to clinical samples, and is not seen only in relation to very severe disorders. Generally, rates of comorbidity are twice the levels expected by chance alone (see Caron & Rutter, 1991, for a discussion). For example, in a community survey of 11-year-old children, Anderson, Williams, Mcgee, and Silva (1987) reported that 7.5 percent of the sample exhibited anxiety disorder and 6.7 percent showed symptoms of attention deficit disorder. By chance alone, the expected rate of comorbid anxiety and attention deficit disorder would be 0.5 percent, but the rate observed was more than double that expected.

This chapter provides a selective review of aspects of psychiatric comorbidity in childhood and adolescence. Alternative models for understanding comorbidity and methodological issues that complicate the interpretation of available data are discussed. The very different approaches to the problems of comorbidity in the *Diagnostic and Statistical Manual of Mental Disorders,* fourth edition (*DSM-IV*) (American Psychiatric Association [APA], 1994) and the *International Classification of Disease,* tenth edition (*ICD-10*) (World Health Organization [WHO], 1990) are summarized. Available data on treatment approaches to comorbid disorders are reviewed and areas for future research are highlighted.

RESEARCH ISSUES AND METHODOLOGICAL PROBLEMS

Surprisingly, the issue of comorbidity has, at least until recently, been a relatively neglected research topic. Understanding psychiatric comorbidity in childhood and adolescence is important for several reasons. The common approach in research studies is to assume a unitary disorder; this assumption, in turn, leads to several important methodological problems. For example, if one assumes that the *pure* disorder is one in which no other conditions are present, a logical implication is that only such cases should be included in research studies. In the absence of data regarding alternative approaches to classification this attempt to study theoretically stringent samples (i.e, cases without comorbidity) may be misleading: The samples selected may not reflect more typical clinical presentations and may prevent investigators from appreciating the importance of comorbid conditions and patterns of relationships among the disorders studied. The attempt, for example, to study pure depression, conduct, attention deficit, and anxiety disorders by effectively eliminating cases in which more than one of these conditions is present makes it impossible for researchers to appreciate the high rates of comorbidity within this group of conditions and the apparent relationships of these conditions to each other. On the other hand methodological problems may also result in overestimated rates of comorbidity—for example, rates are lower when criteria related to severity and impairment are included in epidemiological studies (Weissman, Warner, & Fendrich, 1987). In these cases, diagnostic categories may be developed and defined in ways that make comorbidity inevitable (Cantwell, 1996).

There are several models for understanding patterns of comorbidity in children and adolescents. Comorbidity may represent an aspect of syndrome expression in children, meaning that the presence of any single disorder that interferes with functioning puts the child at increased risk for other, or at least certain other, disorders. For example, a child with a serious developmental disorder such as mental retardation might be at increased risk for diverse behavioral problems and, conversely, serious behavioral disorders might impact the child's development negatively and interfere with learning, thus placing the child at greater risk for developmental disorders. Although good epidemiological data are limited, it seems that children with mental retardation are at three to four times greater risk for developing other psychiatric disorders than are children without mental retardation (Rutter, Tizard, & Whitmore, 1970). Similarly, the presence of a significant sensory impairment such as deafness also is associated with a high prevalence of psychiatric disorder (Hindley, Hill, McGuigan, & Kitson, 1993).

Another possibility is that two different disorders may share the same, or largely overlapping, risk factors, giving the impression of comorbidity when indeed it does not exist (Caron & Rutter, 1991). For example, severe neglect may produce some degree of both mental retardation and attachment disorder. However, such an association may more properly be thought of as the result of a shared major risk factor (neglect) that does not necessarily imply that the two disorders are themselves otherwise fundamentally related.

Another alternative is that conditions viewed as two separate disorders are, in fact, parsimoniously viewed as a single disorder with a more complex phenomenology than currently is appreciated (Caron & Rutter, 1991). Thus, comorbid conduct disorder and depression may represent a distinctive category, as this combination apparently differs in several ways from depression not associated with conduct disorder (Angold & Rutter, 1992). The classification of such conditions remains the topic of some debate, but some conditions clearly share clinical features to a sufficient degree that they deserve special recognition in their own right—for example, schizoaffective disorder.

The usual reliance on categorical rather than dimensional approaches to diagnosis may obscure meaningful patterns of relationship among clinical features. Hierarchical approaches to diagnosis, common in categorical diagnostic systems, may present obvious or more subtle obstacles to the recognition of comorbidity. For example, under the diagnostic system presented in *DSM-III* (APA, 1980), a patient could not, by definition, have autism and schizophrenia, even though the latter condition is relatively common and it seems unlikely that having autism would protect against schizophrenia. On the other hand, if categorical diagnostic criteria are not sufficiently discriminating, artificial and meaningless comorbidity may be diagnosed. As a practical matter, particularly in children, common symptoms such as anxiety, depression, and overactivity are not syndrome specific. Imprecision of diagnostic categories because of such shared features may lead to artificially high estimates of comorbidity, as in the diagnostic system of the *DSM-III-R* (APA, 1987), in which the various anxiety disorders of childhood were defined in such a way as often to exist with each other.

Unfortunately, the attempt to devise more rational diagnostic systems may introduce inadvertent and artificial confoundings to the task of disentangling psychiatric comorbidity in children. For example, Weinstein, Stone, Noam, Grimes, & Schwab-Stone (1989) noted that if *DSM-III* exclusionary rules were strictly applied, 20 percent of cases exhibited comorbidity, in contrast to almost 80 percent of cases when hierarchical exclusionary rules were discarded. As Caron and Rutter (1991) suggest, it seems that the complex exclusionary rules in *DSM-III-R* (APA, 1987) probably led to underestimates of comorbidity.

A further complication is childhood and adolescence itself. Identifying psychopathological conditions is extremely difficult during a period of life when development is proceeding at a very fast pace and when major change is the rule rather than the exception. Thus, in childhood and adolescence, developmental factors confound diagnosis in general and the diagnosis of comorbidity in particular (Nottelman & Jensen, 1995). This reality makes it even more difficult to understand the potentially complex continuities of conditions over time—that is, from childhood to adulthood. Particularly in very young children, diagnostic issues are often quite complex indeed, and a lack of precision in diagnostic systems complicates attempts to clarify aspects of comorbidity in this group. Furthermore, the stability of psychiatric conditions over time is much less in childhood than in adolescence and, in turn, less in early adolescence than in late adolescence (Nottelman & Jensen, 1995). Both the *DSM-IV* (APA, 1994) and *ICD-10* (WHO, 1990) diagnostic systems tend to provide a clinical snapshot in time, and both tend to deemphasize a more developmental orientation toward diagnosis. Thus, what appear to be the manifestations of one condition early in the child's development may in retrospect be appreciated as the first manifestations of another condition. For example, many children who develop Tourette's syndrome are noted to have exhibited marked problems in attention and activity earlier in their development (Leckman, in press). A similar observation can be made with respect to the distinctions between oppositional defiant and conduct disorder (Loeber, Lahey, & Thomas, 1991). One might hope that treatment-specific effects would help to disentangle these dilemmas; however, treatments are generally not highly specific, and treatment response, therefore, is not a particularly strong measure to use in clarifying aspects of comorbidity. Other research strategies, including twin and adoption studies, may ultimately provide clarification of these issues (Caron & Rutter, 1991).

Although there is a general clinical presumption that a single diagnosis should be made whenever possible, this often is not possible. Particularly with disorders in childhood and adolescence, the importance of comorbid conditions has been recognized in the adoption of multiaxial classification systems. Such approaches have certain advantages over uniaxial systems even when such systems allow for assignment of multiple diagnoses (Rutter et al., 1969). A multiaxial approach allows for notation of associated medical conditions and mental handicap as well as for other associated variables. The use of this approach and formal diagnostic criteria in *DSM-III* (APA, 1980) led, in large part, to the increased appreciation of the complex problem of comorbidity in children and adolescents.

APPROACHES TO CLASSIFICATION: *DSM-IV* AND *ICD-10*

The current official diagnostic systems—*DSM-IV* (APA, 1994) and *ICD-10* (WHO, 1990)—share many similarities but differ in important ways in their approaches to comorbid psychiatric conditions. In general, the similarities of the two systems are greater than the differences (Cooper, 1995; Volkmar and Schwab-Stone, 1996). However, some basic differences in the two systems are of particular relevance to the classification of comorbid conditions. The *ICD-10* system provides alternative criteria for research and guidelines for clinical use, whereas the single *DSM-IV* system is meant to be applicable in both contexts. Another major difference relates to the different approaches to comorbidity in the two systems. Although both diagnostic systems allow multiple diagnoses for certain comorbid conditions, multiple diagnoses are preferred in *DSM-IV*. In *ICD-10,* however, certain comorbid conditions are diagnosed through the use of a single category— for example, a single code can be used to specify combinations such as depression and conduct disorder or hyperkinetic conduct disorders in *ICD-10* but not in *DSM-IV*. In the *DSM-IV* system, both diagnoses would be made, if appropriate. As Cantwell and Rutter (1994) point out, data that would convincingly resolve this issue are presently lacking; the risk of the *DSM-IV* approach, of course, is that if this distinction does have some validity, studies that use *DSM-IV* will have failed to appreciate its importance.

Essentially, the *ICD-10* assumes that comorbid conditions such as hyperkinetic conduct disorder or depressive conduct disorder are unique in some important way or ways. Data to address these issues are clearly needed, although some work (e.g., Harrington et al., 1993) does seem to provide a separate category for depressive conduct disorder. The theoretical rationale for use of such mixed diagnoses is relatively clear; that is, it is possible that such cases represent a single disorder with various clinical features (Rutter, Tuma, & Lann, 1988). From a research standpoint, the ability to denote such cases would appear to be of importance at least until the questions of syndrome boundaries have been clearly addressed. From a clinical standpoint, the use of such categories is justified by the tendency of clinicians to make single diagnoses even when multiple diagnoses are present (Rutter & Shaffer, 1980). On the other hand, the reification of mixed categories tends to imply more of a basis for special coding than presently exists. It is possible, if all diagnoses are indeed assigned, to disentangle potential comorbid conditions using *DSM-IV*. Discussion of comorbidity in two rather diverse groups of conditions—mental retardation and the developmental disorders, and the disruptive behavior disorders—illustrates some of these issues.

COMORBIDITY IN THE DEVELOPMENTAL DISORDERS

Several factors complicate the study of comorbid disorders in children with developmental disability. Epidemiological data are often lacking; criteria for diagnostic categories may be difficult to apply particularly in the presence of very severe disability; issues of assessment are complicated; and there is often a failure to appreciate the presence of additional conditions in the face of significant developmental disorder. Unfortunately, clinicians have often assumed implicitly that mental retardation and other developmental disabilities tend to protect individuals from other conditions. In fact, it would be logical to assume that the presence of developmental disabilities would increase the risk for other psychiatric conditions. A series of studies has suggested that psychiatric disorders are increased three- to fourfold in children with mental retardation (see Scott, 1994, for a review). In children with mild mental retardation, rates of disorder are relatively high, probably three times as high as in children of the same age without mental retardation. Rates of associated conditions increase with the degree of mental retardation, so that among individuals with severe mental retardation, half of cases will exhibit significant psychiatric disturbance (Scott, 1994). Among individuals with mental retardation, rates of conduct, affective, and anxiety disorders are proportionally at the same levels as observed in the general population. The frequency of other conditions, however, is markedly increased. These conditions include autism and related disorders, stereotyped movement disorders, and attention deficit disorder. Symptoms of overactivity and stereotyped movements are more common in more handicapped individuals.

Autism and other pervasive disorders are often associated with some degree of mental retardation; in autism, usual rates are in the 70 percent to 80 percent range (Volkmar, 1996). However, in Asperger's disorder and in about 20 percent of individuals with strictly defined autism, the individual functions within the normal range of intelligence (Klin, 1994). Issues of definition and diagnosis are a complication, but in persons with mental retardation the additional burden of a pervasive developmental disorder is substantial (Scott, 1994). As noted by Wing and Gould (1979), the combination of some autisticlike features is relatively common in lower IQ samples and may affect as many as half of individuals with severe mental retardation.

In higher functioning persons with autism and Asperger's disorder, comorbid conditions are sometimes present. The controversy over autism and its relationship to childhood schizophrenia illustrates some of the problems for documentation of comorbidity when diagnostic systems adopt specific exclusionary criteria. In the *DSM-III* (APA, 1980) the validity of autism as a diagnostic category was recognized, and, in response to the early controversies about its continuity with childhood schizophrenia, the two conditions were made exclusionary from each other. However, there was no reason to expect that having autism would protect an individual from developing a rather common major mental illness like schizophrenia, and some such cases have indeed been reported, although not at rates greater than those expected by the frequency of schizophrenia in the general population (Volkmar & Cohen, 1991). Although the continuity of Asperger's syndrome and higher functioning autism remains the topic of some debate (Klin, 1994), several studies have suggested that individuals with Asperger's disorder are at increased risk for psychotic phenomena and possibly for depression as well. Other disorders possibly associated with autism have included obsessive compulsive disorder and Tourette's disorder, although the lack of good epidemiological data and the complexities of diagnosis create difficulties in adequately evaluating reports of such associations.

There is considerable evidence that speech-language problems are frequently associated with behavioral difficulties. Although methodological problems complicate the interpretation of many studies, it does appear that children with speech-language problems are at increased risk for conditions such as attention deficit disorder. There is also some suggestion that the nature of the underlying speech-language problem can be related to the frequency with which children develop such associated conditions. For example, Baker and Cantwell (1982) reported that the rate of psychiatric disorder was close to 30 percent in a sample of children with disorders of speech (articulation, stuttering, and so on), but in children with more persistent language disorder, rates were much higher. Conversely, screening of children attending outpatient child psychiatry clinics has shown that nearly one-third also exhibit a previously unrecognized language disorder of at least moderate severity (Cohen, Devine, & Meloche-Kelly, 1989). Studies of children with learning disorders similarly show relatively high rates of behavior problems, some of which are quite persistent (McKinney, 1989; Richman, Stevenson, & Graham, 1982). For them, the risk for conduct disorder appears to be increased. In the Isle of Wight study (Rutter et al., 1970), 25 percent of 10 year olds with reading problems had conduct problems as well. The persistence of such problems and their meaning remains unclear. For example, it is possible that shared risk factors may account for the association or that either the learning or conduct problems are primary and led to the other condition (Rutter et al., 1970). Similarly, it is possible that the presence of a language disorder leads to repeated experiences of frustration and negative expectations, or that language problems stem from earlier vulnerabilities, which, in turn, may relate to risk, for other conditions. Longitudinal studies (e.g., Hinshaw, 1992) may be useful in clarifying such associations, although Prizant and Wetherby (1990) have rightly noted that relationships of early language and learning problems to subsequent behavioral difficulties may be very difficult to disentangle.

COMORBIDITY IN THE DISRUPTIVE BEHAVIOR, ANXIETY, AND AFFECTIVE DISORDERS

High rates of comorbidity between attention deficit hyperactivity disorder (ADHD) and oppositional defiant (ODD) or conduct disorder (CD) have repeatedly been noted. For example, rates of comorbidity for ADHD and conduct disorder have ranged from 30 percent to 50 percent; for ADHD and mood disorders, 15 percent to 75 percent; for ADHD and anxiety disorders, 25 percent; and for conduct disorder and depression, up to 50 percent (Anderson, Williams, McGee, & Silva, 1987; Biederman et al., 1991). Similarly, Kovacs, Gatsonis, Paulauskas, and Richards (1989) reported high rates of anxiety disorders with various depressive disorders; overall, 41 percent of cases also exhibited an anxiety disorder in addition to depression. As noted by McArdle, O'Brien, and Kolvin (1995), pervasive overactivity has the strongest links to conduct disorder. Woolston et al. (1989) have reported high rates of multiple comorbid disorders in psychiatrically hospitalized children; in this study it was common for both internalizing and externalizing disorders to be present simultaneously. Interestingly, there was a trend for children with both internalizing and externalizing disorders to have higher adaptive functioning than children with only externalizing disorders.

Unfortunately, the significance of these associations has not usually been clear. Recurrent changes in taxonomy are only one part of the problem (Lahey et al., 1990). It is possible that the apparently high rates of comorbidity are actually artifactual and represent artificial distinctions drawn within what is essentially one condition (see Achenbach, 1990/1991). The problem, however, is not simply one of overreliance on categorical diagnostic approaches; Biederman and colleagues (1993) reported that a widely used dimensional assessment instrument could be employed to identify cases of ADHD with and without comorbid diagnoses. On the other hand, some data suggest that the combination of conduct disorder and depression does differ from depression without conduct disorder—for example, in terms of lower risk for depression in adulthood (Harrington, Fudge, Rutter, Pickles, & Hill, 1991) and with lower rates of affective disorder in the family (Puig-Antich et al., 1989). Similarly, the course and prognosis of depression associated with anxiety disorders seems no different from that of depression alone, whereas the combination of depression and conduct disorder does seem to differ (Angold & Rutter, 1992).

In secondary analyses of epidemiological data obtained in Puerto Rico, Bird, Gould, and Staghezza (1993) noted high rates of comorbidity for symptoms of ADD, conduct problems, anxiety disorder, and depression. In essentially all comparisons, rates of comorbidity among any two of the four diagnostic groups was higher than expected by chance alone. As the number of comorbid diagnoses increased, so did the proportion of children receiving clinical services.

IMPLICATIONS FOR TREATMENT

There are several important implications of psychiatric comorbidity for clinical work with children and adolescents. Probably most important is that the high rates of comorbidity observed in epidemiological studies almost certainly are lower than rates actually observed in clinical settings. On the one hand this should not be surprising; children and adolescents with multiple problems would more likely be referred for evaluation and treatment than would patients with single problems. On the other hand, clinicians frequently think in terms of single diagnoses and often fail to observe comorbidity when it is present. For example, the behavioral difficulties of children with conduct or attentional problems may be so compelling that specific developmental disorders are missed. Although the meaning of specific patterns of comorbidity remains to be established, certain patterns are of interest either because they have so commonly been recognized or have important public health implications. As an example, the association of conduct disorder, depression, and substance abuse is particularly important because of the patient's increased risk for suicide. The study of comorbid conditions is also important because of the potential for continuity of a disorder into adulthood. Biederman and colleagues (1993) reported on the continuity of attention deficit hyperactivity disorder into adulthood, noting that the condition was associated with diverse other conditions.

Recognition of the problem of comorbidity in children and adolescents is also reflected in the growing trend toward combination pharmacotherapies (Wilens, Spencer, Biederman, Wozniak, & Connor, 1994). Thus, multiple agents have been used in the treatment of depression associated with attention deficit or conduct disorder (Wilens et al., 1994). Comorbid anxiety and depression or anxiety and attention deficit disorder may also respond to a combination of agents. Children with pervasive developmental disorders or schizophrenia associated with depression or anxiety may respond to appropriate pharmacological intervention. As noted by Wilens and colleagues (1994), the use of multiple agents for treatment of comorbid conditions carries both potential risks and benefits. The efficacy and safety of such treatments remains to be established.

As is evident from the nosological confusion about the spectrum of comorbid conditions and syndromic clusters, no treatment protocols can equivocally be applied to these conditions. However, several axioms of clinical common sense apply. First, all treatment must employ a comprehensive and integrated approach. The child with his or her various symptoms lives in a complex developmental context of family, school, and neighborhood. A child with a disruptive behavior disorder, a mood disorder, an anxiety disorder, a specific developmental disorder, and a parent-child problem cannot be adequately treated with a single modality, be it one or more medications or a type of psychotherapy. Instead, such a child requires multimodal assessment and intervention at the individual, family, school, and systems levels. Such a child might benefit from pharmacotherapy to ameliorate symptoms of inattention, impulsivity, anxiety, and depression; from focused psychotherapy to address low self-esteem and inadequate social coping skills; from family therapy to improve the parents' parenting skills and communication styles; and special educational services to identify and accommodate specific difficulties in learning and behavior. More multimodal, integrated interventions are required for the readily identifiable, neuropsychiatric developmental clusters occurring with specific conditions. Examples of these are Tourette's disorder that may be accompanied by obsessive compulsive disorder, attention deficit hyperactivity disorder, and/or oppositional defiant disorder; and pervasive developmental disorder not otherwise specified that may occur with attention deficit hyperactivity disorder, oppositional defiant disorder, and/or specific developmental disorder or cognitive impairment. Simply because a disorder or syndrome complex has neuropsychiatric developmental origins is no reason to avoid using psychosocial and educational interventions.

The second basic principle of treatment is to establish a hierarchy of symptom amelioration so that treatment goals can be focused and prioritized. For example, if the family functioning and/or educational placement of a patient are problematic, individual treatment of any sort is not likely to be effective. Thus, while pharmacotherapy and/or individual psychotherapy may be indicated, they must be implemented in conjunction with these other treatment modalities.

The third treatment principle is to match interventions with well-established symptom indicators. The poorly defined nature of comorbid syndromes creates diagnostic confusion for the clinician. This confusion may tempt the clinician to lump together a variety of symptoms into a proposed single underlying disorder, which is then treated. For example, the child with pervasive developmental disorder syndrome might display temper tantrums, mood lability, and episodes of aggression and depression. A clinician might be tempted to explain these diverse symptoms as resulting from a single underlying neuropsychiatric syndrome, such as bipolar disorder. With this reductionistic assumption, the clinician would probably treat the child for the single disorder instead of attempting a more comprehensive but complex intervention approach.

SUMMARY AND DIRECTIONS FOR FUTURE RESEARCH

Given the complex interrelationships of behavior and development, it is probably not surprising that rates of psychiatric comorbidity in children and adolescents are relatively high. Although present data, in important respects, are somewhat limited, there is no doubt that certain conditions are much more frequently noted together in children than would be expected on the basis of chance alone. At the same time, issues in research methods, sample studies, and definitions of disorders have acted to limit knowledge in this area.

Various potential models of comorbidity in childhood and adolescence have been identified but, with very few exceptions, data that would confirm one or another of these alternative hypotheses have been lacking. It is possible and probably likely that different comorbid associations will reflect different causal relationships. At the present time, it seems particularly important not to foreclose any options in this regard. Both clinical and research work in this area should avoid premature closure of issues—for example, by selecting against comorbid conditions in research studies. The use of alternative assessment procedures, such as using dimensions of function/dysfunction may be helpful in this regard.

Given the importance of developmental factors in the expression of diverse syndromes, careful attention to multidimensional/multiaxial diagnostic procedures is particularly important. Some conditions in childhood are of relatively brief duration, but others clearly are lifelong. Unfortunately, categorical diagnostic systems that employ complex exclusionary criteria tend to promote the misconception that having a single disorder acts, in some unspecified way, to protect a person against other disorders. The high rates of psychopathology among individuals with mild mental retardation may present an important potential area for research in this regard as the disorders observed in this group are not fundamentally different from those observed in the general population.

Although current categorical diagnostic systems generally are more alike than different, the few areas of difference in their treatment of comorbid conditions are noteworthy. It remains unclear which approach to the diagnosis of comorbidity will ultimately predominate. From the standpoint of treatment, certain comorbid combinations are of particular interest either because of their clinical significance, their importance for research, or the opportunity they present for new pharmacological approaches. It is also important to note that issues in the classification of disorders of adjustment and of subthreshold disorder present a relatively neglected topic of research in which aspects of comorbidity may have been underappreciated (Cantwell, 1996).

REFERENCES

Achenbach, T.M. (1990/1991). "Comorbidity" in child and adolescent psychiatry: Categorical and quantitative perspectives. *Journal of Child and Adolescent Psychopharmacology, 1,* 271–278.

American Psychiatric Association. (1980). *Diagnostic and statistical manual of mental disorders* (3rd ed.). Washington, DC: Author.

American Psychiatric Association. (1987). *Diagnostic and statistical manual of mental disorders* (3rd ed., rev.). Washington, DC: Author.

American Psychiatric Association. (1994). *Diagnostic and statistical manual of mental disorders* (4th ed.). Washington, DC: Author.

Anderson, J.C., Williams, S., McGee, R., & Silva, P.A. (1987). DSM-III disorders in preadolescent children: Prevalence in a large sample from the general population. *American Journal of Psychiatry, 44,* 69–76.

Angold, A., & Rutter, M. (1992). Effects of age and pubertal status on depression in a large clinical sample. *Development and Psychopathology, 4,* 5–28.

Baker, L., & Cantwell, D.P. (1982). Psychiatric disorders in children with different types of communication disorders. *Journal of Communication Disorders, 15,* 113–126.

Biederman, J., Newcorn, J., & Sprich, S. (1991). Comorbidity of attention deficit disorder with conduct, depressive, anxiety, and other disorders. *American Journal of Psychiatry, 148,* 564–577.

Biederman, J., Faraone, S.V., Doyle, A., Lehman, B.K., Kraus, I., Perrin, J., & Tsuang, M.T. (1993). Convergence of the Child Behavior Checklist with structured interview-based psychiatric diagnosis of ADHD children with and without comorbidity. *Journal of Child Psychology and Psychiatry, 34,* 1241–1251.

Bird, H.R., Gould, M.S., & Staghezza, B.M. (1993). Patterns of diagnostic comorbidity in a community sample of children aged 9 through 16 years. *Journal of the American Academy of Child and Adolescent Psychiatry, 32,* 361–369.

Cantwell, D.P. (1996). Classification of child and adolescent psychopathology. *Journal of Child Psychology and Psychiatry, 37,* 3–12.

Cantwell, D.P., & Rutter, M. (1994). Classification: Conceptual issues and substantive findings. In M. Ruitter, E. Taylor, & L. Hersov (Eds.), *Child and adolescent psychiatry: Modern approaches* (3rd ed., pp. 3–21). London: Blackwell.

Carlson, C.L. (1986). Attention deficit disorder without hyperactivity. In B. Lahey & A. Kazdin (Eds.), *Advances in clinical child psychology* (Vol. 9, pp. 152–175). New York: Plenum Press.

Caron, C., & Rutter, M. (1991). Comorbidity in child psychopathology: Concepts, issues, and research strategies. *Journal of Child Psychology and Psychiatry, 32,* 1063–1080.

Cohen, N.J., Devine, M., & Meloche-Kelly, M. (1989). Prevalence of unsuspected language disorder in a child psychiatric population. *Journal of the American Academy of Child and Adolescent Psychiatry, 28,* 107–111.

Cooper, J. (1995). On the publication of the *diagnostic and statistical manual of mental disorders:* Fourth edition *(DSM-IV). British Journal of Psychiatry, 166,* 4–8.

Harrington, R., Fudge, H., Rutter, M., Pickles, A., & Hill, J. (1991). Adult outcome of childhood and adolescent depression. I. Psychiatric status. *Archives of General Psychiatry, 47,* 465–473.

Harrington, R., Fudge, H., Rutter, M., Bredenkamp, D., Grothues, C., & Pridham, J. (1993). Child and adult depression: A test of continuities with family study data. *British Journal of Psychiatry, 30,* 434–439.

Hindley, P.A., Hill, P.D., McGuigan, S., & Kitson, N. (1993). Psychiatric disorder in deaf and hearing impaired children and young people: A prevalence study. *Journal of Child Psychology and Psychiatry, 35,* 917–934.

Hinshaw, S.P. (1992). Externalizing behavior problems and academic underachievement in childhood and adolescence: Causal relationships and underlying mechanisms. *Psychological Bulletin, 111,* 127–155.

Kashani, J.H., Beck, N.C., Hoeper, E.W., and Associates. (1987). Psychiatric disorders in a community sample of adolescents. *American Journal of Psychiatry, 144,* 584–589.

Klin, A. (1994). Asperger's syndrome. *Child and Adolescent Psychiatry Clinics of North America, 3,* 131–148.

Kovacs, M., Gatsonis, C., Paulauskas, S.K., & Richards, C. (1989). Depressive disorders in childhood IV: A longitudinal study of comorbidity with and risk for anxiety disorders. *American Journal of Psychiatry, 46,* 776–782.

Kovacs, M., Gatsonis, C., Pollock, M., & Parrone, P.L. (1994). A controlled prospective study of *DSM-III* adjustment disorder in childhood: Short term prognosis and long-term predictive validity. *American Journal of Psychiatry, 51,* 535–541.

Lahey, B.B., Loeber, R., Stouthamer-Loeber, M., Christ, M.A., Green, S., Russo, M.K., Frick, P.J., & Dulcan, M. (1990). Comparison of *DSM-II* and *DSM-III-R* diagnoses for prepubertal children: Changes in prevalence and validity. *Journal of the American Academy of Child and Adolescent Psychiatry, 29,* 620–626.

Leckman, J.F. (in press). Tic disorders. *Journal of Child Psychology and Psychiatry.*

Loeber, R., Lahey, B.B., & Thomas, C. (1991). Diagnostic conundrum of oppositional defiant disorder and conduct disorder. *Journal of Abnormal Psychology, 100,* 379–390.

McArdle, P., O'Brien, G., & Kolvin, I. (1995). Hyperactivity: Prevalence and relationship with conduct disorder. *Journal of Child Psychology and Psychiatry, 36,* 279–303.

McKinney, J.D. (1989). Longitudinal research on the behavioral characteristics of children with learning disabilities. *Journal of Learning Disabilities, 22,* 141–150.

Nottelman, E.D., & Jensen, P.S. (1995). Comorbidity of disorders in children and adolescents: Developmental perspectives. *Advances in Clinical Child Psychology, 17,* 109–155.

Prizant, B.M., & Wetherby, A.M. (1990). Towards an integrated view of early language and communication development and social-emotional development. *Topics in Language Disorders, 10,* 1–16.

Puig-Antich, J., Goetz, D., Davies, M., Kaplan, T., Davies, S. et al. (1989). A controlled family history study of prepubertal major depressive disorders. *Archives of General Psychiatry, 46,* 406–418.

Richman, N., Stevenson, J., & Graham, P.J. (1982). *Preschool to school: A behavioural study.* London: Academic Press.

Rutter, M. (1989). Annotation: Childhood psychiatric disorders in *ICD-10*. *Journal of Child Psychology and Psychiatry, 30,* 449–513.

Rutter, M., Lebovichi, S., Eisenberg, L., Sneznevskij, A.V., Sadound, R., Brooke, E., & Lin, T.Y. (1969). A triaxial classification of mental disorders in childhood. *Journal of Child Psychology and Psychiatry, 10,* 41–61.

Rutter, M., & Shaffer, D. (1980). *DSM-III:* A step forward or back in terms of the classification of child psychiatric disorder? *Journal of the American Academy of Child and Adolescent Psychiatry, 10,* 371–394.

Rutter, M., Tizard, J., & Whitmore, K. (1970). *Education, health, and behaviour.* London: Longman.

Rutter, M., Tuma, A.H., & Lann, I.S. (Eds.). (1988). *Assessment and diagnosis in child psychopathology.* New York: Guilford Press.

Scott, S. (1994). Mental retardation. In M. Rutter, E. Taylor, & L. Hersov (Eds.), *Child and adolescent psychiatry: Modern approaches* (3rd ed., pp. 616–646). London: Blackwell.

Volkmar, F.R. (1996). Autism and the pervasive developmental disorders. In M. Lewis (Ed.), *Child and adolescent psychiatry: A comprehensive textbook* (2nd ed., pp. 489–497). Baltimore: Williams & Wilkins.

Volkmar, F.R., & Cohen, D.J. (1991). Co-morbid association of autism and schizophrenia. *American Journal of Psychiatry, 148,* 1705–1707.

Volkmar, F.R., & Schwab-Stone, M. (1996). Annotation: *DSM-IV. Journal of Child Psychology and Psychiatry, 37,* 779–784.

Weinstein, S.R., Stone, K., Noam, G.G., Grimes, K., & Schwab-Stone, M. (1989). *Comparison of DISC with clinician's DSM-III diagnoses in psychiatric inpatients.* Location: Publisher.

Weissman, M., Warner, V., & Fendrick, M. (1987). Applying impairment criteria to children's psychiatric diagnosis. *Journal of the American Academy of Child and Adolescent Psychiatry, 29,* 789–795.

Wilens, T.E., Spencer, T., Biederman, J., Wozniak, J., & Connor, D. (1994). Combined pharmacotherapy: An emerging trend in pediatric psychopharmacology. *Journal of the American Academy of Child and Adolescent Psychiatry, 34,* 110–112.

Wing, L. (1977). The use of case registers in child psychiatry and mental retardation. In P. Graham (Ed.), *Epidemiological approaches in child psychiatry* (pp. 31–44). London: Academic Press.

Wing, L., & Gould, J. (1979). Severe impairments of social interaction and associated abnormalities in children: Epidemiology and classification. *Journal of Autism and Developmental Disorders, 9,* 11–29.

Woolston, J.L., Rosenthal, S.L., Riddle, M.A., Sparrow, S.S., Cicchetti, D., & Zimmerman, L.D. (1989). Childhood comorbidity of anxiety/affective disorders and behavior disorders. *Journal of the American Academy of Child and Adolescent Psychiatry, 28,* 707–713.

World Health Organization. (1990). Mental and behavioural disorders: Diagnostic criteria for research. (Draft). *International classification of diseases* (10th ed.). Geneva: World Health Organization.

14

Comorbidity in the Elderly
Implications for Diagnosis and Treatment

GARY J. KENNEDY
MARY ALICE O'DOWD

The interplay of mental and physical illness, social factors, and the accumulation of years make comorbidity the rule rather than the exception in geriatric practice (Table 14-1). For both causality and course of illness, mental and physical health are inseparable in aged persons (Katz, 1996). However, several concepts from the literature, including geriatric syndromes, comprehensive geriatric assessment, the functional approach to treatment, and the theory of excess disability help to clarify this bewildering array of etiologies and treatment options. The discussion of treatment presented here focuses on late-life conditions encountered in the clinic, hospital, community, and nursing home in which comorbidity seems most frequent.

GERIATRIC SYNDROMES

Frequently, conditions of old age are encountered for which the conventions of etiology and diagnostic nomenclature are an insufficient guide to treatment. Cognitive impairment, incontinence, deficits in hearing or vision, osteopenia (osteoporosis and fractures), falls, impaired mobility, pressure

TABLE 14-1
Situations and Conditions in Which
Mental and Physical Comorbidity Should Be Suspected

Sociodemographic situations
  •Bereaved, socially isolated seniors and those older than 75
  •Nursing home residents
Common cardiac and vascular conditions
  •Myocardial infarction, stroke
Common neurologic conditions
  •Parkinson's disease, the dementias
Recent onset of other physically disabling conditions
  •Hip fracture, trauma
Psychiatric disorders
  •Late onset (after age 55) mania or psychosis
  •Dysthymia
  •Minor depression
  •Major depression, especially when recurrent or psychotic
  •Mixed anxiety and depression
  •Adjustment disorder with depressed or anxious mood
Suicidal ideas, self-neglect, self-injurious behaviors, elder abuse and neglect

Source: Adapted from G.J. Kennedy (1994). The geriatric syndrome of late life depression. *Psychiatric Services, 46,* 43–48. Reproduced with permission.

ulcers, malnutrition and polypharmacy are the most commonly cited geriatric syndromes (Beck, 1989). The syndrome terminology reflects the multifactorial etiology typical of these conditions and the multidimensional treatment required to return the older person to optimum function.

A major change in the clinical approach to old age depression occurred in the 1990s (Karasu et al., 1993; National Institutes of Health Consensus Development Panel, 1992), resulting in an expanse of therapeutic indications, treatments, outcomes, and end points that is best captured by the geriatric syndrome concept. The syndromal approach also resolves much of the conflict between epidemiologic (Myers, Weissman, et al., 1984) and clinical (Kermis, 1986) studies of depression in old age.

COMORBIDITY OF MENTAL
AND PHYSICAL ILLNESS IN OLD AGE

As many as 30 percent of elderly primary care patients demonstrate significant depressive symptomatology (Katz, Curil, & Nemetz, 1988). Close to half that number meet criteria for a depressive disorder (Rapp, Parisi, & Walsh, 1988). Hypnotics and antianxiety agents are more often prescribed for older adults with depressive symptoms than are antidepressants. Not surprisingly, depressive symptoms tend to persist in the routine care context (Kennedy, Kelman, & Thomas, 1991). Depressive symptoms among older adults lead them to utilize outpatient services and nursing facilities at a higher rate than would be expected for the level of disability associated with their medical conditions (Kelman & Thomas, 1990). Depression amplifies physical disability, and even minor depression may be more disabling than most chronic physical conditions (Wells et al., 1989). As many as one quarter of those initially diagnosed as having a minor depression experience a major depressive disorder within the subsequent 24 months (Wells, Burnam, Rogers, Hays, & Camp, 1992). More important, the disability of depression may be avoidable (Strain et al., 1991).

For patients who have suffered a stroke, more than half of them experience major depression within six months after the stroke, a development that interferes substantially with their rehabilitation (Parikh, Lipsey, Robinson, & Price, 1987). Twenty percent of Parkinson patients develop a major depressive episode, and 20 percent develop dysthymia frequently combined with anxiety (Menza, Robertson-Hoffman, & Bonapace, 1993). Depressive disorders are also common in dementia patients (Rovner, Broadhead, Spencer, Carson, & Folstein, 1989) as well as in their caregiving family members (Gallagher, Rose, Rivera, Losett, & Thompson, 1989). Dementia is the most prevalent mental illness in nursing homes followed by depression, and dementia complicated by depression (Rovner, German, Broadhead, Morris, & Brant, 1990).

Although older adults are more likely than younger adults to develop a major depressive episode following bereavement (Zisook, Shuchter, & Sledge, 1994), physical illness and disability explain substantially more of the variance in the prevalence and course of depressive symptoms among older community residents than do sociodemographic, life event, and interpersonal factors (Kennedy, Kelman, & Thomas, 1991). Katz (1996) summarizes two general theories regarding the biological origins of depression in late life. First, subclinical cerebrovascular disease may induce depressive symptoms through neurohumoral or structural brain changes. Second, systemic illness may induce depression through cytokine-mediated changes in behavior that allow the sick individual time to return to physiologic equilibrium by reducing conative activity.

COMORBIDITY OF DEPRESSION
WITH ANXIETY DISORDERS

Among physically healthy older community residents without cognitive disorders, agoraphobia may be more common than depression. Minor depression and the mixed syndrome of depression with anxiety affect more than 1 percent of older community residents (Blazer, Woodbury, et al., 1989). Also, there is considerable comorbidity of depression with generalized anxiety disorder and phobias in older persons (Flint, 1994). Subsyndromal anxiety and anxiety comorbid with psychiatric and medical disorders are also significant (Smith, Sherrill, & Colenda, 1995). Anxiety may be evidence of poor recovery from a previous episode of depression (Blazer, Hughes, & Fowler, 1989). In summary, the bulk of evidence indicates that when anxiety and depression are concurrent, the primary diagnosis in late life is a depressive disorder, whether encountered in the community, the clinic (Blazer, Hughes, & Fowler, 1989), or in the nursing home (Parmalee, Katz, & Lawton, 1993).

COMORBIDITY AND SUICIDE

Although a depressive episode is present in the majority of older adults who commit suicide (Conwell, Melanie, & Caine, 1990), physical illness plays a critical role (Mackensie & Popkin, 1987). Twenty percent of older individuals who kill themselves have seen a physician within 24 hours of their deaths. Although the physicians recall only vague physical complaints and denial of mental symptoms, the patients' families recall difficulties with depression, alcohol, and prescription drugs (Clark, 1992). The profile of suicidal risk, presented in Table 14-2, indirectly indicates the components of treatment. Mental illness, suicidal intent, physical disability, social isolation, alcohol abuse, firearms in the home—all need attention. Suicidal intent should be distinguished from the older person's preparations for death; the latter may be age appropriate, such as making burial arrangements, writing a last will and testament, coming to terms with a terminal illness. However, the older person who describes acts that will lead to his or her death should be considered depressed until proven otherwise.

COMPREHENSIVE GERIATRIC ASSESSMENT

Because late-life mental illness is so closely associated with functional disability, the functionally oriented approach of a comprehensive geriatric as-

TABLE 14-2
Characteristics of Older Adults at Increased Risk for Suicide

Sociodemographic	*Clinical*	*Historical*
White, male	Depression	Previous attempt
Divorced, widowed	Alcoholism	Family history
Lives alone	Chronic pain	Lethality of attempt
Recent life change event	Poor health	Rescued by accident
Anniversary of loss	Disability	Firearms possession
75 or older		Expressed intent

Source: Adapted from Kennedy, G.J., & Lowinger, R. (1993). Psychogeriatric emergencies. In L. Pousada (Ed.), *Clinics in Geriatrics Medicine, 9,* 641–654. Reproduced with permission.

sessment (Winograd, 1992) described in Table 14-3, is very helpful in guiding optimum treatment. The assessment identifies therapeutic avenues, obstacles, and goals. The end point is the most independent level of function attainable, given the person's capacities, support, and setting.

The comprehensive assessment need not be exhausting. Most older adults are brought to the attention of mental health specialists by family, a primary care provider, or a social service agency. Thus, physical examination and laboratory procedures have often been performed prior to the patient's referral. Usually, a patient will not object to the clinician's interviewing a collateral informant. The information such a person can provide may be essential both for assessment and maintenance of a therapeutic regimen, and it may make the work more efficient for the therapist and less burdensome for the patient.

A review of medications—prescribed and over-the-counter—may reveal unfavorable interactions of regimens the patient has difficulty following. Reducing polypharmacy and switching to other medications may improve the older person's mental status and quality of life (Testa, Anderson, Nackley, & Hollenberg, 1993). Nutritional assessment may also be indicated when patients are frail, when their teeth are in disrepair, and when weight loss is a problem. Functional assessment of daily living activities includes a review of patients' capacity to manage personal hygiene, ambulation, shopping, and finances. The clinician should determine how much assistance patients require in these areas and whether they have disabilities that might respond to physical or occupational therapy.

An assessment of social rhythms (Reynolds et al., 1992), the day-to-day flow of both formal and informal socially supportive activities, will indicate the extent to which the patient is isolated or has abandoned social

TABLE 14-3
Comprehensive Geriatric Assessment

History, physical examination, mental status examination including use of cognitive
    screening instrument
Collateral interview, brief patient personality assessment
Survey of prescribed medications, over-the-counter preparations, nutrition
Functional assessment of activities of daily living and sleep habits
Social rhythms assessment
Routine diagnostic procedures
  • Electrocardiogram, complete blood count, urine analysis, triiodothyronine, thyroid
    stimulating hormone, B12, folate, chemistries, liver function, VDRL (skin test and
    chest X-ray for tuberculosis, test for the human immunodeficiency virus may be
    indicated if the VDRL is positive)
Elective procedures to explain treatment resistance or enlighten prognosis
  • Electroencephalogram, computerized axial tomography, magnetic resonance
    imaging, neuropsychological tests, polysomnography

Source: Adapted from Blazer, D. (in press). Geriatric psychiatry. In J. Hales (Ed.), *Textbook of Psychiatry.* Washington, DC: American Psychiatric Press; and Winograd, C.H., (1992). Geriatric assessment: Concepts, components, and settings. In J.E. Morely (Ed.), *Geriatric care* (pp. 212–233). St. Louis: G.W. Manning.

reinforcers of self-esteem while it helps to identify socially meaningful points of intervention and measures of recovery. Finally, elective procedures may be indicated when the patient fails to respond to interventions or when a latent dementia or other central nervous system disorder is suspected. These procedures include neuropsychological evaluation, brain imaging, and electroencephalogram.

COMPREHENSIVE TREATMENT

As shown in Table 14-4 the treatment of comorbid conditions requires an approach composed of definitive, rehabilitative, and supportive components. In the case of depressive illness, the approach spans the course of treatment including the acute, continuation, and maintenance phases. Because late onset mental disorders are so often associated with structural brain changes, they are frequently recurrent. Recurrence prevention is as important as attaining an initial remission of symptoms (Frank, 1994).

The relationships between mental and physical illnesses and disabilities are reciprocal, and interventions must be relevant to the etiology, course, and treatment of each to be fully effective (Gurland, Wilder, & Berkman, 1988). For example, a physical disorder such as hypothyroidism accompa-

TABLE 14-4
Treatment of Depression as a Geriatric Syndrome

When depression is associated with somatic illness, disability, or dementia:
Definitive, restorative (e.g., thyroid replacement)
Rehabilitative (e.g., physical and occupational therapy)
Supportive (e.g., family/caregiver counseling, psychoeducation)
When depression arises de novo or the above approaches seem inadequate:
Psychotherapy
    •Interpersonal or cognitive-behavioral, marital, family, group
Pharmacotherapy of unipolar disorders
    •Nortriptyline (therapeutic levels, mild anticholinergic effect)
    •Sertraline (not sedative, no cardiovascular or cognitive risks)
    •Nefazodone (mild sedative, no cardiovascular or cognitive risks)
    •Trazadone (sedating, hypotensive but not anticholinergic)
    •Tranylcypromine (hypotensive, not anticholinergic or sedating)
    •Bupropion (not sedating but associated with seizures, weight loss)
    •Buspirone (for anxiety with depression)
    •Methylphenidate (rapid onset of action, for frail, apathetic elderly)
Pharmacotherapy of bipolar disorder or to augment unipolar regimen
    •Valproic acid (therapeutic levels)
When depression occurs with psychosis or fails to respond to combinations of the above:
Haloperidol, perphenazine (extrapyramidal effect, no cardiovascular risk)
Thioridazine (no extrapyramidal effects, but hypotensive, sedative)
When depression is life threatening or fails to respond to combinations of the above:
Electroconvulsive therapy, twice weekly, over three to five weeks

Source: Adapted from Kennedy, G.J. (1994). The geriatric syndrome of late life depression. *Psychiatric Services, 46,* 43–48.

nied by depression should be treated definitively with thyroid replacement. However, treatment of the depression should not be withheld until the somatic disorder remits. Rather, the decision to treat the depression should be based on the extent to which the person's function is impaired as well as the intensity of the dysphoria. The cause of the depression may be obvious, but when recovery is not spontaneous or the condition is emotionally painful, interventions are justified.

Antidepressant medication and/or psychotherapy may be sufficient treatment when depression occurs without comorbid conditions. Often, interventions in the environment and with the caregivers will also be required. A patient's social isolation may be lessened by referring or returning the patient to a senior citizen or religious center, hiring a home health aide or companion, or helping the family to schedule a more reliable pattern of visits to their elderly relative. Occupational therapy to help the patient improve his or her hygiene and nutrition may be critical to the restoration of self-worth and pride in appearance. Physical and occupational therapy are particularly useful when apraxia complicates stroke or dementia. A speech pathologist may be essential if aphasia interferes with rehabilitation of mood and interpersonal skills. If the patient cannot benefit from the restorative approach, the focus turns to the caregiver to help maintain the patient's independence and well-being.

Psychotherapies

The indications for psychotherapy and psychoeducation clearly go beyond medication noncompliance, comorbidity, and social isolation. Pharmacotherapy, combined with psychotherapy, appears to minimize attrition from treatment and recurrence of depression (Reynolds et al., 1992). Interpersonal psychotherapy (IPT) and cognitive-behavioral psychotherapy (CBT) have been developed and written into manuals specifically for research in depression. Among older persons, the benefits of CBT have more often been demonstrated with physically healthy, cognitively intact, community residents than with elderly patients with multiple difficulties (Teri, Curtis, Gallager-Thompson, & Thompson, 1994). Cognitive group therapy may be particularly appropriate for geriatric patients (Yost, Beutler, & Corbishley, 1986).

Depression may degrade marital and family relations (Coyne, 1976). Problems with intimacy, communication, and individuality common to marital therapy among younger couples may be difficult to resolve in older couples without attending to each partner's need for concrete social services or medication (Greenberg & Kennedy, 1991). Treatment of sexual dysfunction among older persons with mental illness is beyond the scope of this chapter but should not be neglected with patients of advanced years. Because depression can recur despite medication compliance in older patients, a family psychoeducational approach is often helpful, to engage the family as a multigenerational treatment modality for the older patient's depression (Papolos, 1994).

Antidepressants

Side effect profile, availability of therapeutic drug levels, and patient characteristics rather than differences in effectiveness dictate the choice of antidepressants. Because the antidepressant effect may be delayed in the elderly (Perel, 1994), considerable skill is necessary to sustain the patient's and family's collaboration. However, a patient's anxiety, agitation, and sleep disturbance may be reduced within days of beginning therapy. Treatment maintained at acute phase levels achieves the lowest recurrence rate (Georgotas, McCue, Cooper, Nagachandran, & Chang, 1988).

Nortriptyline is the most extensively studied antidepressant for older adults. It is both adrenergic and serotonergic, may be effective in doses as low as 10 mg daily, and is mildly sedative with a moderate to low risk of hypotension, arrhythmia, and amnesia (Salzman, 1994). Nortriptyline is unique among antidepressants in that it possesses a therapeutic window (50–150 mg/ml) a clinician can use to determine whether a patient's lack of response is due to too little drug, whether the drug has failed, or whether the dose should not be increased further because of the risk of toxicity. The patient might begin taking a soluble fiber laxative with the first prescription to prevent constipation. Alternatively, the reversible monoamine oxidase inhibitor tranylcypromine may be useful when anticholinergic and proarrhythmic effects must be avoided entirely (Jenike, 1985). The patient must follow precautions for diet and medications, and the clinician must monitor for hypotension, which can be a problem.

Trazodone (25 mg initial dose) may be preferable when sleep disturbance or agitation are the patient's most salient problems. It is a beneficial antidepressant but hypotension and sedation limit its effectiveness. The newer agent nefazadone (50 mg twice daily) has serotonergic reuptake inhibitor properties, is free of amnestic and arrhythmic effects, and is less sedative than trazodone.

The selective serotonergic agent sertraline (up to 200 mg daily) may be better for lethargic or demented, frail and hypotensive patients. For the depression of Parkinson's disease, and especially for the frail patient who can tolerate no side effects, the selectively noradrenergic bupropion (75 mg twice daily) is a reasonable choice. Bupropion and sertraline are stimulatory and free of cardiac and cognitive toxicity (Karasu et al., 1993). Alternatively, methylphenidate (5–15 mg after breakfast and lunch) may be prescribed and has the advantage of rapid onset of therapeutic activity.

Medication for Bipolar Disorder

The use of lithium for bipolar disorder or to augment the response of antidepressants is problematic in the elderly, partly because of their reduced renal function and structural brain changes. Also, lithium may be toxic to this population, even at therapeutic levels that would be normal in the younger patient (Parfrey, Ikeman, Anglin, & Cole, 1983). The anticonvulsant valproic acid (Maletta, 1992) is increasingly considered the first choice for augmentation and treatment of mania. A therapeutic level is available and although hepatic toxicity is a risk, it is infrequent.

Antipsychotics

When psychosis is present, a low dose of haloperidol (0.5 mg) or perphenazine (2 mg) should be added to nortriptyline, trazodone or tranylcypromine. Thioridazine (10 mg) is less likely to provide extrapyramidal side effects than haloperidol, but because of its sedative and hypotension propensities, it should be added only when sertraline or bupropion is already in place. Haloperidol, perphenazine, and thioridazine each are available as liquid concentrates that allow for precise dose titration and ease of administration. Monotherapy in the treatment of psychotic depression is not good practice. However, when psychosis occurs as a complication of dementia or is a brief reaction within the context of personality disorder, resperidone (0.5 mg initially) may be preferable for frail seniors who may not tolerate the sedative or hypotensive effects of thioridazine. There are insufficient data on which to base a recommendation of resperidone for psychotic depression or bipolar disorder.

Electroconvulsive Therapy

Age-related factors increase the value of electroconvulsive therapy (ECT) for geriatric major depression (Myers, Kalayum, & Mei-tal, 1984). It may be particularly useful in cases of medication inefficacy or intolerance, imminent suicidal risk, or morbid nutritional status. Advanced age, concurrent antidepressants, and cardiovascular compromise increase the risk of adverse reactions to ECT, with cardiovascular complications being the most frequent events. The cognitive impairment associated with ECT includes temporary postictal confusion, transient anterograde or retrograde amnesia, and, less commonly, permanent amnestic syndrome in which events surrounding the treatment are forgotten (American Psychiatric Association Task Force on ECT, 1990). Treatments may be limited to twice weekly and applied unilaterally to the patient's nondominant hemisphere to minimize confusion. However, bilateral treatment may be more effective (Sackeim et al., 1993). Single treatment maintenance ECT can be administered over intervals of several weeks to months (Hay & Hay, 1992) and may offer higher rates of sustained recovery than is obtained with complete cessation of treatment.

TREATMENT OF COMORBID BEHAVIORAL DISTURBANCES IN DEMENTIA

The number and effectiveness of medications to lessen the cognitive impairment of dementia remain limited (Patel, 1995). However, there are approaches, both pharmacologic and otherwise, to reduce the comorbid disability of behavioral disturbances caused by depression, psychosis, anxiety, and sleep disorders, which occur in a substantial minority of persons with dementia and are more prominent in middle to later stages of decline (Teri et al., 1992). Reifler and Larson's (1988) concept of reducible, excess disability in dementia follows a rule of halves. One half of demented persons are affected by the comorbid physical or mental illness that adds to their impairment. Half that number can experience temporary benefits from treatment of the concurrent condition. The benefits will last a year or more in half that group.

Problem behaviors are an expression of the caregiving context, the caregiver's capacities, and the patient's disease. The etiology may be multifactorial, but not all factors can be changed. Making the patient's behavior less of a problem is usually a more realistic goal than outright elimination of the behavior. The risk/benefit/burden ratio of treatment is a critical concern for both the patient and caregivers. Conflicts over patient and caregiver rights may be avoided through recognition of the shared nature of autonomy in the context of dementia. Once the patient is dependent on others, the autonomy of those others becomes a shared concern and common focus of clinical attention. Interventions are justified for behavior that is disagreeable to others with whom the patient resides or depends upon.

Agitation

A common problem with a variety of etiologies is agitation. When the change in behavior is abrupt, delirium due to acute illness or change in medication should be suspected. However, sleep deprivation and placement in unfamiliar or chaotic surroundings can also induce confusion in an elderly patient that is indistinguishable from delirium. Sometimes patients respond to explanations for their confusion, but potentially harmful behavior such as attempts to remove intravenous lines or life supports may require psychotropic medications or physical restraints.

Depression, anxiety, psychosis, and pain can also cause agitation (Greenwald et al., 1989). Age-related impairments in hearing and vision and faulty or missing glasses or hearing aids add to the problem. Patients who cannot express their needs due to aphasia may also become agitated. Their inability to comprehend spoken cues may interfere with efforts to reassure them. Frontal lobe degeneration degrades patient judgment and the capacity to sequence appropriate steps to gain attention or comfort. If the clinician will explain the impediments to communication that the patient is experiencing, this knowledge may lessen staff and family frustration and justify the time and patience they must spend to reduce if not prevent the patient's agitation.

Screaming

Possibly the most distressing form of agitation for caregivers is screaming by the patient (Cohen-Mansfield, Werner, & Marx, 1990). The patient is often unable to explain the behavior or identify an unmet need. The caregivers must infer possible causes, which include pain, fecal or urinary urgency, constipation, anxiety, depression, psychosis, sensory isolation, boredom, lack of exercise, and cortical disinhibition. Often the patient's screaming can be reduced in frequency and volume without resorting to sedation if caregivers make brief checks for toileting, snacks, or physical stimulation. Once such checks are incorporated into the staff routine, they are not burdensome. Caregivers generally prefer a little unpleasant vocalization to a patient sedated with psychotropics.

Sundowning

Increased confusion with the onset of evening hours, or *sundowning,* can usually be managed by recognizing that changes in the environmental routine trigger the patient's problem behavior. Some patients become troubled at the change of shifts in the nursing home or hospital as a response to the increase in stimulation. Others may be bothered by the reduction in stimulation as the work day winds down and daylight fades. In either situation, providing the optimum of stimulation is preferable to medication. Snacks, brief personal contact, or music are some of the alterations in the care routine that alleviate sundowning. Caregivers should also be sure that any hearing or visual impairments in the patient have been addressed to the degree possible. When suspiciousness or agitation becomes disruptive, however, and it is not lessened by modulating the environment, antipsychotic medication may be necessary.

Psychotic Phenomena

It is important for clinicians to distinguish persistent false beliefs or perceptions from transitory illusions that result from impairments in vision, hearing, and cortical deficits due to the patient's dementia (Wragg & Jeste, 1989). When a patient briefly mistakes one family member for another, the lapse can be upsetting for the family but rarely leads to disturbed behavior. However, when a patient refuses to attend a day care center, admit a home health aide, or allow health maintenance procedures, he or she may be suffering from paranoia rather than expressing a reasoned preference. Paranoia can also take the form of delusional accusations of infidelity. When patients act on their delusions through seclusiveness, threats, accusations, or assault, antipsychotic medication will be necessary. Usually psychotic demented patients retain enough regard for an empathic physician that they will consent to medication to restore sleep, alleviate stress, or help them control their temper. Patients can be informed that family or nursing staff will place liquid medication in their juice or cereal each morning if they agree. Consent need not be renewed with each dose. In cases of refusal, the concept of shared autonomy, or negotiated consent should be recalled (Moody, 1988).

Sleep Disturbance

Disturbances in sleep are common in dementia and problematic in that both the patient's and the caregiver's sleep are disrupted. A review of the patient's sleep patterns, length of time spent in bed, and daytime activities may identify the possibilities for changing the sleep schedule, adding exercise, or prescribing medication. If physical discomfort awakens the patient, an analgesic at bedtime may help. The frequency of nighttime urination may be reduced by withholding fluids after six P.M. Although such behavioral interventions are the mainstay of treatment, it is the caregiver's behavior that must be modified if the demented person's sleep is to improve. And the burdens and benefits of treatment need to be estimated for both the patient and caregiver. Sedation is an obvious solution but predisposes the patient to falling.

Hypersomnia is less often a problem than insomnia. For patients who sleep too much, coffee or tea may be useful. Other patients who are apathetic or nap too frequently may benefit from low dose methylphenidate (5–15 mg after breakfast or lunch).

Indiscreet or Unwelcome Sexual Behavior

Behavior described as sexual acting out may be the result of lack of privacy or an appropriate partner. However, when sexual advances are unwelcome or when self-stimulation is not managed discreetly, more may be required than directing the patient to a private area. The problem should be discussed directly with the patient at the time of the behavior and disapproval indicated for the circumstances surrounding the act, not the impulse. A matter-of-fact approach by the clinician with family and staff also helps alleviate their reluctance to discuss the issue. Modeling openness and a willingness to help the patient regain control is preferable to a punitive attitude. Pathological sexuality in dementia is more often the result of the disinhibition of frontal lobe pathology than of willfulness. Staff and family will be less morally outraged once the neurologic basis of the behavior is explained to them.

Therapy with medroxyprogesterone or conjugated estrogen have been used to lessen sexual aggression in males with dementia. Psychotropic medications used for this purpose should be reserved for incidents of assaultiveness or masturbatory self-mutilation.

Difficulties with Personal Care

Efforts to assist patients with feeding, bathing, and transfer from bed to chair or toilet are sometimes met with assaultive behavior, particularly when the patient and caregiver form an unfamiliar pair. Assaultiveness results from primitive protective reflexes and disinhibition resulting from the dementia. Apraxia, aphasia, and agnosia, common in Alzheimer's disease and worsened by impairments in vision and hearing, degrade the patient's capacity to carry out or comprehend simple motor tasks or to recognize the caregiver.

Staff should be made aware that the objectionable behavior results from neurologic deficits and protective responses rather than malice. Given time, staff will become accustomed to the patient's needs and develop an effective strategy for addressing them. Using two persons to help bathe a patient, or placing mittens on the patient's hands may prevent him or her from scratching or assaulting the helper. Physical or chemical restraints often result in more rather than less time and effort required by caregivers. Time saved by a team approach to problem bathers compensates for the added personnel.

Willful Behavior and Personality Disorders

Staff and family often mistakenly attribute the demented person's behavior to willfulness. However, individuals with the dramatic-impulsive cluster of personality disorders (histrionic, borderline, narcissistic, antisocial) may also develop dementia. Distinguishing their impulsiveness, extreme emotionality, or manipulations from the impaired judgment and emotional lability of dementia may be difficult. A long-standing lack of regard for others' feelings further limits the capacity of these patients to appreciate the consequences of their behavior. Strained interpersonal relations throughout adulthood is the key historical finding, suggesting that limit setting and confrontation may be more effective with these patients than psychotropic medications. Because the behavior is part of an established pattern, staff should adjust their expectations accordingly.

MEDICATIONS TO LESSEN BEHAVIORAL DISTURBANCES

Start low, go slow is the key to safe prescribing for older adults. However, to control behavioral disturbance, it is equally important to monitor efficacy and side effects with patience and perseverance. Older persons vary greatly in their tolerance of psychotropic medications and some require doses more frequently encountered with young adults. Mechanical restraints should be used only as an emergency procedure while awaiting the effects of sedation to take hold. For the patient, such restraints can cause anxiety, a struggle, and undesirable physiologic consequences (Evans & Strumph, 1993).

Sedatives

A short-acting benzodiazepine (lorazepam 0.5 mg oral or intramuscular) can help the patient through procedures such as CAT scan or MRI. For sleep disturbance, low doses of the sedating antidepressant trazodone (25 mg) may be effective, but hypotension will ensue as the dose is increased (Houlihan et al., 1994). The sedating antipsychotic thioridazine, again in low doses (10 mg), may also be beneficial.

Antidepressants and Antipsychotics

Antidepressants and antipsychotics are discussed earlier in this chapter, during the discussion of depression. Both types of medications are used frequently when symptoms of depression or psychosis complicate dementia. The considerations dictating the choice of specific agents are the same whether the condition is depression or dementia. However, most patients with a behavioral disturbance complicating dementia will not require combined treatment with both antidepressant and antipsychotic medications.

Antianxiety Agents

Antidepressants are frequently effective in combating anxiety. Nortriptyline and nefazadone may be less sedating than the benzodiazepines and therefore less likely to impair patients' awareness. However, frail patients who cannot tolerate any degree of sedation may be given buspirone (5 mg daily), which is also free of amnestic and hypnotic effects.

Antiaggression Agents

Although antipsychotics have long been the main treatment of aggression, valproate (125 mg initially) has gained increasing recognition as an antiaggression agent as well as a mood stabilizer. It is relatively free of adverse reactions and is not amnestic, arrhythmogenic, or hypotensive, but it should be monitored with therapeutic levels (Maletta, 1992). Antiadrenergic agents (beta-blockers) have also been advocated for this purpose but are more likely to compromise cardiovascular function.

PERSONALITY DISORDERS AND COMORBIDITY

Personality disorders may predispose individuals to anxiety or mood disorders and may complicate their course and treatment (Costa & McCrue, 1994). Personality disorder in the context of old age affective disorders may be more closely linked to disability rather than severity of depressive symptoms (Abrams, Rosendahl, Card, & Alexopoulos, 1994). As a result, clinicians may need to adjust their expectations for older persons who recover from an episode of depression but seem unable to return to their previous level of function.

Differential Diagnosis

Personality disorders are distinguished from a change in personality resulting from delirium, dementia, bereavement, or catastrophic illness. Personality change due to general medical condition may be diagnosed if a persistent, disabling disturbance in personality is the direct physiological consequence of the condition and is not better explained by other mental illness, dementia, or delirium. Traumatic brain injury, stroke, seizure disorders, neurologic conditions, and endocrinopathies are examples of conditions that may significantly change personality. Emotional lability, disinhibition of sexual and other impulses, aggressive speech and behavior, apathy and indifference, suspiciousness or paranoid thinking, and combinations of the above may be used to specify the type of personality change.

Treatment

Although a personality disorder is lifelong, the events that bring the disorder to clinical attention may be more episodic and modifiable. When the event represents irrevocable change, such as a long-term nursing home admission, adaptation need not be ideal to be acceptable. The goal is to help the patients and their immediate community regain equilibrium. Interactions stylized to fit the patient's character can be tailored to the presenting problem.

In Cluster A, the paranoid, schizoid, or schizotypal person may become intolerably anxious or transiently psychotic when interpersonal barriers are breached. Demands for trust or intimacy occasioned by hospitalization, nursing home admission, medical or legal procedures, bereavement, retirement, or the onset of disability require an empathic but dispassionate stance by medical staff and caregivers. Staff acknowledgment of the real difficulties with trust and intimacy behind the patient's paranoid accusations can allow an element of trust without joining in the paranoia. Schizoid, aloof persons need respite from interpersonal stimulation, and this need should be respected. The patient's social withdrawal and lack of feeling or responses are explained to staff as self-protective rather than unappreciative or bigoted. A conservative rather than aggressive care plan may be more acceptable to the schizoid person who initially refuses services even when he or she is obviously ill.

For the overly dramatic, impulsive disorders of Cluster B (histrionic, narcissistic, borderline, or antisocial), the intensity of patient affect, particularly anger, need not cause alarm. The feelings are intense but short-lived, and the therapist should not overreact. This attitude will help patients choose less problematic ways to express their feelings or moderate the intensity of these displays. When impulsiveness leads to self-destructive behavior or objectionable acts, these patients need confrontation and limit-setting to regain control. Insight into how the behavior is ultimately self-defeating or unacceptable is praiseworthy, but managing the behavior is the more immediate concern. Containing or minimizing objectionable behaviors may be a more reasonable goal than outright elimination.

For patients with Cluster B disorders, therapists should be alert to their propensity for seeing individual caregivers as either rescuers or persecutors. This phenomenon is not impossible to repair but is difficult to prevent. Communication between all parties providing services to the person keeps the care team from taking sides according to the roles assigned by the patient. When difficult treatment decisions arise, a team meeting with the patient and family can avoid fragmentation into adversarial camps. A behavioral contract can be drawn up in the meeting, specifying the team's expectations of the patient and contingencies if these expectations are not met. Family and staff agree to provide a consistent approach across disciplines and work shifts to prevent the patient from using manipulation in playing one person against another. Environmental modifications may also be necessary to contain impulsiveness or countermanipulations.

Patients with Cluster C (avoidant, dependent, obsessive compulsive) disorders may become inflexible and noncompliant with medical treatment if they become overly anxious. Identifying sources of their anxiety and preferred types of comfort (reassurance, information, direction, medication) can guide the management of their anxiety.

Psychotropic Medications

Psychotropic medications are indicated when a major depressive or anxiety disorder develops and when episodic psychosis or sleep disturbance occurs. Short-term use of low dose antipsychotics is helpful when suspiciousness, rage or impulsiveness reach psychotic proportions.

SOMATOFORM DISORDERS

Because seniors with somatoform disorders will also have concurrent physical conditions, a sort-out rather than rule-out approach to treatment is more effective. Older persons may have a number of concerns about their health, but it is the obsessive pursuit of examinations, physician attention, and anger that characterize hypochondriasis, which may be difficult to distinguish from depression. In somatization disorder, patients typically lack the anger of persons with hypochondriacal orders but they share the pattern of seeing one physician after another and seeking medical procedures. Conversion disorder represents a failure of voluntary motor or sensory function that is psychologically based but not consciously effected. Conversion disorder often resolves spontaneously once the precipitating conflict or event subsides, but it may become chronic, confining the patient to a wheelchair or leaving the patient dependent on others for activities of daily living. *DSM-IV* criteria for pain disorder identify pain as the predominant complaint, disproportionate to any anatomical findings. The diagnosis is difficult in late life because of the frequency with which arthritis and vascular disease cause pain and dysfunction and the age-related reduction in the physiologic signs that accompany pain.

Treatment

The principles of treatment are similar across the somatoform disorders. Symptoms are taken at face value, with no intimation that they are imaginary, or that they are signs of immaturity or attention seeking. Depression or the abuse of prescribed analgesics, sedatives, or alcohol, if present, are therapeutic priorities that require treatment even if the symptoms of the somatoform disorder remain unexplained.

Referral by a physician to a mental health specialist will be interpreted by the patient as lack of concern or abandonment if not handled cautiously. However, a tardy referral, after the patient has undergone invasive or disfiguring and unnecessary procedures, is equally problematic. Referral should be presented to the patient as an adjunct to primary care rather than an alternative. Labeling the need for consultation as the physician's rather than the patient's need will facilitate the process. Finding a mutually agreed-upon reason for the consultation is essential. Stress reduction; behavioral therapy to minimize analgesic dependence; diagnosis and treatment recommendations for depression, anxiety, or sedative dependence are examples.

The therapist should seek to establish and maintain a supportive, empathic relationship through regularly scheduled rather than as needed appointments. The promise of constancy is more important than cure when forging a therapeutic alliance with these patients. Even though the hypochondriacal patient may disparage the therapist, a sustained relationship is nonetheless possible; in time, it can lead to a sense of security and a reduction in both symptoms and hostility. Establishing this relationship requires tact, tolerance, and acknowledgment of the frustration engendered when symptoms remain despite effort and expense on the patient's part. Protection of these patients from unnecessary, invasive procedures and excessive use of family and health care resources is a major achievement, regardless of whether the incapacity occasioned by a somatoform disorder is fully reduced. To avoid working at cross-purposes and becoming trapped in an unproductive power struggle, the therapist should focus on a rehabilitative approach, reducing the disability first before achieving insight or elimination of complaints. The approach is psychological and behavioral, but the focus is on the physical and functional.

SUBSTANCE ABUSE

In the present cohort of older persons, abuse of alcohol and misuse of prescription and over-the-counter medications, usually sedatives and analgesics, are more common than illicit drug use. One third of alcohol abuse cases in late life emerge for the first time after the age of retirement, and as many as one half of alcoholic male outpatients may also be diagnosed with an additional psychiatric disorder, such as major depression, anxiety, and cognitive disorders (Blow, Cook, Booth, Falcon, & Friedman, 1992). Recent heavy drinking is a significant risk factor for suicide among middle-age and older men (Murphy, Wetzel, Robins, & McEvoy, 1992). Because older persons are more sensitive to the metabolic and cognitive toxicity of alcohol, small amounts may cause significant impairments yet meet the criteria for moderate drinking—for example, two drinks per day for men, one for women. The use of analgesics, so prevalent in late life, compounds the hepatic toxicity of alcohol (Lieber, 1995).

As a result, the frequency with which alcohol contributes to physical and mental comorbidity in late life is underestimated, and because older people's level of intake may seem socially acceptable, their capacity to underestimate the impact of alcohol on their health is increased. Added to denial is social isolation, which may further keep the problem from coming to clinical recognition until a person's unexplained falls, fractures, or noncompliance with prescription medications provoke the clinician's suspicion. Because of physical frailty, the use of disulfiram, even when administration and supervision can be assured, is problematic in old age. Older alcoholics whose mobility is constrained may also find it difficult to attend self-help or Alcoholics Anonymous (AA) groups with the necessary frequency to reinforce abstinence. Age-appropriate AA groups may be difficult to find.

However, the difficulties in recognizing alcohol problems in the aged also suggest reasons for therapeutic optimism. First, older persons are less likely to be physiologically dependent and are less likely to suffer an abstinence syndrome. Second, simple failure of an older person to appreciate the consequences of alcohol use may be more easily overcome than the denial seen in alcohol dependent persons. The patient's family and physician may also be unaware of the risk, and the therapist may be able to assist the patient to remain abstinent by educating other caregivers. Third, if the older person drinks to counter social isolation, loneliness, or boredom, the drinking may be reduced if alternatives are identified and reinforced. These include helping the patient to prepare an appointment calendar of activities and social events; referral to and reinforcement of attendance at a senior center or AA; attendance at religious institutions and engagement in acts of personal devotion; alerting family or friendly visitor organizations of the need for contact.

Fourth, for the alcohol-dependent homebound person, the source of supply (family, friends, home care personnel, liquor store home delivery) must be identified. Finally, treatment of comorbid depression, anxiety, sleep disturbance, or psychosis with the psychotherapy, behavioral paradigms, and medications described elsewhere is critical. Treatment is equally important for persons who medicate the sleep disturbance and physical discomfort of depression with sedatives or analgesics. Obviously, none of these approaches is feasible without the patient's consent and the therapist's optimism and perseverance. The family's involvement, if available, may be the key. In summary, a comprehensive rather than narrowly focused approach offers the best chance of success, whether the problem is alcohol or over-the-counter or prescription medications.

MISCELLANEOUS CONSIDERATIONS

Problems of comorbidity in elder abuse, posttraumatic stress syndrome, and schizophrenia merit at least brief review because of their clinical implications. Comorbid family pathology as well as frailty and dementia in the elder person are part of the profile of risk for elder abuse or neglect. Similarly, those who commit acts of abuse are more often family members with mental illness or substance abuse problems. Thus, elder abuse should be considered a problem in which comorbidity needs to be investigated.

Fifty percent of Engdahl, Speed, Emberly, and Schwartz's (1991) sample of older World War II prisoners of war received a diagnosis of posttraumatic stress disorder; of these, nearly two thirds met criteria for an anxiety or depressive disorder as well. Moreover, the overwhelming stress that provoked the disorder may kindle a vulnerability to comorbid disorders, with the comorbid psychiatric symptoms and disorders—

particularly depression, anxiety and alcohol abuse—becoming increasingly autonomous.

Finally, in schizophrenia, the cognitive impairment associated with negative symptoms worsens in a minority of patients of advanced age but may not be associated with the neuritic tangles and amyloid plaques of Alzheimer's disease (Purohit et al., 1993). However, older schizophrenics seem as likely to experience the age-related decline in cholinergic function and cognitive processing speed as aged persons without dementia. As a result, avoidance of anticholinergic medications is particularly important.

CONCLUSION

Because most studies of late-life mental illness employ restrictive diagnostic definitions, knowledge of mental comorbidity among physically healthy but psychiatrically ill older persons is limited (Caine, Lyness, & King, 1993). The outcome of late-life treatment for psychiatric disorders more often has been based on relieving symptoms than reducing disability or improving quality of life. Without a more global approach to both treatment and outcome, unrecognized comorbidity may limit the potential of seniors to benefit from mental health services (Fogel, 1993). Clinical studies are needed that can examine the variability introduced by physical conditions and mental symptoms that span diagnostic boundaries. Presently, clinicians must rely on experience and theory rather than controlled studies to reduce the loss of independence and well-being of older persons with comorbid conditions.

REFERENCES

Abrams, R.C. (1991). Anxiety and personality disorders. In J. Sadavoy, L. Jarvik, & L. Lazarus (Eds.), *Comprehensive review of geriatric psychiatry.* Washington, DC: American Psychiatric Press Inc.

Abrams, R.C., Rosendahl, E., Card, C., & Alexopolous, G.S. (1994). Personality disorder correlates of late and early onset depression. *Journal of the American Geriatrics Society, 42,* 727–731.

American Psychiatric Association Task Force on ECT. (1990). *The practice of ECT: Recommendations for treatment, training, and privileging.* Washington, DC: American Psychiatric Press.

Beck, J.C. (Ed.). (1989). *Geriatrics review syllabus.* New York: American Geriatrics Society.

Blazer, D.G., Hughes, D.C., & Fowler, N. (1989). Anxiety as an outcome of depression in elderly and middle-aged adults. *International Journal of Geriatric Psychiatry, 4,* 273–278.

Blazer, D., Woodbury, M., Hughes, D.C., George, L.K., Manton, K.G., Bachar, J.R., Fowler, N., & Cohen, H.J. (1989). A statistical analysis of the classification of depression in a mixed community and clinical sample. *Journal of Affective Disorders, 16,* 11–20.

Blow, F.C., Cook, C.A.L., Booth, B.M., Falcon, S.P., & Friedman, M.J. (1992). Age-related psychiatric comorbidities and level of functioning in alcoholic veterans seeking outpatient treatment. *Hospital and Community Psychiatry, 43,* 990–995.

Caine, E., Lyness, J.M., & King, D.A. (1993). Reconsidering depression in the elderly. *American Journal of Geriatric Psychiatry, 1,* 4–20.

Clark, D.C. (1992, December 10). *Remarks.* Conference on the National Suicide Survey, "Too Young to Die," conducted by Empire Blue Cross and Blue Shield and the Gallup Organization, New York.

Cohen, G.D. (1988). *The brain in human aging.* New York: Springer.

Cohen-Mansfield, J., Werner, P., & Marx, M.S. (1990). Screaming in nursing home residents. *Journal of the American Geriatrics Society, 38,* 785–792.

Conwell, Y., Melanie, R., & Caine, E.D. (1990). Completed suicide at age 50 and over. *Journal of the American Geriatric Society, 38,* 640–644.

Costa, P.T., & McCrue, R.R. (1994). Depression as an enduring disposition. In L.S. Schneider, C.F.F. Reynolds, B.D. Lebowitz, & A.J. Ffriedhoff (Eds.), *Diagnosis and treatment of depression in late life* (pp. 155–168). Washington, DC: American Psychiatric Press.

Coyne, J.C. (1976). Depression and the response of others. *Journal of Abnormal Psychology, 85,* 186–193.

Engdahl, B.E., Speed, N., Emberly, R.E., & Schwartz, J. (1991). Comorbidity of psychiatric disorders and personality profiles of American World War II prisoners of war. *Journal of Nervous and Mental Disease, 179,* 181–187.

Evans, L.K., & Strumph, N.E. (1993). Frailty and physical restraints. In Y. Perry, J. Morley, & R. Coe (Eds.), *Aging and musculoskeletal disorders* (pp. 324–333). New York: Springer.

Flint, A.J. (1994). Epidemiology and comorbidity of anxiety disorders in the elderly. *American Journal of Psychiatry, 151,* 640–649.

Fogel, B. (1993). Mental health services and outcome driven health care. *American Journal of Public Health, 83,* 319–321.

Frank, E. (1994). Long-term prevention of recurrence in elderly patients. In L.S. Schneider, C.F.F. Reynolds, B.D. Lebowitz, & A.J. Ffriedhoff (Eds.), *Diagnosis and treatment of depression in late life* (pp. 317–330). Washington, DC: American Psychiatric Press.

Frank, E., Prien, R.F., Jarret, R.B., Keller, M.B., Kupfer, D.J., Lavoir, P., Rush, A.J., & Weissman, M.M. (1991). Conceptualization and rationale for consensus definitions of terms in major depressive disorder: Response, remission, recovery, relapse and recurrence. *Archives of General Psychiatry, 48,* 851–855.

Gallagher, D., Rose, J., Rivera, P., Losett, S., & Thompson, L. W. (1989). Prevalence of depression in family caregivers. *Gerontologist, 29,* 449–456.

Georgotas, A., McCue, R.E., Cooper, T.B., Nagachandran, N., & Chang, I. (1988). How effective and safe is continuation therapy in elderly depressed patients? *Archives of General Psychiatry, 45,* 929–932.

Greenberg, D., & Kennedy, G.J. (1991). Till death do us part: Marital therapy in a geriatric ambulatory practice. *Gerontologist, 31,* 118.

Greenwald, B.S., Kramer-Ginsberg, E., Marin, D.B., Laitman, L.B., Herman, C.K., Mohs, R.C., & Davis, K.L. (1989). Dementia with coexistent major depression. *American Journal of Psychiatry, 14,* 1472–1478.

Gurland, B.J., Wilder, D.E., & Berkman, C. (1988). Depression and disability in the elderly: Reciprocal relations and changes with age. *International Journal of Geriatric Psychiatry, 3,* 163–179.

Harnet, D.S. (1994). Psychopharmacological treatment of depression in the medical setting. *Psychiatric Annals, 24,* 545–551.

Hay, D., & Hay, L. (1992). The role of ECT in the treatment of depression. In C.D. McCann and N.S. Endler (Eds.), *Depression: New directions in theory, research, and practice* (pp. 255–272). Toronto: Wall and Emerson.

Houlihan, D.J., Mulsant, B.H., Sweet, R.A., Rifai, A.H., Pasternak, R., Rosen, J., & Zubenko, G.S. (1994). A naturalistic study of trazodone in the treatment of behavioral complications of dementia. *American Journal of Geriatric Psychiatry, 2,* 78–85.

Jenike, M.A. (1985). *Handbook of geriatric psychopharmacology.* Littleton, MA: PSR Publishing.

Karasu, T.B., Docherty, J.P., Gelenberg, A., Kupfer, A.J., Merriam, A.E., & Shadoan, R. (1993). Practice guidelines for major depressive disorder in adults. *American Journal of Psychiatry, 150,* 4 (supplement).

Katz, I.R. (1996). On the inseparability of mental and physical health in aged persons. *American Journal of Geriatric Psychiatry, 4,* 1–16.

Katz, I.R., Curil, S., & Nemetz, A. (1988). Functional psychiatric disorders in the elderly. In L.W. Lazarus (Ed.), *Essentials of geriatric psychiatry* (pp. 113–137). New York: Springer.

Katz, I.R., Streim, J., & Parmelee, P. (1994). Psychiatric-medical comorbidity: Implications for health services delivery and for research on depression. *Biological Psychiatry, 36,* 141–145.

Kelman, H.R., & Thomas, C. (1990). Transitions between community and nursing home residence in an urban elderly population. *Journal of Community Health, 15,* 105–122.

Kennedy, G.J., Katsnelson, N., Laitman, L., & Alvarez, E. (1995). Psychogeriatric services in certified home health agencies: Guidelines for the psychiatric consultant. *American Journal of Geriatric Psychiatry, 3,* 339–347.

Kennedy, G.J., Kelman, H.R., & Thomas, C. (1991). Persistence and remission of depressive symptoms in late life. *American Journal of Psychiatry, 148,* 174–178.

Kermis, M.D. (1986). The epidemiology of mental disorders in the elderly: A response to the Senate/AARP report. *Gerontologist, 26,* 482–487.

Lieber, C.S. (1995). Medical disorders of alcoholism. *New England Journal of Medicine, 333,* 1058–1065.

Mackensie, T.B., & Popkin, M.K. (1987). Suicide in the medical patient. *International Journal of Psychiatry in Medicine, 17,* 3–22.

Maletta, G.J. (1992). Treatment of behavioral symptomatology of Alzheimer's disease, with emphasis on aggression: Current clinical approaches. *International Psychogeriatrics, 4,* 117–130.

Menza, M.A., Robertson-Hoffman, D.E., & Bonapace, A.S. (1993). Parkinson's disease and anxiety: Comorbidity and depression. *Biological Psychiatry, 34,* 465–470.

Mintzer, O., Flores, L.P., & Milanes, F.J. (1992). Phenomenology and course of psychiatric disorders with combat-related posttraumatic stress disorder. *American Journal of Psychiatry, 149,* 1568–1574.

Molinari, V., & Marmion, J. (1993). Personality disorders in geropsychiatric outpatients. *Psychological Reports, 73,* 256–258.

Moody, H.R. (1988). From informed consent to negotiated consent. *Gerontologist, 28,* 64–70.

Murphy, G.E., Wetzel, R.D., Robins, E., & McEvoy, L. (1992). Multiple risk factors predict suicide in alcoholism. *Archives of General Psychiatry, 49,* 459–463.

Myers, J.K., Kalayum, B., & Mei-tal, V. (1984). Late-onset delusional depression: A distinct clinical entity? *Journal of Clinical Psychiatry, 45,* 347–349.

Myers, J.K., Weissman, M.M., Tischler, G.L., Holzer, C.E., Leat, P.J., Orvaschel, H., Anthony, J.C., Boyd, J.H., Burke, J.D., Kramer, M., & Stoltzman, R. (1984). Six month prevalence of psychiatric disorders in the community. *Archives of General Psychiatry, 41,* 959–967.

National Institutes of Health Consensus Development Panel on Depression in Late Life. (1992). Diagnosis and treatment of depression in late life. *Journal of the American Medical Association, 268,* 1018–1024.

Papolos, D.F. (1994). The family psychoeducational approach: Rationale for a multigenerational treatment modality for major affective disorders. In D.F. Papolos and H. Lackman (Eds.), *Genetic studies of affective disorders: Overview of basic methods, current directions, and critical research issues.* New York: Wiley.

Parfrey, P.S., Ikeman, R., Anglin, D., & Cole, C. (1983). Severe lithium intoxication treated by forced diuresis. *Canadian Medical Association Journal, 129,* 979–980.

Parikh, R.M., Lipsey, J.R., Robinson, R.G., & Price, T.R. (1987). Two-year longitudinal study of post-stroke mood disorders: Dynamic changes in correlates of depression at one and two years. *Stroke, 18,* 579–584.

Parmalee, P.A., Katz, I.R., & Lawton, M.P. (1993). Anxiety and its association with depression among institutionalized elderly. *American Journal of Geriatric Psychiatry, 1,* 46–58.

Patel, S.V. (1995). Pharmacotherapy of cognitive impairment in Alzheimer's disease: A review. *Journal of Geriatric Psychiatry and Neurology, 8,* 81–95.

Perel, J.M. (1994). Geropharmacokinetics of therapeutics, toxic effects and compliance. In L.S. Schneider, C.F.F. Reynolds, B.D. Lebowitz, & A.J. Ffriedhoff (Eds.), *Diagnosis and treatment of depression in late life* (pp. 245–258). Washington, DC: American Psychiatric Press.

Purohit, D.P., Davidson, M., Perl, D.P., Powchik, P., Haroutunian, V.H., Bierer, L.M., McCrystal, J., Losonczy, M., & Davis, K.L. (1993). Severe cognitive impairment in elderly schizophrenic patients: A clinicopathological study. *Biological Psychiatry, 33,* 255–260.

Rapp, S.R., Parisi, S.A., & Walsh, D.A. (1988). Psychologic function and physical health among elderly medical inpatients. *Journal of Consulting and Clinical Psychology, 56,* 851–855.

Reifler, B.V., & Larson, E. (1988). Excess disability in demented elderly outpatients: The rule of halves. *Journal of the American Geriatrics Society, 36,* 82–83.

Reynolds, C.F., Hoch, C.C., Buysee, D.J., Houck, P.R., Schlernitzauer, M., Frank, E., Mazumdar, S., & Kupfer, D. (1992). EEG sleep in spousal bereavement and bereavement-related depression of late life. *Biological Psychiatry, 31,* 69–82.

Reynolds, C.F., Frank, E., Perel, J.M., Imber, S.D., Cornes, C., Morycz, R.K., Mazumdar, S., Miller, M.D., Pollock, B.G., Plifai, A.H., Stack, J.A., George, C.J., Huuck, P.R., & Kupfer, D.J. (1992). Combined pharmacotherapy and psychotherapy in the acute continuation treatment of elderly patients with recurrent major depression: A preliminary report. *American Journal of Psychiatry, 149,* 1687–1692.

Rovner, B.W., Broadhead, J., Spencer, M., Carson, K., & Folstein, M.F. (1989). Depression and Alzheimer's disease. *American Journal of Psychiatry, 146,* 350–353.

Rovner, B.W., German, P.S., Broadhead, J., Morris, R.K., & Brant, L.J. (1990). The prevalence and management of dementia and other psychiatric disorders in nursing homes. *International Psychogeriatrics, 2,* 13–24.

Sackeim, H.A., Prudic, J., Devanand, D.P., Kiersky, J.E., Fitzsimons, L., Moody, B.J., McElhiuey, M.C., Coleman, E.A., & Settembrino, J.M. (1993). Effects of stimulus intensity and electrode placement on the efficacy and cognitive effects of electroconvulsive therapy. *New England Journal of Medicine, 328,* 839–846.

Salzman, C. (1994). Pharmacologic treatment of depression in elderly patients. In L.S. Schneider, C.F.F. Reynolds, B.D. Lebowitz, & A.J. Ffriedhoff (Eds.), *Diagnosis and treatment of depression in late life* (pp. 181–244). Washington, DC: American Psychiatric Press.

Smith, S.L., Sherrill, K.A., & Colenda, C.C. (1995). Assessing and treating anxiety in elderly persons. *Psychiatric Services, 46,* 36–42.

Strain, J.J., Lyons, J.S., Hammer, J.S., Fahs, M., Lebovits, A., Paddison, P.L., Snyder, S., Strauss, E., Burton, R., & Nuber, G. (1991). Cost offset from a psychiatric consultation-liaison intervention with elderly hip fracture patients. *American Journal of Psychiatry, 148,* 1004–1049.

Teri, L., Curtis, J., Gallager-Thompson, D., & Thompson, L.W. (1994). Cognitive-behavioral therapy with depressed older adults. In L.S. Schneider, C.F.F. Reynolds, B.D. Lebowitz, & A.J. Ffriedhoff (Eds.), *Diagnosis and treatment of depression in late life* (pp. 279–292). Washington, DC: American Psychiatric Press.

Teri, L., Rabins, P., Whitehouse, P., Berg, L., Reisberg, B., Sunderland, T., Eichelman, B., & Phelps, C. (1992). Management of behavior disturbance in Alzheimer disease: Current knowledge and future directions. *Alzheimer Disease and Associated Disorders, 6,* 77–88.

Testa, M.A., Anderson, R.B., Nackley, J.F., & Hollenberg, N.K. (1993). Quality of life and antihypertensive therapy in men. *New England Journal of Medicine, 328,* 901–913.

Thomas, C., & Kelman, H.R. (1990). Health services use among the elderly under alternative health service delivery systems. *Journal of Community Health, 15,* 77–92.

Wells, K.B., Burnam, M.A., Rogers, W., Hays, R., & Camp, P. (1992). The course of depression in adult outpatients. *Archives of General Psychiatry, 49,* 788–794.

Wells, K.B., Stewart, A., Hays, R.D., Burnam, M.A., Rogers, W., Daniels, M., Berny, S., Greenfield, S., & Ware, J. (1989). The functioning and well-being of depressed patients: Results from the Medical Outcomes Study. *Journal of the American Medical Association, 262,* 914–919.

Winograd, C.H. (1992). Geriatric assessment: Concepts, components, and settings. In J.E. Morely (ed.), *Geriatric care* (pp. 212–233). St. Louis, MO: G.W. Manning.

Wragg, R.E., & Jeste, V.D. (1989). Overview of depression and psychosis in Alzheimer's disease. *American Journal of Psychiatry, 146,* 577–587.

Yost, E., Beutler, L., & Corbishley, M.A. (1986). *Group cognitive therapy: A treatment approach for depressed older adults.* New York: Pergamon Press.

Zisook, S., Shuchter, S.R., & Sledge, P. (1994). Diagnostic and treatment considerations in depression associated with late-life bereavement. In L.S. Schneider, C.F.F. Reynolds, B.D. Lebowitz, & A.J. Ffriedhoff (Eds.), *Diagnosis and treatment of depression in late life* (pp. 419–430). Washington, DC: American Psychiatric Press.

Author Index

Subject Index